SPECIALTY IMAGING™
GASTROINTESTINAL ONCOLOGY

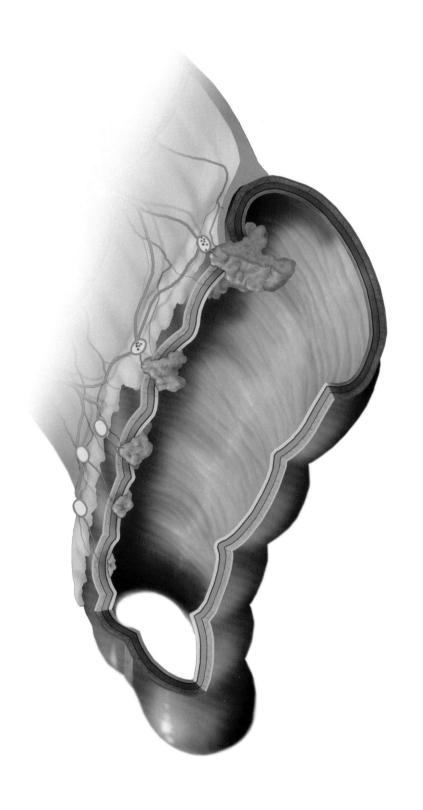

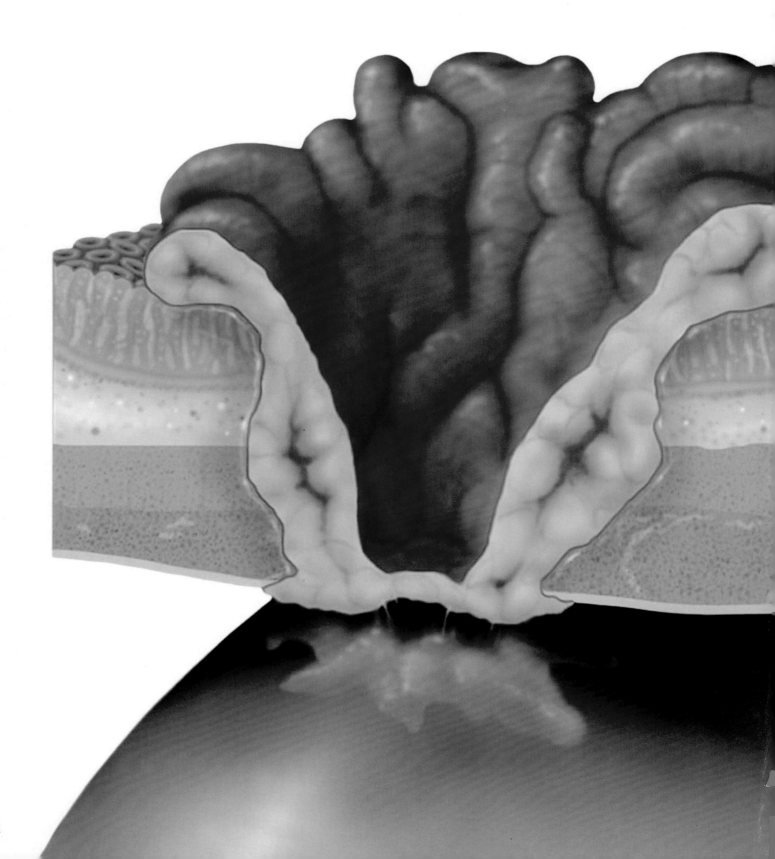

SPECIALTY IMAGING™
GASTROINTESTINAL ONCOLOGY

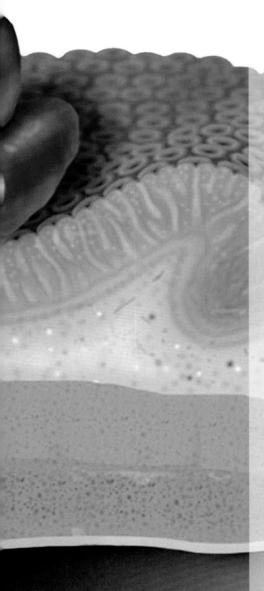

Akram M. Shaaban, MBBCh
Associate Professor of Radiology
University of Utah School of Medicine
Salt Lake City, UT

Maryam Rezvani, MD
Assistant Professor of Radiology
University of Utah School of Medicine
Salt Lake City, UT

Mohamed E. Salama, MD
Assistant Professor
Department of Pathology
University of Utah and ARUP Reference Laboratory
Salt Lake City, UT

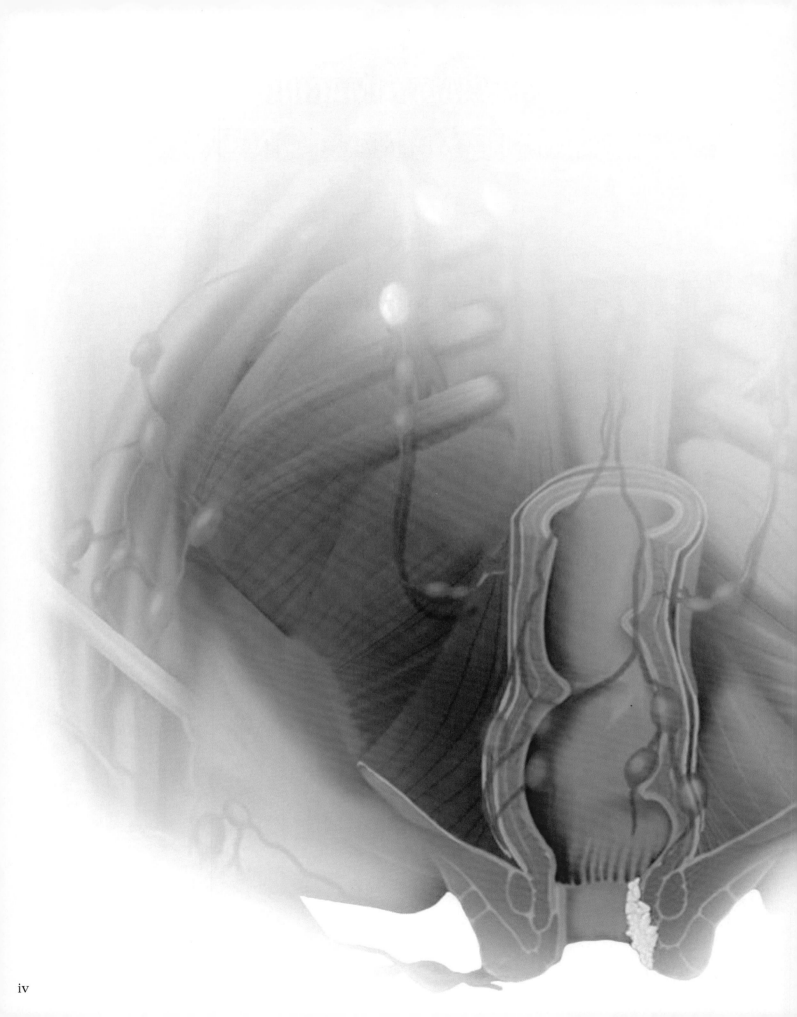

CONTRIBUTING AUTHORS

Jeffrey D. Olpin, MD
Associate Professor of Radiology
University of Utah School of Medicine
Salt Lake City, UT

Marc S. Tubay, MD
Chief of Body MRI Imaging
David Grant Medical Center
Travis Air Force Base, Fairfield, CA

Alex Schabel, MD
Resident
University of Utah School of Medicine
Salt Lake City, UT

Lauren Zollinger, MD
Neuroradiology Fellow
University of Utah Department of Radiology
Salt Lake City, UT

Anita J. Thomas, MD
Assistant Professor
Department of Radiology
Section Head, Nuclear Medicine
Wake Forest University Health Sciences
Winston-Salem, NC

Paige B. Clark, MD
Associate Professor of Nuclear Medicine
Department of Radiology
Wake Forest University Health Sciences
Winston-Salem, NC

AMIRSYS®

Names you know. Content you trust.®

First Edition

Printed in Canada by Friesens, Altona, Manitoba, Canada

ISBN: 978-1-931884-23-5

Notice and Disclaimer

Library of Congress Cataloging-in-Publication Data

Shaaban, Akram M.
  Specialty imaging. Gastrointestinal oncology / Akram M. Shaaban. -- 1st ed.
      p. ; cm.
  Gastrointestinal oncology
  Includes index.
  ISBN 978-1-931884-23-5
  1. Digestive organs--Cancer--Imaging. I. Title. II. Title: Gastrointestinal
oncology.
  [DNLM: 1. Gastrointestinal Neoplasms--diagnosis. 2. Diagnostic Imaging.
WI 149]
  RC280.D5S53 2011
  616.99'43--dc22
                              2010038959

To my parents, I truly owe you everything.
To my wife Inji, son Karim and daughter May, the jewels
of my life, thanks for your
understanding and tremendous support.
AMS

To my parents, Houshmand and Shahla, I dedicate not
just this work but all my efforts in life and faith.
To my sister, Sara, for believing in me and everything
I humbly attempt.
MR

To my wife and best friend, Nahla Heikal, for her
sustaining love and patience.
To my children, Youssef and Farah, for their joy of life.
MES

PREFACE

In *Specialty Imaging: Gastrointestinal Oncology*, Amirsys proudly presents the most up-to-date staging and imaging for gastrointestinal cancers—less than one year after the introduction of the 7th edition of the *AJCC Cancer Staging Manual*. This includes the brand new TNM and prognostic stage grouping for appendiceal cancers (both carcinoma and carcinoid), gastrointestinal stromal tumors (GIST), neuroendocrine tumors, and cancers of the intrahepatic, distal, and perihilar bile ducts. You'll also find the redefined TNM and prognostic stage grouping for cancers of the esophagus, stomach, small intestine, colon and rectum, liver, and gallbladder, along with the newly unified staging system for both endocrine and exocrine pancreatic tumors.

Each lavishly illustrated chapter offers multiple ways to make sense of a particular gastrointestinal cancer. Quick reference tables provide the definitions for TNM and AJCC prognostic groups. Rich drawings illuminate these stages. High-quality images of practically every stage of every tumor demonstrate radiographic appearances. All of these vivid images—more than 1,100 in the volume—are fully annotated to maximize their illustrative potential. Bulleted text distills the pertinent information to the essentials. Whether you are looking for routes of spread, imaging techniques for local staging, or treatment options, you will find it quickly in this easy-to-use yet comprehensive reference.

Like other Amirsys books, *Specialty Imaging: Gastrointestinal Oncology* was designed with you, the reader, in mind. We think you'll find this new volume a handy and wonderfully rich resource that will significantly enhance your practice—and find a welcome place on your bookshelf.

Paula J. Woodward, MD
David G. Bragg, MD and Marcia R. Bragg Presidential Endowed
Chair in Oncologic Imaging
Professor of Radiology
University of Utah School of Medicine
Salt Lake City, UT

ACKNOWLEDGEMENTS

Text Editing

Arthur G. Gelsinger, MA

Katherine Riser, MA

Dave L. Chance, MA

Matthew R. Connelly, MA

Image Editing

Jeffrey J. Marmorstone

Medical Editing

Jonathan Shakespear, MD

Illustrations

Lane R. Bennion, MS

Richard Coombs, MS

Laura C. Sesto, MA

Michael Havranek, MAMS, CMI

Asha Renée Kays, MS

John O. Dorn, MA

Art Direction and Design

Laura C. Sesto, MA

Associate Editor

Ashley R. Renlund, MA

Production Lead

Kellie J. Heap

AMIRSYS®

Names you know. Content you trust.®

TABLE OF CONTENTS

Esophageal Carcinoma   2
Akram M. Shaaban, MBBCh
Anita J. Thomas, MD & Paige B. Clark, MD

Stomach Carcinoma   28
Akram M. Shaaban, MBBCh

Small Intestine Carcinoma   52
Maryam Rezvani, MD

Appendiceal Carcinoma   66
Akram M. Shaaban, MBBCh

Appendiceal Carcinoid   86
Akram M. Shaaban, MBBCh

Colorectal Carcinoma   94
Lauren Zollinger, MD & Akram M. Shaaban, MBBCh

Anal Canal Carcinoma   118
Akram M. Shaaban, MBBCh

Gastrointestinal Stromal Tumor (GIST)   134
Marc Tubay, MD

Neuroendocrine Tumors 154
Akram M. Shaaban, MBBCh

Hepatocellular Carcinoma 180
Jeffrey Olpin, MD

Gallbladder Carcinoma 202
Akram M. Shaaban, MBBCh

Intrahepatic Bile Duct Carcinoma 224
Maryam Rezvani, MD

Perihilar Bile Duct Carcinoma 238
Maryam Rezvani, MD

Distal Bile Duct Carcinoma 258
Maryam Rezvani, MD

Ampulla of Vater Carcinoma 270
Akram M. Shaaban, MBBCh

Endocrine Pancreatic Carcinoma 288
Akram M. Shaaban, MBBCh

Exocrine Pancreatic Carcinoma 308
Alex Schabel, MD & Akram M. Shaaban, MBBCh

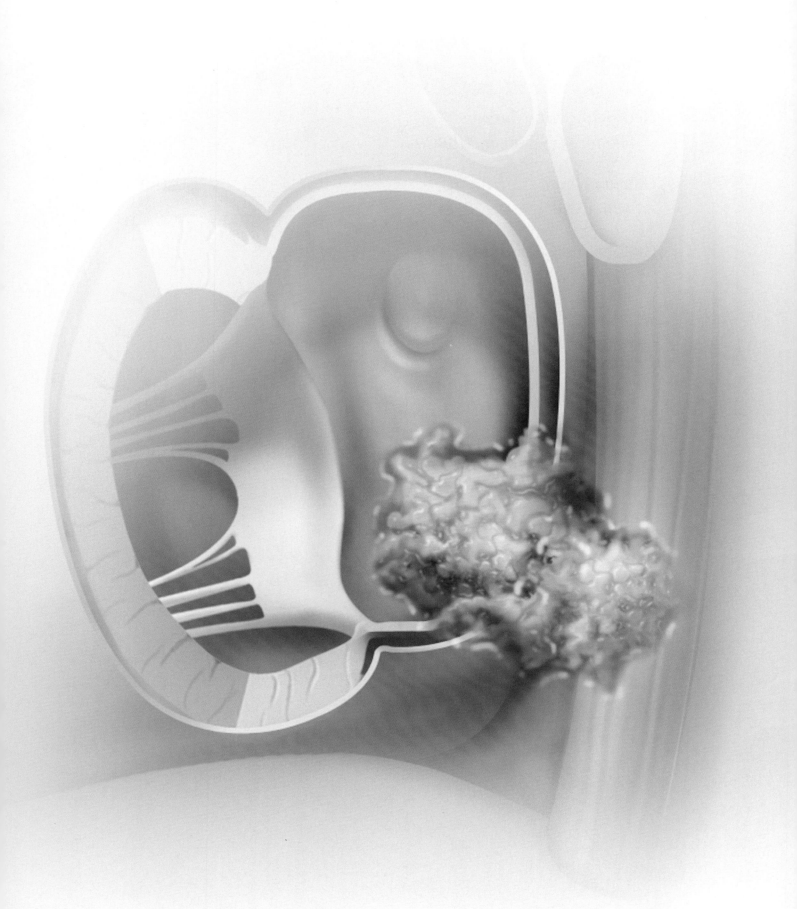

Esophageal Carcinoma

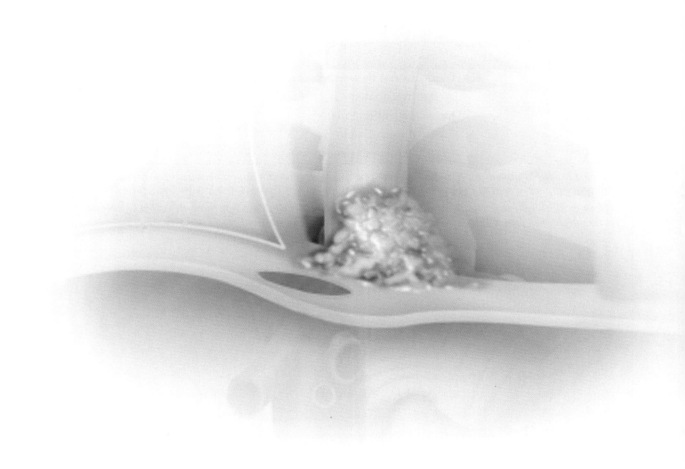

ESOPHAGEAL CARCINOMA

(T) Primary Tumor

Adapted from 7th edition AJCC Staging Forms.

TNM	Definitions
TX	Primary tumor cannot be assessed
T0	No evidence of primary tumor
Tis	High-grade dysplasia*
T1	Tumor invades lamina propria, muscularis mucosae, or submucosa
T1a	Tumor invades lamina propria or muscularis mucosae
T1b	Tumor invades submucosa
T2	Tumor invades muscularis propria
T3	Tumor invades adventitia
T4	Tumor invades adjacent structures
T4a	Resectable tumor invading pleura, pericardium, or diaphragm
T4b	Unresectable tumor invading other adjacent structures, such as aorta, vertebral body, trachea, etc.

(N) Regional Lymph Nodes

NX	Regional lymph nodes cannot be assessed
N0	No regional lymph node metastasis
N1	Metastasis in 1-2 regional lymph nodes
N2	Metastasis in 3-6 regional lymph nodes
N3	Metastasis in ≥ 7 regional lymph nodes

(M) Distant Metastasis

M0	No distant metastasis
M1	Distant metastasis

(G) Histologic Grade

GX	Grade cannot be assessed; stage grouping as G1
G1	Well differentiated
G2	Moderately differentiated
G3	Poorly differentiated
G4	Undifferentiated; stage grouping as G3 squamous

At least maximal dimension of the tumor must be recorded; multiple tumors require the T(m) suffix. Number must be recorded for total number of regional nodes sampled and total number of reported nodes with metastasis.

*High-grade dysplasia includes all noninvasive neoplastic epithelia that was formerly called carcinoma in situ, a diagnosis that is no longer used for columnar mucosae anywhere in the gastrointestinal tract.

ESOPHAGEAL CARCINOMA

AJCC Stages/Prognostic Groups for Adenocarcinoma

Adapted from 7th edition AJCC Staging Forms.

Stage	T	N	M	G
0	Tis	N0	M0	G1, GX
IA	T1	N0	M0	G1-2, GX
IB	T1	N0	M0	G3
	T2	N0	M0	G1-2, GX
IIA	T2	N0	M0	G3
IIB	T3	N0	M0	Any G
	T1-2	N1	M0	Any G
IIIA	T1-2	N2	M0	Any G
	T3	N1	M0	Any G
	T4a	N0	M0	Any G
IIIB	T3	N2	M0	Any G
IIIC	T4a	N1-2	M0	Any G
	T4b	Any N	M0	Any G
	Any T	N3	M0	Any G
IV	Any T	Any N	M1	Any G

AJCC Stages/Prognostic Groups for Squamous Cell Carcinoma[1]

Adapted from 7th edition AJCC Staging Forms.

Stage	T	N	M	G	Location[2]
0	Tis	N0	M0	G1, GX	Any location
IA	T1	N0	M0	G1, GX	Any location
IB	T1	N0	M0	G2-3	Any location
	T2-3	N0	M0	G1, GX	Lower, X
IIA	T2-3	N0	M0	G1, GX	Upper, middle
	T2-3	N0	M0	G2-3	Lower, X
IIB	T2-3	N0	M0	G2-3	Upper, middle
	T1-2	N1	M0	Any G	Any location
IIIA	T1-2	N2	M0	Any G	Any location
	T3	N1	M0	Any G	Any location
	T4a	N0	M0	Any G	Any location
IIIB	T3	N2	M0	Any G	Any location
IIIC	T4a	N1-2	M0	Any G	Any location
	T4b	Any N	M0	Any G	Any location
	Any T	N3	M0	Any G	Any location
IV	Any T	Any N	M1	Any G	Any location

[1]*Or mixed histology including a squamous component or NOS.*

[2]*Location of the primary cancer site is defined by the position of the upper (proximal) edge of the tumor in the esophagus.*

ESOPHAGEAL CARCINOMA

Tis

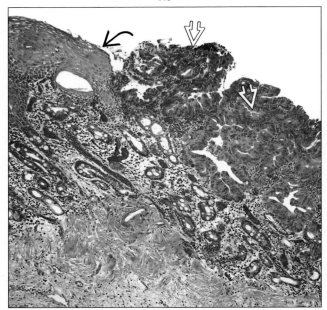

H&E stained section shows esophageal mucosa with high-grade dysplasia. In the left upper corner, there is normal squamous surface epithelium ➡. High-grade dysplasia ➡ is evident with distortion and complexity of the glandular architecture that reaches to the luminal surface. (Original magnification 40x.)

Tis

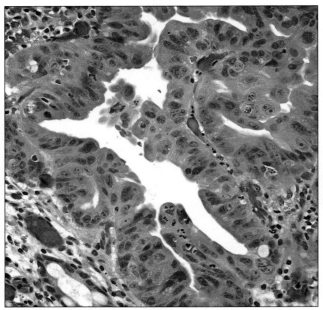

Higher magnification of the previous image shows nuclear aberrations including stratification, nuclear pleomorphism, and hyperchromasia, as well as prominent nucleoli. Architectural complexity including cellular tufting into the lumen is also evident. (Original magnification 500x.)

T1a

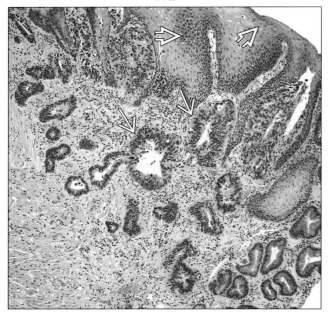

H&E stained section of esophageal mucosa shows unremarkable surface squamous mucosa ➡ and moderately differentiated adenocarcinoma, arranged in acini ➡, invading into the muscularis propria. (Original magnification 100x.)

T1a

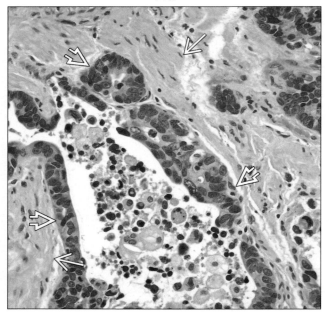

Higher magnification of the previous image shows malignant cells ➡ with gland formation invading into bundles of muscularis mucosae ➡. (Original magnification 400x.)

T2

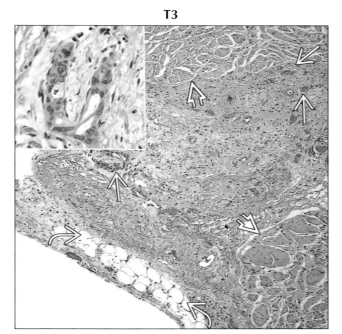

H&E stained section of an esophageal resection specimen shows denuded esophageal mucosa at the luminal aspect ⮊. *The invasive esophageal carcinoma cells* ⮊ *invade through, but not beyond, the muscularis propria. (Original magnification 20x.)*

T2

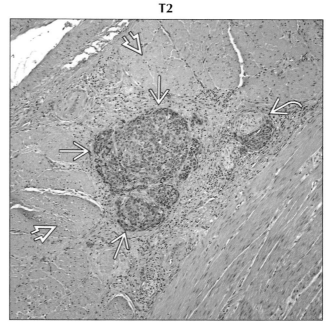

Higher magnification of the previous image shows a cluster of esophageal carcinoma ⮊ *invading into the surrounding thick eosinophilic muscle bundles of the muscularis propria* ⮊. *Note the perineural invasion with the neoplastic cells around a nerve* ⮊. *(Original magnification 100x.)*

T3

H&E stained section shows esophageal carcinoma ⮊ *extending beyond the muscularis propria* ⮊ *into the fibrofatty tissue* ⮊ *of the adventitia. (Original magnification 40x.) The inset shows a higher magnification of the invasive neoplastic cells arranged in gland formation.*

T4b

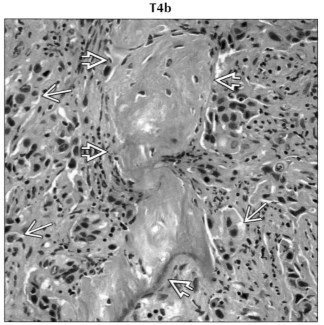

Photomicrograph shows esophageal carcinoma ⮊ *extending to invade a vertebral body. Bony trabecula* ⮊ *is seen surrounded by tumor. Unresectable tumor invading other adjacent structures is classified as T4b. (Original magnification 400x.)*

ESOPHAGEAL CARCINOMA

T1a

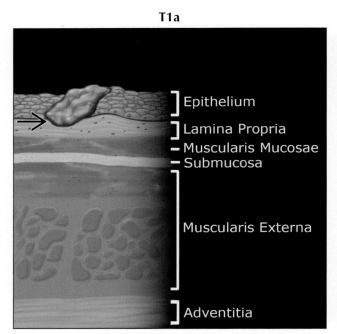

Graphic shows tumor invading lamina propria ⮕.

T1b

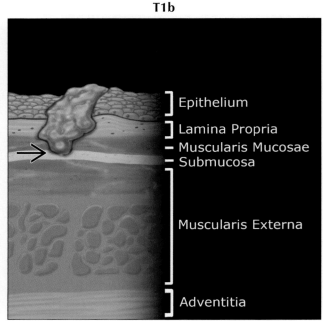

Graphic shows tumor extending into submucosa ⮕.

T2

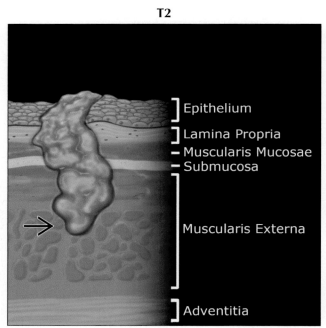

Graphic shows tumor invading muscularis propria ⮕.

T3

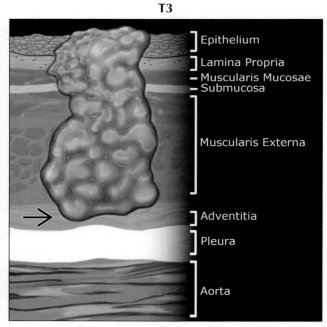

Graphic shows tumor extending to adventitia ⮕.

T3

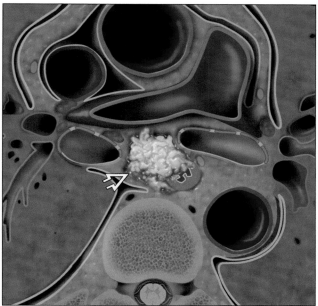

Graphic illustrates T3 tumor ⮒ invading through the adventitia and into the mediastinal fat, without invading the surrounding mediastinal structures.

T4a

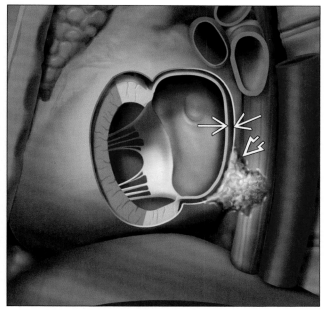

Graphic illustrates T4a tumor ⮒ invading the pericardium, separated from the heart by a thin epicardial fat layer ⮒. T4a tumors are potentially resectable.

T4a

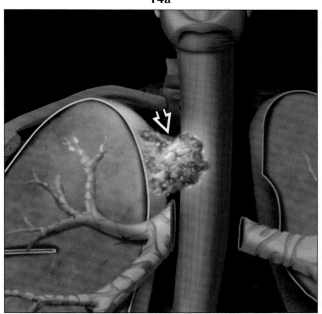

Graphic illustrates T4a tumor ⮒ invading the pleura.

T4a

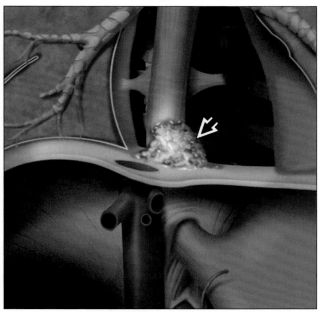

Graphic illustrates T4a tumor ⮒ invading the diaphragm.

T4b

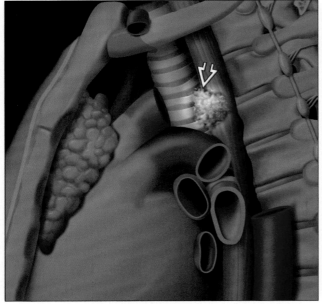

Graphic illustrates T4b tumor ➡ invading the trachea. T4b tumors are not resectable.

T4b

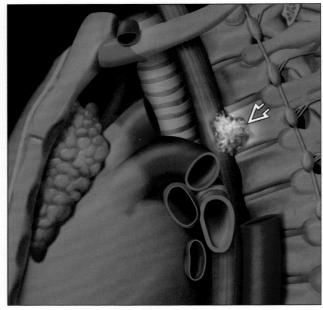

Graphic illustrates T4b tumor ➡ invading a vertebral body.

T4b

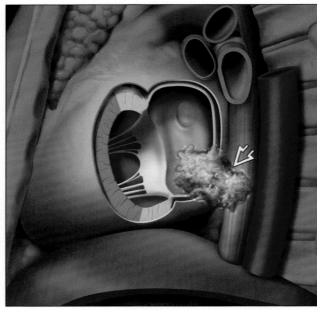

Graphic illustrates T4b tumor ➡ invading through the pericardium and into the heart.

Regional Nodal Drainage of Esophageal Carcinoma

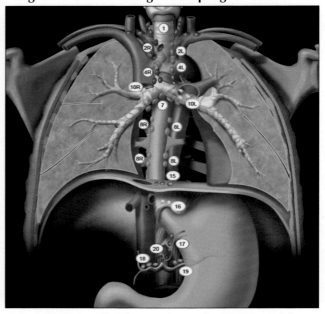

1) Supraclavicular, 2R) right upper paratracheal (UPT), 2L) left UPT, 4R) right lower paratracheal (LPT), 4L) left LPT, 7) subcarinal, 8M) middle paraesophageal (PO), 8L) left lower PO, 8R) right lower PO, 10R) right tracheobronchial (TB), 10L) left TB, 15) diaphragmatic, 16) paracardial, 17) left gastric, 18) common hepatic, 19) splenic, and 20) celiac nodes.

ESOPHAGEAL CARCINOMA

Regional Nodal Drainage of Esophageal Carcinoma (Right Side)

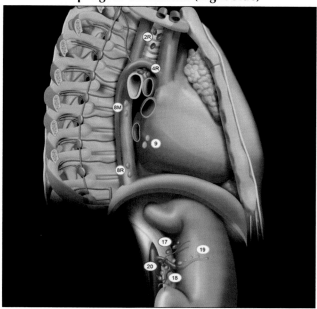

2R) Right upper paratracheal, 4R) right lower paratracheal, 8M) middle paraesophageal, 8R) right lower paraesophageal, 9) pulmonary ligament, 17) left gastric, 18) common hepatic, 19) splenic, and 20) celiac nodes.

Regional Nodal Drainage of Esophageal Carcinoma (Left Side)

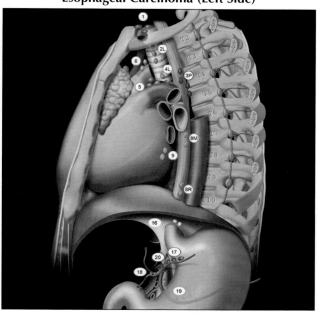

1) Supraclavicular, 2L) left upper paratracheal (PT), 3P) posterior mediastinal, 4L) left lower PT, 5) aortopulmonary, 6) anterior mediastinal, 8M) middle paraesophageal (PE), 8L) left lower PE, 9) pulmonary ligament, 15) diaphragmatic, 16) paracardial, 17) left gastric, 18) common hepatic, 19) splenic, and 20) celiac nodes.

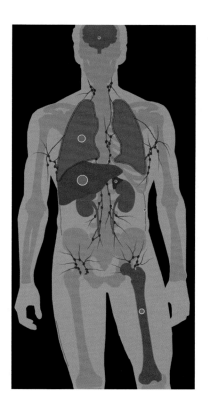

METASTASES, ORGAN FREQUENCY

Liver	35%
Lung	20%
Bone	9%
Adrenal gland	5%
Peritoneum	2%
Brain	2%

ESOPHAGEAL CARCINOMA

OVERVIEW

Classification
- Adenocarcinoma (AC) ≈ 50%
- Squamous cell carcinoma (SCC) ≈ 50%
  - SCC variants
    - Basaloid carcinoma
    - Spindle cell carcinoma
    - Verrucous carcinoma
    - Lymphoepithelioma-like carcinoma
- Other esophageal cancers
  - Melanoma
  - Malignant stromal tumors
  - Carcinoid
  - Lymphoma
  - Other rare carcinomas

PATHOLOGY

Routes of Spread
- Direct spread
  - No anatomic barrier to prevent rapid local extension of tumor into mediastinum
    - Esophageal wall lacks serosa and is attached to neighboring structures by only loose connective adventitia
  - Esophageal cancer can easily spread to adjacent structures in neck or thorax, including
    - Upper esophagus → trachea, thyroid gland, larynx
    - Middle esophagus → trachea, bronchi, aorta, lung, pericardium
    - Lower esophagus → aorta, lung, pericardium, diaphragm
- Lymphatic spread
  - Extensive lymphatic drainage system that consists of 2 lymphatic plexuses
    - First arises in mucosa
      - Pierces muscular layer and drains to regional lymph nodes
    - Second arises in muscular layer
  - Flow of lymph in upper 2/3 of esophagus tends to be upward, whereas that in distal 1/3 tends to be downward
    - Tumors in upper esophagus are more likely to metastasize to cervical or mediastinal nodes
    - Tumors in distal esophagus are more likely to metastasize to abdominal lymph nodes
  - All lymphatic channels intercommunicate, and there is bidirectional flow in tracheal bifurcation
    - Lymphatic fluid from any portion of esophagus may move to any other portion and may spread to any region of thorax or draining nodal bed
  - Nodal stations as described by AJCC
    - 1: Supraclavicular nodes
      - Above suprasternal notch and clavicles
    - 2R: Right upper paratracheal nodes
      - Between intersection of caudal margin of innominate artery with trachea and lung apex
    - 2L: Left upper paratracheal nodes
      - Between top of aortic arch and lung apex
    - 3P: Posterior mediastinal nodes
      - Upper paraesophageal nodes, above tracheal bifurcation
    - 4R: Right lower paratracheal nodes
      - Between intersection of caudal margin of innominate artery with trachea and cephalic border of azygous vein
    - 4L: Left lower paratracheal nodes
      - Between top of aortic arch and carina
    - 5: Aortopulmonary nodes
      - Subaortic and paraaortic nodes lateral to ligamentum arteriosum
    - 6: Anterior mediastinal nodes
      - Anterior to ascending aorta or innominate artery
    - 7: Subcarinal nodes
      - Caudal to tracheal carina
    - 8M: Middle paraesophageal nodes
      - From tracheal bifurcation to caudal margin of inferior pulmonary vein
    - 8L: Lower paraesophageal nodes
      - From caudal margin of inferior pulmonary vein to esophagogastric junction
    - 9: Pulmonary ligament nodes
      - Within inferior pulmonary ligament
    - 10R: Right tracheobronchial nodes
      - From cephalic border of azygous vein to origin of right upper lung bronchus
    - 10L: Left tracheobronchial nodes
      - Between carina and left upper lung bronchus
    - 15: Diaphragmatic nodes
      - Lying on dome of diaphragm and adjacent to or behind its crura
    - 16: Paracardial nodes
      - Immediately adjacent to gastroesophageal junction (GEJ)
    - 17: Left gastric nodes
      - Along course of left gastric artery
    - 18: Common hepatic nodes
      - Along course of common hepatic artery
    - 19: Splenic nodes
      - Along course of splenic artery
    - 20: Celiac nodes
      - At base of celiac artery
- Hematogenous spread
  - Most common sites, in descending order of frequency of occurrence
    - Liver
    - Lungs
    - Bones
    - Adrenal glands
    - Kidneys
    - Brain
- Pleural or peritoneal seeding
  - Pleural seeding follows tumor extension to parietal pleura
  - Peritoneal seeding is usually secondary to abdominal or retroperitoneal lymph node metastases

General Features
- Comments
  - Determination of tumor location is important
    - For surgical planning
    - Site of primary tumor can affect tumor stage in case of SCC

- T2-3 N0 M0 tumor in lower esophagus is stage IB, while similar tumor in upper or middle esophagus is stage IIA
  - Tumor location is best expressed as distance from incisors as measured endoscopically
  - Esophageal anatomical divisions
    - Cervical esophagus
      - Bordered superiorly by hypopharynx and inferiorly by thoracic outlet (at level of sternal notch)
      - Typically 15-20 cm from incisors
      - Thickening of esophageal wall begins above sternal notch
      - Related to trachea, carotid sheath, and vertebrae
    - Upper thoracic esophagus
      - Bordered superiorly by thoracic outlet (at level of sternal notch) and inferiorly by lower border of azygos vein
      - Typically 20-25 cm from incisors
      - Thickening of esophageal wall begins between sternal notch and azygos vein
      - Related to trachea, arch vessels, great veins, and vertebrae
    - Middle thoracic esophagus
      - Bordered superiorly by lower border of azygos vein and inferiorly by inferior pulmonary vein
      - Typically 25-30 cm from incisors
      - Thickening of esophageal wall begins between azygos vein and inferior pulmonary vein
      - Related to pulmonary hilum, descending thoracic aorta, pleura, and vertebrae
    - Lower thoracic esophagus
      - Bordered superiorly by inferior pulmonary vein and inferiorly by stomach, including GEJ
      - Typically 30-40 cm from incisors
      - Thickening of esophageal wall begins below inferior pulmonary vein
      - Related to pericardium, descending thoracic aorta, and vertebrae
    - Abdominal esophagus
      - Tumors of GEJ or those whose epicenter is within proximal stomach (5 cm of gastric cardia) with extension to GEJ are grouped with esophageal carcinoma
- Genetics
  - Adenocarcinoma
    - Probable with Barrett esophagus
      - Frequent chromosome loss/gain/amplification
  - Squamous cell carcinoma
    - High predisposition in patients with nonepidermolytic palmoplantar keratoderma (tylosis)
      - Rare
      - 95% risk of esophageal SCC by 70 years of age
      - Autosomal dominant
      - Abnormal 17q25 chromosome
- Etiology
  - Adenocarcinoma
    - Associated with gastroesophageal reflux
      - Obesity may contribute by increasing intraabdominal pressure
      - Weekly symptoms = 8x increased risk of AC
    - Barrett esophagus

- More than 95% of ACs develop in association with Barrett esophagus
- Normally mucosa changes from squamous to columnar at GEJ
- Progressive columnar metaplasia of distal esophagus
- Overall prevalence of AC in patients with Barrett esophagus is 5-28%
  - Associated with prior radiation therapy (breast, mediastinal cancer)
  - Squamous cell carcinoma
    - Esophagus normally lined with stratified squamous epithelium
      - Carcinoma develops from progression of premalignant or dysplastic precursor lesions
      - Carcinomas associated with dysplasia more likely to be multifocal
    - Tobacco use
      - Tobacco carcinogens in saliva contact esophageal mucosa
      - Higher quantity and duration of smoking → higher risk
    - Alcohol abuse
      - Chronic irritation of esophageal mucosa
    - Synergetic effect of alcohol and tobacco use
    - Associated with low socioeconomic status, chronic irritation (tobacco, alcohol, chemicals, bacteria), caustic injury, prior radiation (breast, mediastinum)
    - Increased incidence in patients with esophageal achalasia
- Epidemiology & cancer incidence
  - Increasing incidence and mortality since 1975, with dramatic increase in AC
  - Estimated 16,470 new cases of esophageal AC and SCC diagnosed in USA in 2009
  - 6th leading cause of cancer death worldwide
    - Estimated 14,530 deaths in USA in 2009
  - Lifetime risk: 0.8% for men; 0.3% for women
    - AC: M:F = 7:1
    - SCC: M:F = 3:1
  - Highest incidence in USA among African-American men
    - 13 per 100,000
  - Mean age at diagnosis is 67 years old
  - Esophageal AC as common as SCC in USA
    - Incidence of AC is rapidly increasing since 1970s
    - Incidence of SCC is stable to declining
  - Esophageal SCC more common worldwide than AC
    - Responsible for as much as 90% of cases
  - Large geographic variation in incidence: High incidence in northern China
- Associated diseases, abnormalities
  - Predisposing conditions
    - Chronic stasis
    - Lye strictures
    - Head and neck tumors
    - Celiac disease
  - Complications
    - Tracheoesophageal fistula
    - Bleeding from erosion into vessels
  - In patients with esophageal SCC, head and neck cancers as well as dysplastic lesions are frequently observed

ESOPHAGEAL CARCINOMA

Gross Pathology & Surgical Features

- Adenocarcinoma
  - Masses or nodules in esophageal mucosa, usually in distal 1/3 of esophagus
  - Patterns
    - Polypoid (5-10%)
    - Infiltrating (40-50%)
    - Fungating (20-25%)
    - Flat (10-15%)
- Squamous cell carcinoma
  - Superficial lesions
    - White/gray plaques on mucosal surface
  - 3 patterns found in deeper lesions
    - Polypoid (60%)
      - Protrudes into esophageal lumen
    - Ulcerative (25%)
      - May erode into aorta, trachea, pericardium
    - Infiltrative (15%)
      - Causes luminal narrowing of esophagus, may ulcerate
  - Location
    - Proximal 1/3 (10-20%)
    - Middle 1/3 (50-60%)
    - Distal 1/3 (30%)

Microscopic Pathology

- H&E
  - Adenocarcinoma
    - Well differentiated
      - Tumor cells cuboidal to columnar in shape, contain irregular nucleoli and variable amount of eosinophilic or clear cytoplasm
    - Moderately differentiated
      - Tumor cells arranged in solid nests or clusters, may display cribriform pattern and show stratification
    - Poorly differentiated
      - Often diffusely infiltrate esophageal wall, arranged in sheets with poorly formed glandular lumina
  - Squamous cell carcinoma
    - Well differentiated
      - Intracellular bridges and abundant keratinization
    - Moderately differentiated
      - Higher number of primitive basaloid cells, only focal keratinization
    - Poorly differentiated
      - No keratinization, contains large pleomorphic cells
    - May see various degrees of differentiation within single tumor
- Special stains
  - Lugol iodine may identify areas of dysplasia

IMAGING FINDINGS

Detection

- Endoscopy
  - Gold standard for diagnosis of esophageal carcinoma
  - Endoscopic biopsy establishes histologic diagnosis
- Esophagogram (barium swallow)
  - Imaging appearances
    - Annular constriction
      - Irregular stricture
    - Polypoid
      - Intraluminal filling defect
    - Infiltrative
      - May cause luminal narrowing
    - Ulcerated mass
      - Central collection of barium
- CECT
  - Irregular, thick, enhancing esophageal wall
    - Normal distended esophageal wall is usually < 3 mm thick
    - Any wall thickness > 5 mm is considered abnormal
    - Wall thickening is usually asymmetric
  - Luminal narrowing, usually eccentric
  - Proximal esophageal dilatation
- PET/CT
  - Higher sensitivity than CT in detection of primary esophageal cancer
    - Helpful in detection of esophageal tumors in patients with metastases of unknown origin

Staging

- **Local disease**
  - **Endoscopic ultrasound (EUS)**
    - Most accurate imaging modality available for primary tumor staging (T staging)
      - Accurately predicts depth of invasion in 80-90% of patients
      - Can differentiate between T1, T2, and T3 disease
    - 7.5 and 12 MHz
      - Esophageal wall is visualized as 5 alternating layers of differing echogenicity
      - 1st hyperechoic layer: Interface between balloon and superficial mucosa
      - 2nd hypoechoic layer: Lamina propria and muscularis mucosae
      - 3rd hyperechoic layer: Submucosa
      - 4th hypoechoic layer: Muscularis propria
      - 5th hyperechoic layer: Interface between serosa and surrounding tissues
    - 20 MHz
      - 9 layers can be distinguished
    - Improved accuracy with higher T stage
      - T1 (75-82%)
      - T2 (64-82%)
      - T3 (89-94%)
      - T4 (88-100%)
    - Limitations
      - Operator dependent
      - Stenotic tumors may prevent passage of endoscope
      - Risk of perforation in patients with malignant stricture
      - Insensitive for deep lymph nodes
  - CECT
    - Limited in determining depth of esophageal wall infiltration
    - Unable to adequately differentiate between T1, T2, and T3 disease
    - Accuracy of CT for assessment of T stage is lower than that of endoscopic US

- Accuracy of 49–59% for CECT vs. 76–89% for EUS
- Exclusion or confirmation of T4 disease is most important role of CT in evaluating local disease
- CT criteria for local invasion include
  - Loss of fat planes between tumor and adjacent mediastinal structures
  - Displacement or indentation of other mediastinal structures
- Aortic invasion is suggested by
  - ≥ 90° of aorta in contact with tumor
  - Obliteration of triangular fat space between esophagus, aorta, and spine adjacent to primary tumor
- Tracheobronchial invasion is suggested by
  - Displacement of trachea or bronchus
  - Indentation of tracheal or bronchial posterior wall by tumor
  - Tracheobronchial fistula or tumor extension into airway lumen is definite sign of tracheobronchial invasion
- Pericardial invasion is suspected if there is
  - Pericardial thickening
  - Pericardial effusion
  - Heart indentation with loss of pericardial fat plane
- Performance of CECT for detection of mediastinal invasion
  - Sensitivity (88-100%)
  - Specificity (85-100%)
- Tracheobronchial, aortic, or pericardial involvement
  - ○ PET/CT
    - Limited value in assessing T stage
      - Depth of tumor invasion cannot be resolved
      - Possible relationship between degree of FDG uptake in primary tumor and depth of tumor invasion
- **Regional adenopathy**
  - ○ Nodal staging depends on number of involved nodes
    - In 6th edition of AJCC cancer staging manual, locoregional lymph nodes were defined on basis of location of primary esophageal tumor
      - Nodes away from primary tumor were considered M disease
      - Celiac nodes were considered M1a disease in patients with primary tumor in lower esophagus
    - In 7th edition of AJCC cancer staging manual
      - Regional nodes are redefined as extending from periesophageal cervical nodes to celiac nodes
      - Celiac nodes are considered regional nodes
      - N is subclassified according to number of involved regional nodes
  - ○ EUS
    - Criteria for metastatic nodes on EUS
      - Short axis > 10 mm
      - Round
      - Homogeneous, hypoechoic, central echo
      - Clear border
    - Superior to CT in detecting lymph node metastases
      - Accuracy ranges from 72-80%

- Improved accuracy with EUS-guided biopsy
  - ○ CECT
    - Less accurate than EUS and biopsy
    - Determining involvement of nodes depends on nodal size
      - Intrathoracic and abdominal lymph nodes > 1 cm in diameter
      - Supraclavicular lymph nodes with short axis > 5 mm
    - Limitations
      - Micrometastasis may be found in normal sized nodes
      - Some enlarged nodes may be reactive
    - Performance of CECT for detection of regional adenopathy
      - Sensitivity (30–60%)
      - Specificity (60-80%)
      - Accuracy (46-58%)
    - Performance of CECT for detection of abdominal nodes
      - Sensitivity (42%)
      - Specificity (93%)
  - ○ PET/CT
    - Performance depends on location of lymph nodes in relation to primary tumor
      - Intense uptake of FDG by primary tumor may obscure uptake in adjacent regional lymph nodes
    - Better performance for nodes away from primary tumor
      - Sensitivity of up to 90%
    - PET may confirm that enlarged node is likely metastatic
    - Sensitivity and specificity: 30-57% and 85-90%
      - FDG PET is more sensitive than CT for depicting nodal metastases in patients with esophageal SCC
      - FDG PET is slightly less specific than CT for depicting metastases
      - Low specificity of FDG PET for depiction of nodal metastasis compared with that of CT is caused mainly by high rate of false-positive hilar node interpretations
- **Distant metastases**
  - ○ Liver, lung, bone, peritoneum, nonregional lymph nodes, brain
  - ○ EUS
    - No role in evaluation of distant metastases
  - ○ CECT
    - Liver metastases
      - Ill-defined hypoattenuating lesions
    - Lung metastases
      - Single or multiple nodules
      - Presence of primary lung carcinoma needs to be ruled out in patients with solitary pulmonary metastasis
  - ○ PET/CT
    - Added value for staging over CECT alone
      - In patients with no metastases suspected, PET/CT detects metastases in up to 15%
    - Hypermetabolic activity in liver, lung, bone, peritoneum, nonregional lymph nodes, brain
- **Pleural or peritoneal seeding**

ESOPHAGEAL CARCINOMA

○ Pleural seeding is usually unilateral, may also be bilateral
○ CT demonstrates pleura-based nodules, pleural effusion, and irregular pleural thickening
○ Peritoneal seeding is usually secondary to abdominal or retroperitoneal lymph node metastases
  ▪ Should be suspected when ascites or nodular peritoneal lesions develop

Restaging
• Imaging recommendations
  ○ PET/CT
    ▪ Added value in differentiating tumor recurrence from post-treatment changes
      – Post-treatment changes may include fibrosis and inflammation, making CT appearance nonspecific
    ▪ Most sensitive method of differentiating chemotherapy responders from nonresponders
    ▪ Perform no sooner than 3-4 weeks after completion of chemoradiation
• Restaging important after neoadjuvant chemotherapy to determine if patient is surgical candidate
• May identify complications of therapy
  ○ Esophagitis
  ○ Tracheoesophageal fistula

CLINICAL ISSUES

Presentation
• Most common: Dysphagia for solids
• Later: Dysphagia for liquids, odynophagia, weight loss
• If local invasion: Aspiration (tracheoesophageal fistula), bleeding (aortoesophageal fistula)
• If metastases: Lymphadenopathy (Virchow node, left supraclavicular fossa), hepatomegaly, pleural effusion

Cancer Natural History & Prognosis
• More than 1/2 of patients present with unresectable disease/metastasis
• Survival rates at 5 years
  ○ Overall (14%)
  ○ Stage 0 (> 95%)
  ○ Stage I (50-80%)
  ○ Stage IIA (30-40%)
  ○ Stage IIB (10-30%)
  ○ Stage III (10-15%)
  ○ Stage IV: Median survival < 1 year
• Predictors of poor prognosis
  ○ Higher stage
  ○ Higher age
  ○ Weight loss > 10% body mass
  ○ Dysphagia
  ○ Large tumors
  ○ Lymphatic micrometastases
  ○ Esophageal AC has better long-term prognosis after resection than does SCC
    ▪ Overall 5-year survival rate is 47% for AC vs. 37% for SCC group

Treatment Options
• Major treatment alternatives

○ Endoscopic mucosal resection (EMR) for superficial cancer controversial
  ▪ Mostly used with < 2 cm, flat M1-M2 mucosal lesions arising in Barrett esophagus
  ▪ Requires close follow-up with endoscopy
  ▪ Long-term outcomes unknown
○ Photodynamic therapy (PDT)
  ▪ Photosensitizing drug injected into tumor
  ▪ Tumor exposed to specific wavelength of light through endoscope
  ▪ Nonthermal phototoxic reaction → cell death
○ Radiation therapy (RT)
  ▪ Used for palliation
○ Perioperative chemotherapy
  ▪ Probable small survival benefit vs. surgery alone
○ Concurrent chemoradiation (CRT)
  ▪ Chemotherapy helps sensitize cancer to RT, plus treats micrometastases
  ▪ Radiation therapy plus cisplatin and 5-fluorouracil
  ▪ Higher toxicity than RT alone
  ▪ Increases survival over RT alone
  ▪ 5-year survival ~ 26%
  ▪ May turn out to be a definitive nonoperative treatment (data better for SCC vs. AC)
○ Neoadjuvant CRT + esophagectomy
  ▪ Increased survival over CRT alone
  ▪ Standard of care in USA for localized disease
○ Transthoracic esophagectomy (Ivor-Lewis)
  ▪ Laparotomy plus right thoracotomy to create anastomosis in upper chest or neck
  ▪ Lymphadenectomy under direct visualization
  ▪ Complications: Anastomosis leak, cardiopulmonary complications
○ Transhiatal esophagectomy
  ▪ Anastomosis created in neck, avoids thoracotomy
  ▪ Fewer complications vs. transthoracic esophagectomy
• Major treatment roadblocks
  ○ Toxicity from concurrent CRT
    ▪ Esophageal mucositis
    ▪ Hematologic suppression
  ○ Complications from esophagectomy
    ▪ Operative mortality (8-20%)
      – Lower end of mortality rate in centers that perform > 19 per year; 2% in high volume centers
    ▪ Long-term quality of life issues
      – Swallowing disorders
      – Indigestion/heartburn
• Treatment options by stage
  ○ Stage 0
    ▪ Esophagectomy preferred
    ▪ EMR and PDT if unable to undergo surgery
  ○ Stage I
    ▪ Esophagectomy
    ▪ EMR and PDT if unable to undergo surgery
  ○ Stage IIA
    ▪ Esophagectomy
  ○ Stage IIB
    ▪ Multimodality approach (chemotherapy and radiation) offers best chance for survival benefit in patients able to tolerate

- Chemotherapy may help manage micrometastasis and sensitize tissue for radiation
  - Stage III
    - Multimodality approach
  - Stage IV
    - Palliative treatment, may include radiation therapy and chemotherapy
    - Palliative interventional techniques include balloon dilatation and stents

REPORTING CHECKLIST

T Staging
- Depth of tumor invasion
  - EUS most sensitive for determining tumor depth
  - CT
    - Not useful for differentiation between T1 and T2
    - Look for signs of mediastinal invasion
      - T3: Tumor invades adventitia and extends into mediastinal fat
      - T4a: Resectable tumor invading pleura, pericardium, or diaphragm
      - T4b: Unresectable tumor invading aorta, vertebral body, trachea

N Staging
- Regional lymph nodes
  - EUS most sensitive
- N1: Metastasis in 1-2 regional lymph nodes
- N2: Metastasis in 3-6 regional lymph nodes
- N3: Metastasis in ≥ 7 regional lymph nodes

M Staging
- Most common sites: Liver, lung, bones, adrenals, kidneys, brain
- CECT and PET/CT most sensitive
  - PET/CT upgrades disease in approximately 15%

SELECTED REFERENCES

1. American Joint Committee on Cancer: AJCC Cancer Staging Manual. 7th ed. New York: Springer. 103-15, 2010
2. Morita M et al: Alcohol drinking, cigarette smoking, and the development of squamous cell carcinoma of the esophagus: epidemiology, clinical findings, and prevention. Int J Clin Oncol. 15(2):126-34, 2010
3. Rice TW et al: 7th edition of the AJCC Cancer Staging Manual: esophagus and esophagogastric junction. Ann Surg Oncol. 17(7):1721-4, 2010
4. Kim TJ et al: Multimodality assessment of esophageal cancer: preoperative staging and monitoring of response to therapy. Radiographics. 29(2):403-21, 2009
5. van Vliet EP et al: Staging investigations for oesophageal cancer: a meta-analysis. Br J Cancer. 98(3):547-57, 2008
6. Hofstetter W et al: Proposed modification of nodal status in AJCC esophageal cancer staging system. Ann Thorac Surg. 84(2):365-73; discussion 374-5, 2007
7. Kim TJ et al: Postoperative imaging of esophageal cancer: what chest radiologists need to know. Radiographics. 27(2):409-29, 2007
8. Cerfolio RJ et al: The accuracy of endoscopic ultrasonography with fine-needle aspiration, integrated positron emission tomography with computed tomography, and computed tomography in restaging patients with esophageal cancer after neoadjuvant chemoradiotherapy. J Thorac Cardiovasc Surg. 129(6):1232-41, 2005
9. Downey RJ et al: Whole body 18FDG-PET and the response of esophageal cancer to induction therapy: results of a prospective trial. J Clin Oncol. 21(3):428-32, 2003
10. Glickman JN: Section II: pathology and pathologic staging of esophageal cancer. Semin Thorac Cardiovasc Surg. 15(2):167-79, 2003
11. Morita M et al: Risk factors for multicentric occurrence of carcinoma in the upper aerodigestive tract-analysis with a serial histologic evaluation of the whole resected-esophagus including carcinoma. J Surg Oncol. 83(4):216-21, 2003
12. Yoon YC et al: Metastasis to regional lymph nodes in patients with esophageal squamous cell carcinoma: CT versus FDG PET for presurgical detection prospective study. Radiology. 227(3):764-70, 2003
13. Lightdale CJ: Esophageal cancer. American College of Gastroenterology. Am J Gastroenterol. 94(1):20-9, 1999
14. Noh HM et al: CT of the esophagus: spectrum of disease with emphasis on esophageal carcinoma. Radiographics. 15(5):1113-34, 1995
15. Quint LE et al: Incidence and distribution of distant metastases from newly diagnosed esophageal carcinoma. Cancer. 76(7):1120-5, 1995

ESOPHAGEAL CARCINOMA

Adenocarcinoma, Stage IA (T1 N0 M0 G2)

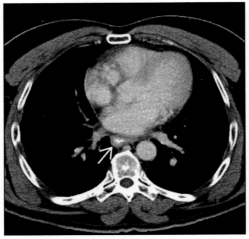

Adenocarcinoma, Stage IA (T1 N0 M0 G2)

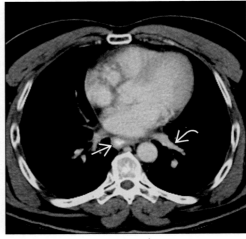

(Left) Axial CECT in a 47-year-old man with long history of Barrett esophagus, who was found to have adenocarcinoma during a routine EGD, shows minimal esophageal wall thickening ➡ without obvious mass. *(Right)* Axial PET/CT in the same patient shows an eccentric area of increased metabolic activity ➡. The upper end of the lesion is above the level of the lower border of the inferior pulmonary vein ➡, making this a middle thoracic lesion.

Adenocarcinoma, Stage IA (T1 N0 M0 G2)

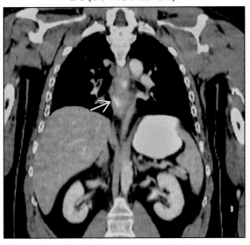

Adenocarcinoma, Stage IA (T1 N0 M0 G2)

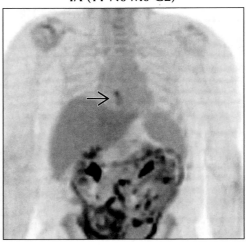

(Left) Coronal PET/CT in the same patient shows the area of increased metabolic activity in the middle to distal thoracic esophagus ➡. *(Right)* Coronal PET shows subtle area of increased metabolic activity in the middle to distal thoracic esophagus ➡. Although tumor location does not affect the staging of adenocarcinoma, it is still important for surgical planning and because many tumors are detected on imaging before histological diagnosis.

Adenocarcinoma, Stage IB (T2 N0 M0 G2)

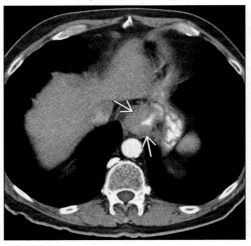

Adenocarcinoma, Stage IB (T2 N0 M0 G2)

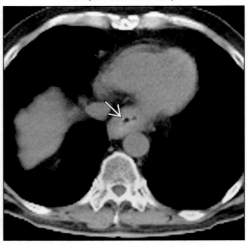

(Left) Axial CECT in a 75-year-old man with history of heartburn shows thickening of the wall of the distal esophagus ➡. *(Right)* Axial PET/CT in the same patient shows increased metabolic activity ➡ limited to the distal esophagus. Pathology showed a T2 adenocarcinoma, grade 2. This is one of the situations in which the tumor grade can affect its stage; if this were grade 3 adenocarcinoma, it would be classified as stage IIA.

ESOPHAGEAL CARCINOMA

Squamous Cell Carcinoma, Stage IIA (T3 N0 M0 G2)

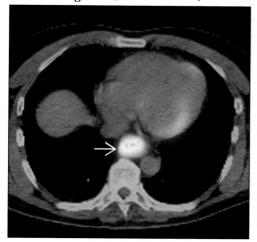

Squamous Cell Carcinoma, Stage IIA (T3 N0 M0 G2)

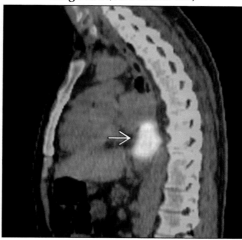

(Left) Axial PET/CT in a 53-year-old man, who presented with dysphagia and was found to have esophageal carcinoma on EGD, shows increased metabolic activity of the diffusely thickened lower thoracic esophagus ➡. (Right) Sagittal PET/CT in the same patient shows increased metabolic activity of the lower esophageal mass ➡. T3 squamous cell carcinoma, grade 2 or 3, in the lower abdominal esophagus is stage IIA, while similar lesions in the upper or middle esophagus are stage IIB.

Adenocarcinoma, Stage IIB (T3 N0 M0)

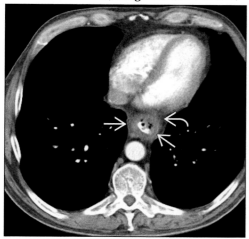

Adenocarcinoma, Stage IIB (T3 N0 M0)

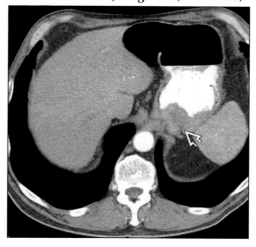

(Left) Axial CECT in a 55-year-old man with history of gastroesophageal reflux shows distal thoracic esophageal circumferential wall thickening ➡. Hazy interface with the periesophageal fat ➡ suggests adventitial invasion. (Right) Axial CECT in the same patient shows tumor invading the gastric cardia ➡. A T3 N0 M0 lower esophageal adenocarcinoma is stage IIB, regardless of histological grade, whereas T3 N0 M0 squamous cell carcinoma is stage IB if G1 and stage IIA if G2-3.

Adenocarcinoma, Stage IIB (T3 N0 M0)

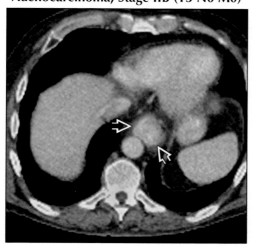

Adenocarcinoma, Stage IIB (T3 N0 M0)

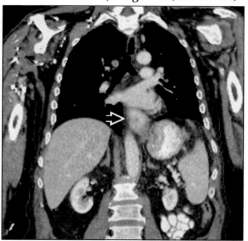

(Left) Axial PET/CT in the same patient shows significant increase in metabolic activity of the lower esophageal mass ➡. (Right) Coronal PET/CT in the same patient shows the hypermetabolic lower esophageal mass ➡. No nodal or distant metastases were found.

ESOPHAGEAL CARCINOMA

Adenocarcinoma, Stage IIB (T3 N0 M0)

Adenocarcinoma, Stage IIB (T3 N0 M0)

(Left) Upper GI barium examination in a patient who presented with painful dysphagia shows irregular stricture ➡ of the lower thoracic esophagus giving pseudoachalasia appearance. *(Right)* Upper GI barium examination in the same patient shows the irregularity and nodularity ➡ of the distal esophagus in the region of stricture.

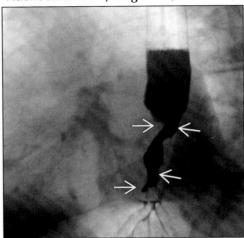

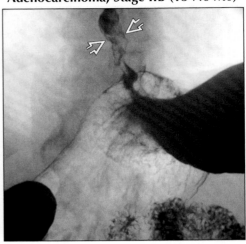

Adenocarcinoma, Stage IIB (T3 N0 M0)

Adenocarcinoma, Stage IIB (T3 N0 M0)

(Left) Axial CECT in the same patient shows circumferential esophageal wall thickening ➡ with tumor extending into the paraesophageal fat ➡ without invasion of the surrounding structures. Note the distended azygos vein ➡ next to the aorta. *(Right)* Sagittal CECT in the same patient shows esophageal wall thickening ➡. The proximal end of the tumor ➡ is above the level of the inferior pulmonary vein; its location is therefore middle esophagus.

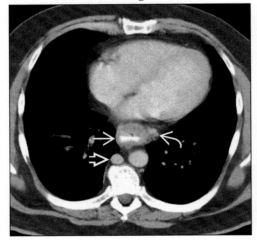

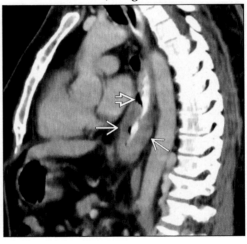

Adenocarcinoma, Stage IIB (T3 N0 M0)

Adenocarcinoma, Stage IIB (T3 N0 M0)

(Left) Axial PET/CT in the same patient shows increased metabolic activity within the thick-walled esophagus ➡. *(Right)* Coronal PET/CT in the same patient shows diffuse increase in metabolic activity within the region of esophageal wall thickening ➡.

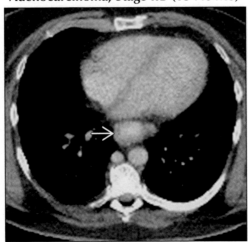

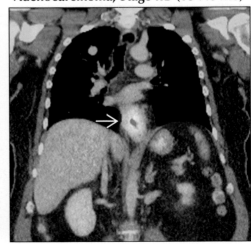

Adenocarcinoma, Stage IIB (T2 N1 M0)

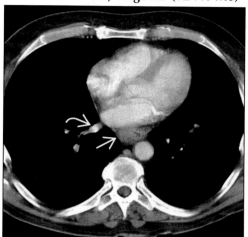

Adenocarcinoma, Stage IIB (T2 N1 M0)

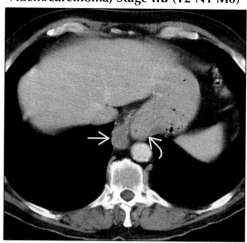

(Left) Axial CECT in a 63-year-old man shows circumferential esophageal wall thickening ➡ that extends above the level of the lower border of the inferior pulmonary vein ➡, making it a middle thoracic esophageal tumor. CECT cannot differentiate between T1 and T2 and sometimes even T3 tumor, as T staging depends on the depth of tumor invasion. *(Right)* Axial CECT in the same patient shows an enlarged diaphragmatic lymph node ➡ adjacent to the GEJ ➡.

Adenocarcinoma, Stage IIB (T2 N1 M0)

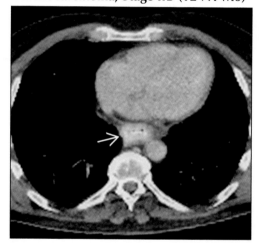

Adenocarcinoma, Stage IIB (T2 N1 M0)

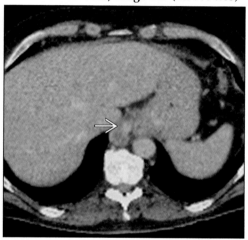

(Left) Axial PET/CT in the same patient shows increased metabolic activity in the area of circumferential wall thickening ➡. *(Right)* Axial PET/CT in the same patient shows increased metabolic activity within the enlarged diaphragmatic lymph node ➡.

Adenocarcinoma, Stage IIB (T2 N1 M0)

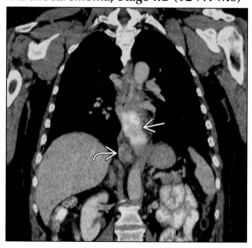

Adenocarcinoma, Stage IIB (T2 N1 M0)

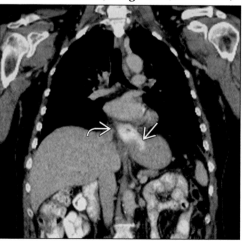

(Left) Coronal PET/CT in the same patient shows increased metabolic activity within the middle and distal thoracic esophagus ➡, as well as mild increased activity within the diaphragmatic lymph node ➡. *(Right)* Coronal PET/CT in the same patient shows increased metabolic activity in the abdominal esophagus ➡ and extending into the gastric cardia ➡.

ESOPHAGEAL CARCINOMA

Squamous Cell Carcinoma, Stage IIB (T2 N1 M0)

Squamous Cell Carcinoma, Stage IIB (T2 N1 M0)

(Left) Axial NECT in a 62-year-old man who presented with dysphagia shows circumferential thickening of the wall of the lower thoracic esophagus ➡ (below the level of the pulmonary vein). *(Right)* Axial NECT in the same patient shows fullness in the region between the esophagus and aorta ➡, as well as a small paraesophageal node ➢.

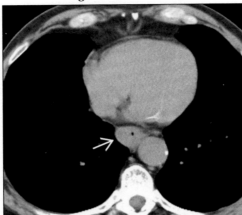

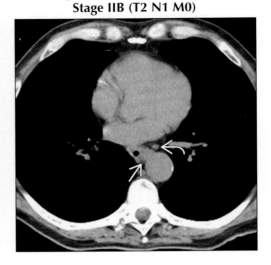

Squamous Cell Carcinoma, Stage IIB (T2 N1 M0)

Squamous Cell Carcinoma, Stage IIB (T2 N1 M0)

(Left) Axial PET/CT in the same patient shows mild increased metabolic activity within the esophagus ➢. *(Right)* Axial PET/CT in the same patient shows increased uptake ➡ in the area of fullness seen on NECT. This was due to metastatic lymph node, which was confirmed at surgery. The paraesophageal node ➢ does not show increased metabolic activity and was negative for malignancy on histological examination.

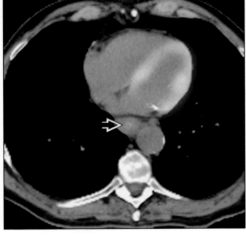

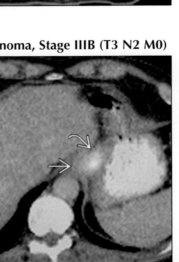

Adenocarcinoma, Stage IIIB (T3 N2 M0)

Adenocarcinoma, Stage IIIB (T3 N2 M0)

(Left) Axial PET/CT in a 45-year-old man, who presented with dysphagia and was found to have abdominal esophageal adenocarcinoma, shows increased metabolic activity in the distal esophagus ➡ with extension to the gastric cardia ➢. *(Right)* Axial PET/CT in the same patient shows increased metabolic activity within 2 small celiac nodes ➢. Celiac nodes are considered regional lymph nodes in the new 7th edition AJCC staging system (2010).

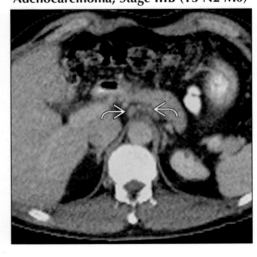

ESOPHAGEAL CARCINOMA

Adenocarcinoma, Stage IIIC (T4b N0 M0)

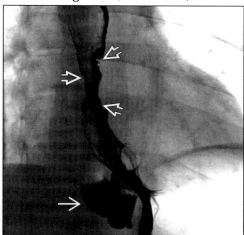

Adenocarcinoma, Stage IIIC (T4b N0 M0)

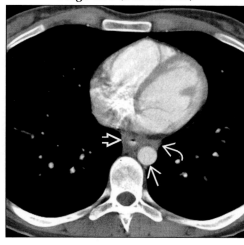

(Left) Oblique view from an esophagogram shows an irregular sticture of the lower thoracic esophagus ➡ in this 35-year-old woman with long history of paraesophageal hernia ➡, reflux esophagitis, and Barrett esophagus. (Right) Axial CECT in the same patient shows circumferential esophageal wall thickening ➡ and abnormal paraesophageal soft tissue ➡ with > 90° contact with the descending thoracic aorta ➡ suggesting aortic involvement. This was confirmed at surgery.

Squamous Cell Carcinoma, Stage IIIC (T4b N1 M0)

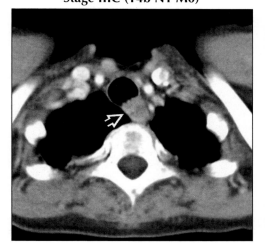

Squamous Cell Carcinoma, Stage IIIC (T4b N1 M0)

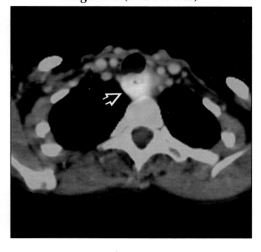

(Left) Axial CECT in a 57-year-old man who presented with dysphagia shows circumferential thickening of the wall of the esophagus ➡ with tumor invading into the posterior wall of the trachea. Unresectable tumor invading surrounding structures, e.g., trachea, vertebrae, or aorta, is designated T4b. (Right) Axial PET/CT in the same patient shows diffuse thickening of the cervical esophagus with circumferential increase in metabolic activity ➡.

Squamous Cell Carcinoma, Stage IIIC (T4b N1 M0)

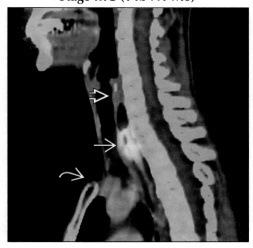

Squamous Cell Carcinoma, Stage IIIC (T4b N1 M0)

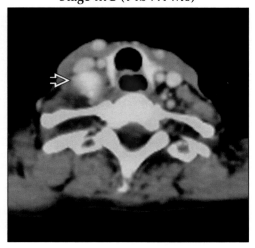

(Left) Sagittal PET/CT in the same patient shows esophageal mass ➡ in the cervical esophagus (below the hypopharynx ➡ and above the sternal notch ➡). The mass is extremely hypermetabolic, which may correlate with deep tumor invasion within the esophageal wall. (Right) Axial PET/CT in the same patient shows an enlarged hypermetabolic cervical lymph node ➡.

ESOPHAGEAL CARCINOMA

(Left) Axial CECT in a 62-year-old man who presented with dysphagia shows circumferential thickening of the wall of the lower thoracic esophagus ➡. The maximum normal thickness of esophageal wall is 5 mm. **(Right)** Axial CECT in the same patient shows an enlarged subaortic lymph node ➢.

Adenocarcinoma, Stage IIIC (T3 N3 M0)

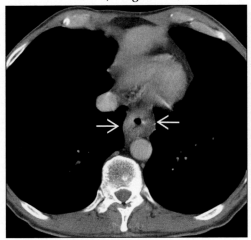

Adenocarcinoma, Stage IIIC (T3 N3 M0)

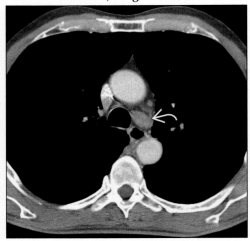

(Left) Axial PET/CT in the same patient shows marked metabolic activity of the primary lower thoracic esophageal tumor ➡. **(Right)** Axial PET/CT in the same patient at a lower level shows increased metabolic activity of left ➢ and right ➡ paraesophageal lymph nodes.

Adenocarcinoma, Stage IIIC (T3 N3 M0)

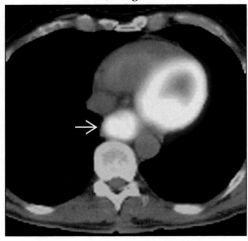

Adenocarcinoma, Stage IIIC (T3 N3 M0)

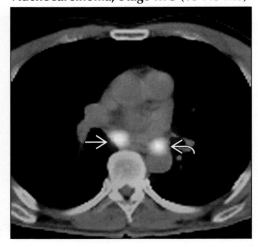

(Left) Coronal PET/CT in the same patient shows the hypermetabolic primary lower thoracic esophageal tumor ➡ in addition to metabolically active subaortic ➢ and diaphragmatic ➡ lymph nodes. **(Right)** Coronal CECT in the same patient shows metabolically active subcarinal ➡ and left paraesophageal lymph nodes. The presence of 7 or more metastatic nodes makes this N3 disease.

Adenocarcinoma, Stage IIIC (T3 N3 M0)

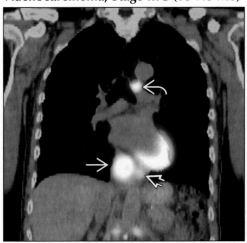

Adenocarcinoma, Stage IIIC (T3 N3 M0)

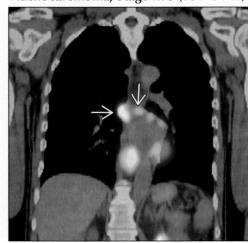

ESOPHAGEAL CARCINOMA

Squamous Cell Carcinoma, Stage IV (T2 N1 M1)

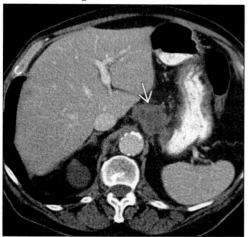

Squamous Cell Carcinoma, Stage IV (T2 N1 M1)

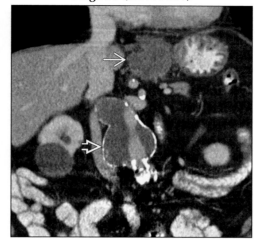

(Left) Axial CECT shows a low-attenuation mass ⮞ in the region of the gastrohepatic ligament in this 72-year-old man, in whom routine CECT for evaluation of aortic aneurysm demonstrated a mass adjacent to the gastroesophageal junction. *(Right)* Coronal CECT in the same patient shows an irregular mass in the region of the gastrohepatic ligament ⮞. Note the abdominal aortic aneurysm ⮞.

Squamous Cell Carcinoma, Stage IV (T2 N1 M1)

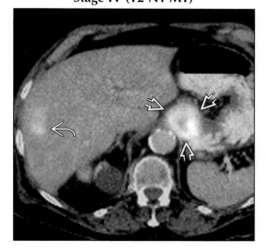

Squamous Cell Carcinoma, Stage IV (T2 N1 M1)

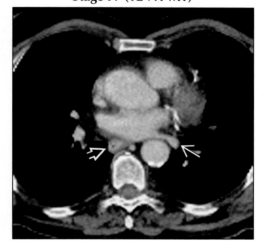

(Left) Axial PET/CT in the same patient shows an enlarged, metabolically active gastrohepatic lymph node ⮞, as well as a metabolically active hepatic metastatic lesion ⮞. *(Right)* Axial PET/CT in the same patient shows increased metabolic activity ⮞ in the middle thoracic esophagus (starting above the level of inferior pulmonary vein ⮞). The esophageal lesion invaded into the muscularis propria and thus is classified T2.

Squamous Cell Carcinoma, Stage IV (T2 N1 M1)

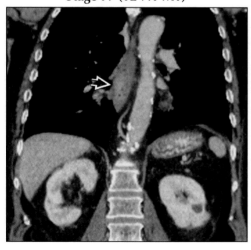

Squamous Cell Carcinoma, Stage IV (T2 N1 M1)

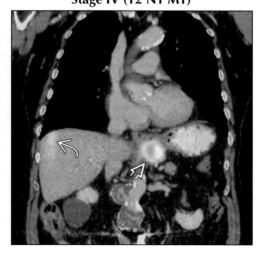

(Left) Coronal PET/CT in the same patient shows a metabolically active primary esophageal tumor ⮞. *(Right)* Coronal PET/CT in the same patient shows a large, metabolically active gastrohepatic node ⮞ and a hepatic metastatic lesion ⮞. This case emphasizes that regional nodal metastases from esophageal carcinoma may occur anywhere from periesophageal cervical nodes to celiac nodes, due to extensive intercommunicating esophageal lymphatic drainage.

ESOPHAGEAL CARCINOMA

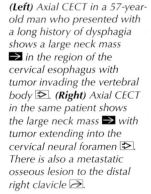

(Left) Axial CECT in a 67-year-old woman who presented with dysphagia shows circumferential thickening ➡ of the wall of the middle thoracic esophagus (between the azygos vein and the pulmonary vein) as well as a right hilar enlarged lymph node ➡. *(Right)* Axial CECT in the same patient shows enlarged subaortic lymph node ➡.

Squamous Cell Carcinoma, Stage IV (T3 N2 M1)

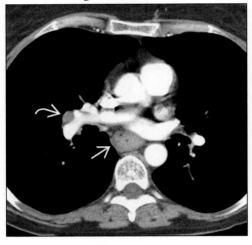

Squamous Cell Carcinoma, Stage IV (T3 N2 M1)

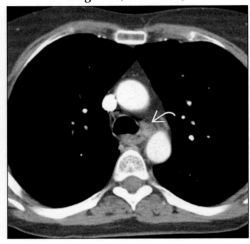

(Left) Axial CECT in the same patient shows enlarged right supraclavicular lymph nodes ➡. *(Right)* Axial CECT, lung window algorithm, in the same patient shows multiple pulmonary nodules ➡, 1 of which is cavitary ➡. Cavitation in pulmonary nodules is a frequent feature of pulmonary metastases from primary squamous cell esophageal carcinoma.

Squamous Cell Carcinoma, Stage IV (T3 N2 M1)

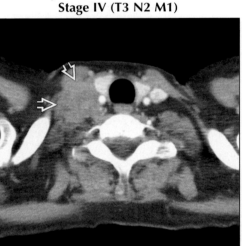

Squamous Cell Carcinoma, Stage IV (T3 N2 M1)

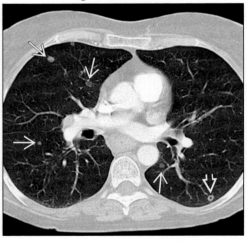

(Left) Axial CECT in a 57-year-old man who presented with a long history of dysphagia shows a large neck mass ➡ in the region of the cervical esophagus with tumor invading the vertebral body ➡. *(Right)* Axial CECT in the same patient shows the large neck mass ➡ with tumor extending into the cervical neural foramen ➡. There is also a metastatic osseous lesion to the distal right clavicle ➡.

Squamous Cell Carcinoma, Stage IV (T4b N0 M1)

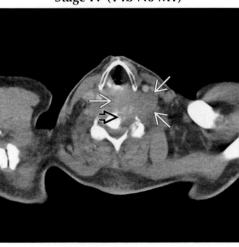

Squamous Cell Carcinoma, Stage IV (T4b N0 M1)

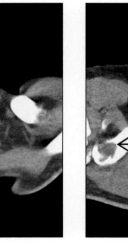

ESOPHAGEAL CARCINOMA

Recurrent Esophageal Carcinoma

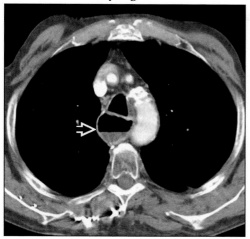

Recurrent Esophageal Carcinoma

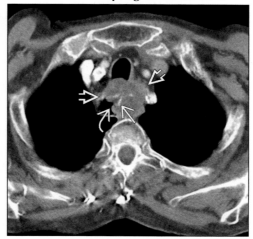

(Left) Axial CECT in a 75-year-old man who underwent esophagectomy and gastric pull-up a year earlier shows the intrathoracic stomach ⮕ with a fluid level. *(Right)* Axial CECT in the same patient at the level of esophagogastric anastomosis shows a large mass ⮕ infiltrating into the superior mediastinum and protruding into the gastric lumen ⮕. Notice the surgical sutures ⮕.

Recurrent Esophageal Carcinoma

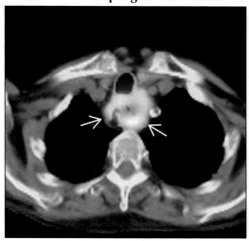

Recurrent Esophageal Carcinoma

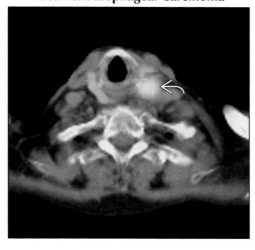

(Left) Axial PET/CT in the same patient shows a hypermetabolic mass ⮕ arising at the site of esophagogastric anastomosis. *(Right)* Axial PET/CT in the same patient at the level of the lower neck shows a metastatic, hypermetabolic, left side neck lymph node ⮕.

Recurrent Esophageal Carcinoma

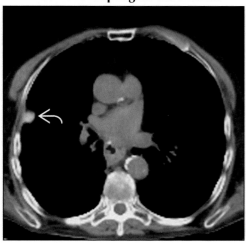

Recurrent Esophageal Carcinoma

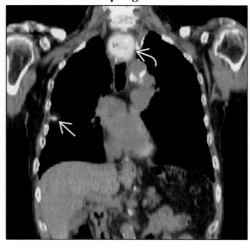

(Left) Axial PET/CT in the same patient shows a hypermetabolic, metastatic, pleural-based pulmonary nodule ⮕. *(Right)* Coronal PET/CT in the same patient shows the recurrent anastomotic tumor ⮕ and the pulmonary parenchymal metastatic nodule ⮕.

ESOPHAGEAL CARCINOMA

Metastatic Disease Following Esophagectomy

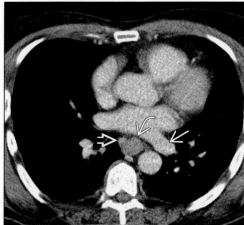

Metastatic Disease Following Esophagectomy

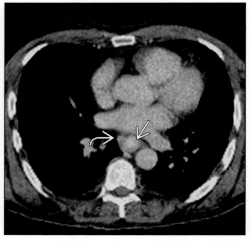

(Left) Axial CECT in a 57-year-old man who presented with dysphagia shows circumferential esophageal wall thickening ➡ starting above the level of the inferior pulmonary vein ➡. There is also a small periesophageal lymph node ⊟. *(Right)* Axial PET/CT in the same patient shows increased metabolic activity within the middle thoracic esophagus ➡ and subtle increased activity within the periesophageal lymph node ➡.

Metastatic Disease Following Esophagectomy

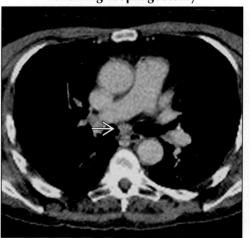

Metastatic Disease Following Esophagectomy

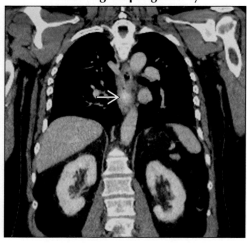

(Left) Axial PET/CT in the same patient shows slight increase in metabolic activity within a subcarinal lymph node ➡. *(Right)* Coronal PET/CT in the same patient shows the increased metabolic activity within the middle thoracic esophagus ➡. Biopsy revealed squamous cell carcinoma. The patient underwent esophagectomy, and the surgical staging was stage IIIA (T2 N2 M0).

Metastatic Disease Following Esophagectomy

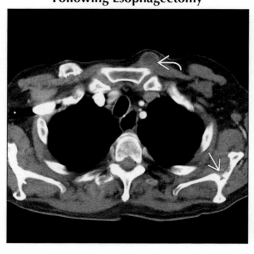

Metastatic Disease Following Esophagectomy

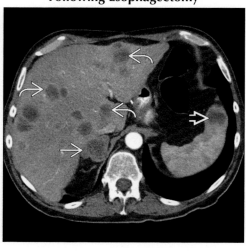

(Left) Axial CECT in the same patient 6 months after esophagectomy shows a metastatic low-attenuation lesion within the left pectoralis muscle ➡ and destructive lesion of the left scapula ➡. *(Right)* Axial CECT in the same patient shows widespread low-attenuation, ill-defined metastatic lesions within the liver ➡, a large metastatic lesion of the right adrenal gland ➡, and a hypoattenuating lesion within the spleen ⊟.

ESOPHAGEAL CARCINOMA

Recurrent Local and Metastatic Disease Following Esophagectomy

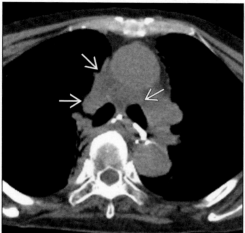

Recurrent Local and Metastatic Disease Following Esophagectomy

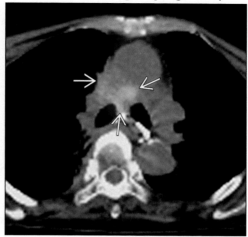

(Left) Axial NECT shows abnormal ill-defined soft tissue mass ➡️ replacing the mediastinal fat in this 66-year-old man who underwent esophagectomy for stage IIB adenocarcinoma of the middle esophagus and presented 1 year later with superior vena caval obstruction. *(Right)* Axial PET/CT in the same patient shows increased metabolic activity within the mediastinal mass ➡️ due to metastatic disease.

Recurrent Local and Metastatic Disease Following Esophagectomy

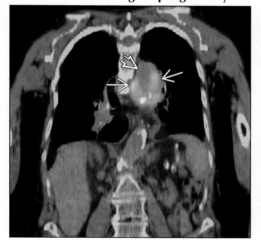

Recurrent Local and Metastatic Disease Following Esophagectomy

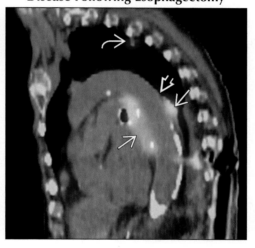

(Left) Coronal PET/CT in the same patient shows increased metabolic activity of the abnormal soft tissue ➡️ encasing the descending thoracic aorta ➡️. *(Right)* Sagittal PET/CT in the same patient shows increased metabolic activity of the abnormal soft tissue ➡️ encasing the descending thoracic aorta ➡️, as well as a pleural-based hypermetabolic nodule ➡️.

Recurrent Local and Metastatic Disease Following Esophagectomy

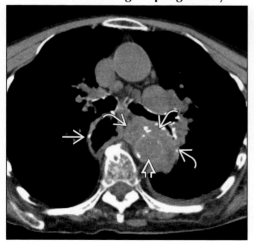

Recurrent Local and Metastatic Disease Following Esophagectomy

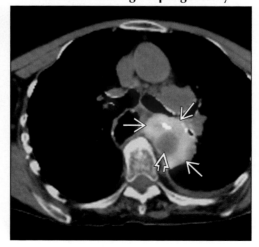

(Left) Axial NECT in a 77-year-old woman, 12 months after esophagectomy for stage IIB esophageal adenocarcinoma (T3 N0 M0), shows gastric pull-up ➡️ and abnormal soft tissue ➡️ encasing the thoracic aorta ➡️. *(Right)* Axial PET/CT in the same patient shows increased metabolic activity of the abnormal soft tissue ➡️ encasing the descending thoracic aorta ➡️.

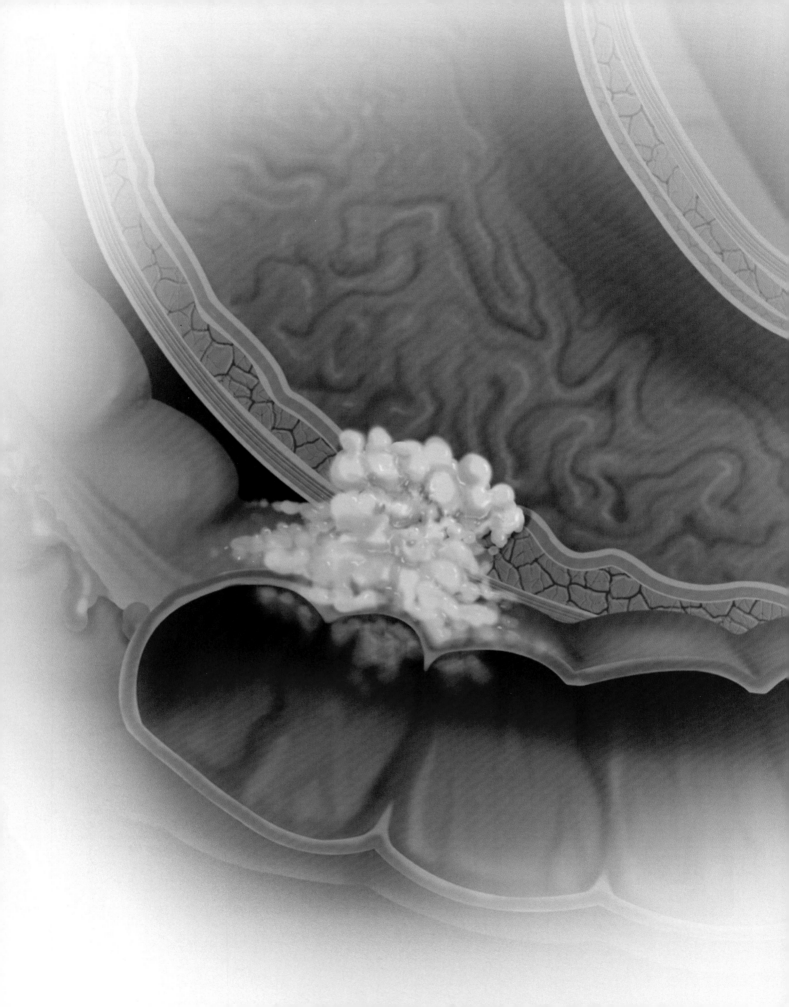

Stomach Carcinoma

STOMACH CARCINOMA

(T) Primary Tumor	Adapted from 7th edition AJCC Staging Forms.
TNM	*Definitions*
TX	Primary tumor cannot be assessed
T0	No evidence of primary tumor
Tis	Carcinoma in situ: Intraepithelial tumor without invasion of the lamina propria
T1	Tumor invades lamina propria, muscularis mucosae, or submucosa
T1a	Tumor invades lamina propria or muscularis mucosae
T1b	Tumor invades submucosa
T2	Tumor invades muscularis propria[1]
T3	Tumor penetrates subserosal connective tissue without invasion of visceral peritoneum or adjacent structures[2]
T4	Tumor invades serosa (visceral peritoneum) or adjacent structures[2]
T4a	Tumor invades serosa (visceral peritoneum)
T4b	Tumor invades adjacent structures

(N) Regional Lymph Nodes	
NX	Regional lymph node(s) cannot be assessed
N0	No regional lymph node metastasis[3]
N1	Metastasis in 1-2 regional lymph nodes
N2	Metastasis in 3-6 regional lymph nodes
N3	Metastasis in ≥ 7 regional lymph nodes
N3a	Metastasis in 7-15 regional lymph nodes
N3b	Metastasis in ≥ 16 regional lymph nodes

(M) Distant Metastasis	
M0	No distant metastasis
M1	Distant metastasis

[1]*A tumor may penetrate the muscularis propria with extension into the gastrocolic or gastrohepatic ligaments, or into the greater or lesser omentum, without perforation of the visceral peritoneum covering these structures. In this case, the tumor is classified T3. If there is perforation of the visceral peritoneum covering the gastric ligaments or the omentum, the tumor should be classified T4.*

[2]*The adjacent structures of the stomach include the spleen, transverse colon, liver, diaphragm, pancreas, abdominal wall, adrenal gland, kidney, small intestine, and retroperitoneum. Intramural extension to the duodenum or esophagus is classified by the depth of the greatest invasion in any of these sites, including the stomach.*

[3]*A designation of pN0 should be used if all examined lymph nodes are negative, regardless of the total number removed and examined.*

STOMACH CARCINOMA

AJCC Stages/Prognostic Groups

Adapted from 7th edition AJCC Staging Forms.

Stage	T	N	M
0	Tis	N0	M0
IA	T1	N0	M0
IB	T2	N0	M0
	T1	N1	M0
IIA	T3	N0	M0
	T2	N1	M0
	T1	N2	M0
IIB	T4a	N0	M0
	T3	N1	M0
	T2	N2	M0
	T1	N3	M0
IIIA	T4a	N1	M0
	T3	N2	M0
	T2	N3	M0
IIIB	T4b	N0	M0
	T4b	N1	M0
	T4a	N2	M0
	T3	N3	M0
IIIC	T4b	N2	M0
	T4b	N3	M0
	T4a	N3	M0
IV	Any T	Any N	M1

STOMACH CARCINOMA

Tis

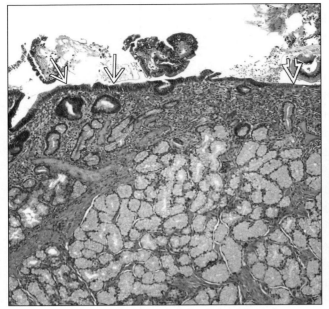

Low magnification of H&E stained section shows a flat lesion with dysplasia of the surface epithelium ➡. Note the abrupt demarcation between the dark blue dysplastic cells and the normal epithelium on the right ➡. (Original magnification 40x.)

Tis

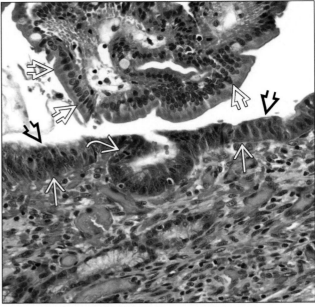

Higher magnification shows neoplastic cells ➡ with hyperchromatic, crowded, and stratified cells that are limited to the basement membrane ➡ and a mitotic figure ➡. Compare the neoplastic cells to the normal epithelium of the floating mucosal fragment ➡. (Original magnification 500x.)

T1

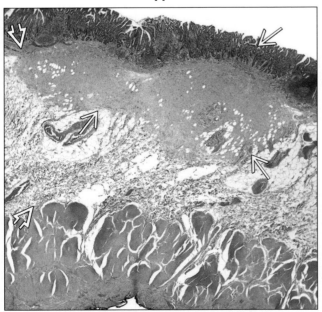

H&E stained section shows invasive gastric carcinoma ➡ that involves lamina propria and extends to invade the upper portion of the submucosa ➡. (Original magnification 20x.)

T1

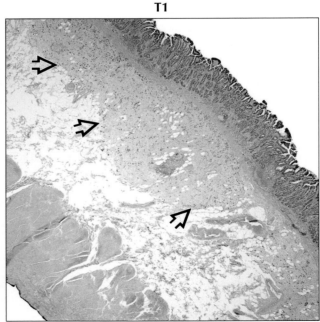

Section from the same specimen stained with cytokeratin immunohistochemical stain highlights (in brown) the invasive carcinoma cells ➡. (Original magnification 20x.)

T1

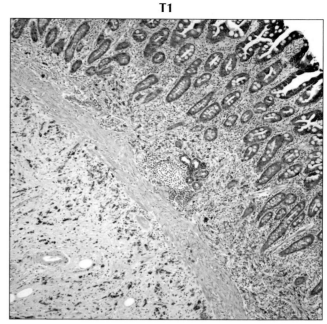

Higher magnification of H&E stained section of invasive gastric adenocarcinoma shows the neoplastic cells in the lamina propria extending through the muscularis mucosae and into the submucosa. (Original magnification 100x.)

T1

Identical high magnification image stained with cytokeratin immunohistochemical stain highlights (in brown) the invasive carcinoma cells in both the lamina propria and the submucosa.

T2

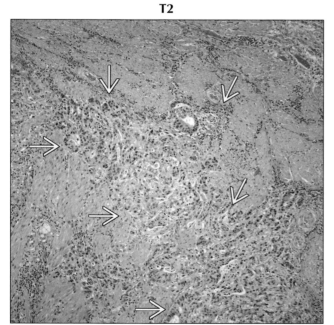

H&E stained section shows invasive gastric adenocarcinoma ➡ extending into the muscle bundles of the muscularis propria. (Original magnification 100x.)

T4

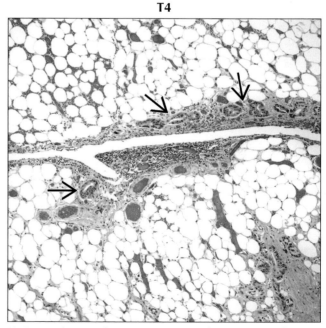

H&E stained section from invasive gastric adenocarcinoma shows the neoplastic glands ➡ invading serosa and extending to involve the fibrofatty connective tissue of the omentum. The fat cells are the round (clear/white) spaces. (Original magnification 100x.)

STOMACH CARCINOMA

T1a

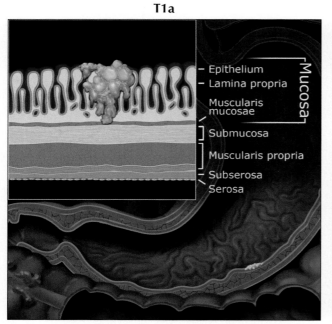

Graphic illustrates T1a tumor, which invades lamina propria or muscularis mucosae.

T1b

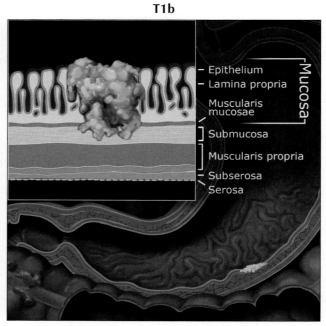

Graphic illustrates T1b tumor, which invades the submucosal layer.

T2

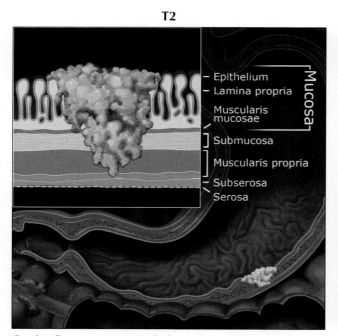

Graphic illustrates T2 tumor, which invades muscularis propria.

T3

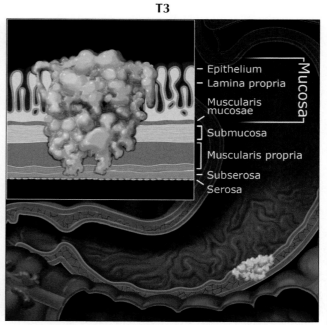

Graphic illustrates T3 tumor, which invades subserosal connective tissue without invasion of visceral peritoneum or adjacent structures.

T3

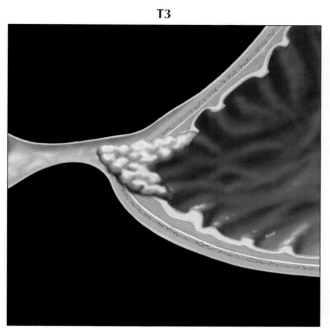

Graphic illustrates T3 tumor, which invades into the subperitoneal space between the peritoneal layers of the gastric ligaments without invasion of visceral peritoneum.

T4a

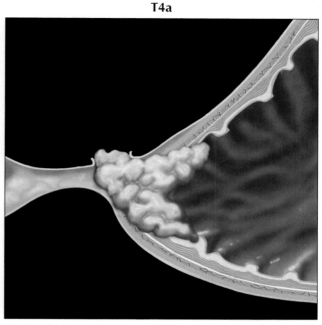

Graphic illustrates T4a tumor, which invades into the subperitoneal space between the peritoneal layers of the gastric ligaments and penetrates through the visceral peritoneum into the peritoneal space.

T4a

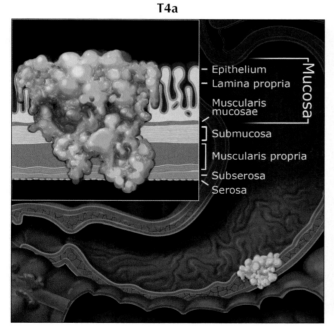

Graphic illustrates tumor that invades serosa (visceral peritoneum) without extension to adjacent structures, consistent with T4a disease.

T4b

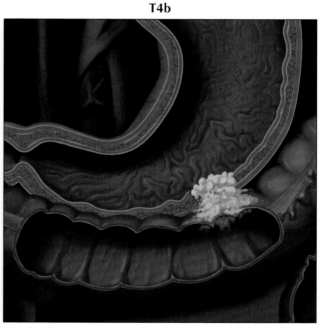

Graphic illustrates tumor invading the transverse colon. Invasion of adjacent structures, which also include the spleen, liver, diaphragm, pancreas, abdominal wall, adrenal gland, kidney, small intestine, and retroperitoneum, constitutes T4b disease.

Nodal Stations of the Stomach

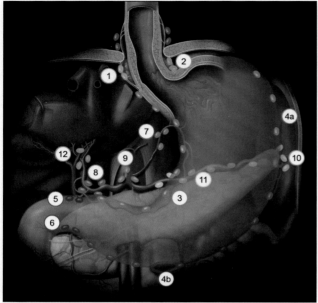

Graphic shows the nodal stations of the stomach: Perigastric nodes of lesser curvature (1, 3, and 5); perigastric nodes of greater curvature (2, 4, and 6); left gastric nodes (7); nodes along common hepatic artery (8); nodes along celiac artery (9); nodes along splenic artery (10 and 11); and hepatoduodenal nodes (12).

N1

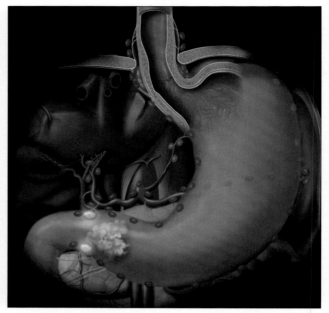

Graphic illustrates N1 disease, defined as metastases in 1-2 regional nodes.

N2

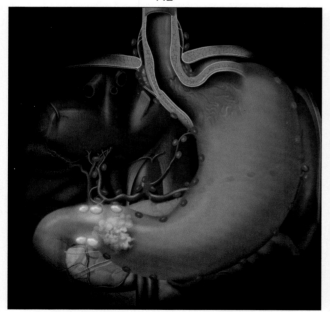

Graphic illustrates N2 disease, defined as metastases in 3-6 regional nodes.

N3a

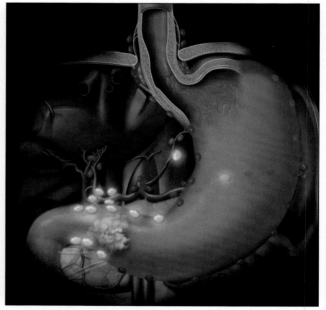

Graphic illustrates N3a disease, defined as metastases in 7-15 regional nodes.

N3b

M1

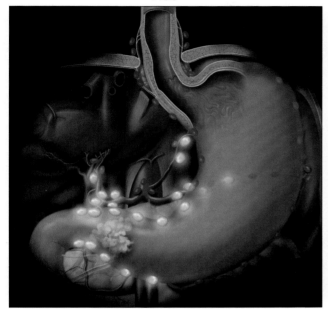

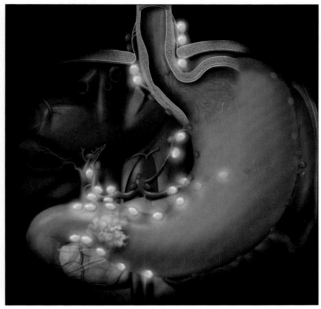

Graphic illustrates N3b disease, defined as metastases in at least 16 regional nodes.

Graphic illustrates involvement of nodes above the diaphragm, which is considered distant metastases (M1).

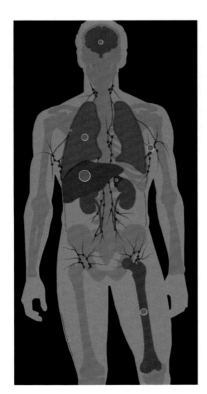

METASTASES, ORGAN FREQUENCY

Liver	37%
Lung	16%
Bone	16%
Lymph nodes	14%
Brain	6%
Adrenal gland	3%
Pleura	2%
Subcutaneous tissues	2%

Other reported sites include breast, kidneys, bone marrow, pericardium, and spine.

STOMACH CARCINOMA

OVERVIEW

General Comments
- Tumors arising at gastroesophageal junction (GEJ) or arising in stomach ≤ 5 cm from and crossing GEJ are staged with esophageal carcinoma

Classification
- Histological classification
  ○ Adenocarcinoma
    ■ Intestinal type
    ■ Diffuse type
  ○ Papillary adenocarcinoma
  ○ Tubular adenocarcinoma
  ○ Mucinous adenocarcinoma
    ■ Substantial amount of extracellular mucin (> 50% of tumor) is retained within tumor
  ○ Signet ring cell carcinoma (> 50% signet ring cells)
  ○ Adenosquamous carcinoma
  ○ Squamous cell carcinoma
  ○ Small cell carcinoma
  ○ Undifferentiated carcinoma
  ○ Other

PATHOLOGY

Routes of Spread
- Submucosal spread
  ○ Main mechanism of transpyloric spread of tumor into duodenum
    ■ Brunner glands believed to prevent direct cancer invasion from gastric mucosa to duodenal mucosa
- Subperitoneal spread
  ○ Tumor may penetrate muscularis propria with extension within subperitoneal space without perforation of visceral peritoneum
    ■ Such tumor is classified T3
  ○ Tumor may spread to adjacent organs between peritoneal layers forming ligaments around stomach
    ■ Spread to left lobe of liver via gastrohepatic ligament (GHL)
      - GHL stretches from cardia and lesser curvature to insert into fissure of ligamentum venosum
      - GHL identified by presence of left and right gastric vessels
    ■ Spread to liver via hepatoduodenal ligament (HDL)
      - HDL is free edge of gastrohepatic ligament, extends from upper aspect of proximal duodenum to liver hilum
      - HDL contains hepatic artery, bile duct, and portal vein
    ■ Spread to spleen via gastrosplenic ligament (GSL)
      - GSL attaches posterolateral wall of fundus and greater curvature to splenic hilum
      - GSL carries short gastric and leftmost parts of left gastroepiploic vessels
    ■ Spread to transverse colon via gastrocolic ligament (GCL)
      - GCL extends from greater curvature to transverse colon and extends anteriorly to form greater omentum, which covers colon and small intestine
      - GCL contains right and most of left gastroepiploic vessels
    ■ Spread to pancreas via lesser sac
- Peritoneal spread
  ○ Tumor invading serosa can seed into peritoneal cavity
  ○ Krukenberg tumors
    ■ Metastatic tumor to ovaries through peritoneal seeding
    ■ Usually bilateral
- Nodal spread
  ○ Perigastric lymph nodes are involved early and later drain into central nodes around celiac axis and superior mesenteric artery
    ■ Tumors along lesser curvature of body and esophagogastric junction (area supplied by left gastric artery) → gastrohepatic ligament nodes → left gastric nodes → suprapancreatic nodes → celiac nodes
    ■ Tumors along lesser curvature of antrum and pylorus (area supplied by right gastric artery) → hepatoduodenal ligament nodes → nodes along hepatic artery → celiac nodes
    ■ Tumors along greater curvature (area supplied by right gastroepiploic artery) → nodes accompanying right gastroepiploic vessels → nodes at gastrocolic trunk or gastroduodenal nodes → superior mesenteric or celiac nodes
    ■ Tumors along greater curvature of body (area supplied by left gastroepiploic artery) → nodes along left gastroepiploic vessels → splenic hilum nodes → celiac nodes
  ○ Risk factors for lymph node metastasis include
    ■ Lymphovascular invasion
    ■ Depth of invasion (submucosa)
    ■ Tumor diameter > 20 mm
    ■ Ulcer or ulcer scar
    ■ Mucinous adenocarcinoma histological type
- Hematogenous spread
  ○ Usually involves liver, lungs, and bones

General Features
- Gastric adenocarcinoma
  ○ Intestinal type
    ■ More common
    ■ Tends to predominate in geographic regions with high incidence of gastric carcinoma, e.g., Japan
    ■ Frequently ulcerative
    ■ Occurs in distal stomach
    ■ Often preceded by prolonged precancerous phase
  ○ Diffuse type
    ■ Incidence is similar in most populations throughout world
    ■ Occurs more often in young patients
    ■ Especially common in cardia
- Etiology
  ○ Known risk factors include
    ■ *Helicobacter pylori* gastric infection
      - 6x increase in risk
    ■ Advanced age
    ■ Male gender
    ■ Diet low in fruits and vegetables
    ■ Diet high in salted, smoked, or preserved foods
    ■ Chronic atrophic gastritis

STOMACH CARCINOMA

- Intestinal metaplasia
- Pernicious anemia
- Gastric adenomatous polyps
- Family history of gastric cancer
- Cigarette smoking
- Ménétrier disease (giant hypertrophic gastritis)
- Familial adenomatous polyposis
  - 0.5% risk of developing gastric carcinoma
- Previous gastric surgery
  - Rationale is that previous gastric surgery alters normal pH of stomach
- Epidemiology & cancer incidence
  - Median age at diagnosis is 71 years
  - Age-adjusted incidence rate is 7.9 per 100,000 per year
    - 11.0 per 100,000 men
    - 5.5 per 100,000 women
  - 4th most common cancer worldwide
    - Estimated 21,130 cases of gastric carcinoma diagnosed in USA in 2009
      - 12,820 men and 8,310 women
  - 2nd leading cause of cancer death worldwide
    - Estimated 10,620 patients died of gastric carcinoma in USA 2009
  - Highest rates of gastric carcinoma in Asia and Eastern Europe
- Associated diseases, abnormalities
  - Chronic atrophic gastritis
  - Pernicious anemia
  - Gastric adenomatous polyps
  - Ménétrier disease (giant hypertrophic gastritis)

Gross Pathology & Surgical Features
- Borrmannthis morphological classification
  - Type I (polypoid): Well-circumscribed polypoid tumors
  - Type II (fungating): Polypoid tumors with marked central infiltration
  - Type III (ulcerated): Ulcerated tumors with infiltrative margins
  - Type IV (infiltrating): Linitis plastica

Microscopic Pathology
- Gastric adenocarcinoma
  - Intestinal type
    - Characterized by cohesive neoplastic cells forming gland-like tubular structures
  - Diffuse type
    - Cell cohesion is absent, so that individual cells infiltrate and thicken stomach wall without forming discrete mass
- Papillary adenocarcinoma
  - Exophytic lesions with elongated slender or plump finger-like processes, in which fibrovascular cores and connective tissue support cells
- Tubular carcinoma
  - Well-defined glandular lumens
- Mucinous carcinoma
  - Sometimes also referred to as colloid carcinoma
  - Contain abundant mucin secreted by tumor cell, creating mucous lakes
- Signet ring cell carcinoma
  - Composed of cells containing unsecreted mucus in cytoplasm to compress nucleus to edge of cell
  - Often demonstrate infiltrative gross appearance

- Some signet ring tumors appear to form a linitis plastica-type tumor by spreading intramurally, usually not involving mucosa

IMAGING FINDINGS

Detection
- Endoscopy
  - Most sensitive and specific diagnostic method in patients suspected of having gastric cancer
  - Allows direct visualization of tumor location, extent of mucosal involvement, and biopsy (or cytologic brushings) for tissue diagnosis
- Double-contrast upper gastrointestinal series
  - 3 major radiographic patterns
    - Malignant ulcer: Radiographic findings include
      - Irregular ulcer crater
      - Distortion or obliteration of surrounding normal areae gastricae
      - Presence of nodular, irregular, radiating folds, which may stop well short of ulcer crater
      - Fused, clubbed, or amputated tips of folds
      - Does not project beyond expected gastric contour when viewed in profile
      - Presence of tumor mass forming an acute angle with gastric wall
    - Polypoid or nodular thickening of gastric wall
    - Diffuse infiltrative pattern (linitis plastica)
      - Diffuse decrease distensibility of stomach
      - Diffuse fold thickening
- CT
  - MDCT has improved detection of gastric carcinoma compared to single slice CT
    - Improved detection rate on thin-sliced MPR images compared to 5 mm slice axial images
    - MDCT allows 3D volume rendering and virtual endoscopic imaging
      - Detection rate of early gastric cancer increases up to 96% when using 3D MDCT
  - Water-filling method with gastric CT allows clear depiction of gastric wall and gastric tumor without overshooting artifacts by air in lumen
  - Appearance on CT parallels gross pathological types
    - Well-circumscribed polypoid tumors
    - Ulcerated tumors with infiltrative margins
    - Linitis plastica
    - Patients with nonvisualized primary lesions on MDCT with optimized imaging protocol have early gastric cancers
      - 98% have stage pT1 confined to mucosa or involving submucosal layer
- FDG PET
  - Water intake just before PET imaging is effective method for suppressing physiological FDG uptake in stomach
  - Variable levels of FDG uptake have been found
  - Mucinous adenocarcinoma, signet ring cell carcinoma, and poorly differentiated adenocarcinomas tend to show significantly lower FDG uptake than do other histologic types

Staging
- **Local disease**

STOMACH CARCINOMA

- Endoscopic ultrasound (EUS), MDCT, and MR have comparable diagnostic accuracy in T staging and in assessing serosal involvement
- EUS
  - Regarded as imaging modality of choice in assessing local invasion of gastric cancer
  - Invasive technique
    - Requires sedation
    - Has recognized procedure- and sedation-related complications, morbidity, and mortality
  - Has limited depth of penetration
    - Well suited for evaluation of local invasion
    - Limited usefulness in overall assessment of more distant spread
  - Potential discrepancy between EUS and histologic findings
    - Normal gastric wall has been described on EUS as consisting of 5-9 layers; histologically, however, it consists of only 5 layers
    - Results from additional echoes produced by interfaces between different histologic layers
    - These ultrasound artifacts → misevaluation of depth of cancer invasion
  - Diagnostic accuracy of EUS for overall T staging varies (65-92.1%)
  - Sensitivity and specificity for assessing serosal involvement varies (77.8-100% and 67.9-100%, respectively)
- CT
  - MDCT has better diagnostic performance than single row CT scanner
    - Faster scanning overcomes breathing artifacts
    - Thinner slices avoid partial volume effect and allow multiplanar reformats
    - Reported accuracy in tumor staging ranges from 43-86% for single detector row CT scanners and from 77-89% for MDCT
  - Addition of MPR significantly improves performance of MDCT in local staging of gastric cancer
  - Advantages of MDCT over EUS
    - Ability to demonstrate regional perigastric disease beyond reach of EUS
    - Ability to demonstrate distant regions, like paraaortic lymph nodes and abdominal organs, such as liver
  - MPR images are superior to axial images for evaluation of craniocaudal extent of tumor
  - Diagnostic accuracy of MDCT for overall T staging varies (73.8-88.9%)
  - Diagnostic accuracy is higher with advanced T disease
    - 45.93% for T1 disease
    - 53.03% for T2 disease
    - 86.49% for T3 disease
    - 85.79% for T4 disease
  - Sensitivity and specificity for assessing serosal involvement varies (82.8-100% and 80-96.8%, respectively)
- MR
  - Diagnostic accuracy of MR for overall T staging varies (71.4-82.6%)

- Sensitivity and specificity for assessing serosal involvement varies (89.5-93.1% and 94.1-100%, respectively)
- PET/CT
  - Not helpful for local staging
- Imaging criteria for T staging
  - T1
    - Tumor invades lamina propria, muscularis mucosae, or submucosa
    - Tumor shows focal thickening of inner gastric wall
    - Visible low-attenuation strip along outer layer of gastric wall
  - T2 and T3
    - Different articles in literature describe imaging findings differentiating T2 and T3
      - Articles are based on 6th edition of AJCC staging system
      - Difficult to radiologically distinguish between T2 and T3 in 7th edition
    - T2
      - Tumor invades muscularis propria
      - Thickened gastric wall with loss or disruption of low-attenuation stripe
      - Smooth outer border and clear fat plane around tumor
    - T3
      - Tumor penetrates subserosal connective tissue without invasion of visceral peritoneum or adjacent structures
      - Tumor shows focal or diffuse transmural thickening of gastric wall
      - Tumor penetrating muscularis propria with extension into gastric ligaments without perforation of visceral peritoneum covering these structures would be classified as T3
  - T4a
    - Tumor invades visceral peritoneum
    - Irregular or nodular outer border &/or infiltration of epigastric fat
      - Tumor perforating visceral peritoneum covering gastric ligaments or omenta is classified as T4a
  - T4b
    - Tumor invades adjacent structures
      - Loss of intervening fat plane between tumor and adjacent structures does not necessarily imply invasion
      - Structures adjacent to stomach are spleen, transverse colon, liver, diaphragm, pancreas, abdominal wall, adrenal gland, kidney, small intestine, and retroperitoneum
- **Nodal disease**
  - Regional lymph nodes are
    - Perigastric nodes, found along lesser and greater curvatures
    - Nodes located along left gastric, common hepatic, splenic, and celiac arteries
  - Involvement of other intraabdominal lymph nodes, such as hepatoduodenal, retropancreatic, mesenteric, and paraaortic, is classified as distant metastasis
  - Regional nodes are considered involved when
    - Short axis diameter is > 6 mm for perigastric nodes

- Short axis diameter is > 8 mm for extraperigastric nodes
- Nearly round shape
- Fatty hilum is absent or eccentric
- Marked or heterogeneous enhancement
- Overall accuracy of MDCT in preoperative N staging is 75.22%
- Regional lymphadenectomy specimen will ordinarily contain at least 15 lymph nodes
- **Distant metastasis**
  - Common sites are liver, lungs, and bones

Restaging
- CT is modality of choice for restaging and follow-up after curative surgery
  - Allows detection of local recurrence, peritoneal implants, and metastatic disease
    - Sensitivity is 89%
    - Specificity is 64%
  - Recurrence at gastric stump or anastomosis appears as nonspecific localized bowel wall thickening
- EUS can be used for local and nodal restaging following neoadjuvant therapy
- PET/CT
  - Sensitivity is 68-75%
  - Specificity is 71-77%
  - Accuracy is 75-83%
  - Negative predictive value is 55-78%
  - Positive predictive value is 86-89%
  - Limitations of PET/CT include
    - Low FDG uptake in signet ring cell carcinoma and mucinous carcinoma
    - Poor spatial resolution for detection of small peritoneal nodules
    - Variability among patients in terms of physiologic peritoneal uptake

CLINICAL ISSUES

Presentation
- Early gastric carcinoma often produces no specific symptoms when it is superficial and potentially surgically curable
  - Up to 50% of patients may have nonspecific gastrointestinal complaints, such as dyspepsia
    - However, gastric cancer is found in only 1-2% of patients with dyspepsia
- Patients may present with
  - Anorexia and weight loss (95%)
  - Vague and insidious abdominal pain
  - Nausea, vomiting, and early satiety
    - May occur with
      - Tumors obstructing gastrointestinal lumen (gastric outlet obstruction)
      - Infiltrative tumors impairing gastric distension
  - Ulcerated tumors may cause bleeding
    - Hematemesis
    - Melena
    - Massive upper gastrointestinal hemorrhage
  - Patients with advanced disease
    - Palpable abdominal mass
    - Cachexia
    - Bowel obstruction
    - Ascites

- Hepatomegaly
- Lower extremity edema
- Carcinoembryonic antigen (CEA) and CA-19.9 serum levels may be elevated in patients with advanced gastric cancers
  - Only approximately 1/3 of all patients with stomach carcinoma have abnormal CEA &/or CA-19.9 levels

Cancer Natural History & Prognosis
- Stage of gastric carcinoma at diagnosis
  - Stage I (20%)
  - Stage II (19%)
  - Stage III (34%)
  - Stage IV (27%)
- Survival depends on the tumor stage
  - Overall survival rate for gastric carcinoma is approximately 15-20%
  - 5-year survival for gastric carcinoma
    - Stage IA (70.8%)
    - Stage IB (57.4%)
    - Stage IIA (45.5%)
    - Stage IIB (32.8%)
    - Stage IIIA (19.8%)
    - Stage IIIB (14.0%)
    - Stage IIIC (9.2%)
    - Stage IV (4.0%)

Treatment Options
- Stage 0, I, and II
  - More than 90% of patients with stage 0 disease treated by gastrectomy with lymphadenectomy will survive beyond 5 years
  - 1 of following surgical procedures
    - Distal subtotal gastrectomy
      - Tumor is not in fundus or at cardioesophageal junction
    - Proximal subtotal gastrectomy or total gastrectomy, both with distal esophagectomy
      - Tumor involves cardia
    - Total gastrectomy
      - Tumor involves stomach diffusely or arises in body of stomach and extends to within 6 cm of cardia or distal antrum
  - Regional lymphadenectomy is recommended with all of above procedures
  - Postoperative chemoradiation therapy for patients with stages IB and II
- Stages III and IV
  - Radical surgery
    - Curative resection procedures are confined to patients who, at time of surgical exploration, do not have extensive nodal involvement
    - All patients with tumors that can be resected should undergo surgery
    - As many as 15% of selected stage III and IV patients can be cured by surgery alone, particularly if lymph node involvement is minimal (< 7 lymph nodes)
  - Postoperative chemoradiation therapy
  - Perioperative chemotherapy

STOMACH CARCINOMA

REPORTING CHECKLIST

T Staging
- EUS, MDCT, and MR have comparable diagnostic accuracy in T staging and in assessing serosal involvement
- T1
  - Focal thickening of inner gastric wall with visible low-attenuation strip along outer layer of gastric wall
- T2 and T3
  - Difficult to radiologically distinguish T2 and T3 based on 7th edition AJCC staging system
  - Thickened gastric wall with loss or disruption of low-attenuation stripe with smooth outer border and clear fat plane around tumor
- T4a
  - Irregular or nodular outer border &/or infiltration of epigastric fat
- T4b
  - Tumor invades adjacent structures

N Staging
- CT, PET/CT, EUS, and MR can be used for nodal staging
- Perigastric nodes and nodes located along left gastric, common hepatic, splenic, and celiac arteries are considered regional nodes
- Other intraabdominal lymph nodes, such as hepatoduodenal, retropancreatic, mesenteric, and paraaortic, as well as extraabdominal nodes are classified as distant metastasis

M Staging
- Commonly to liver, lungs, and bones

SELECTED REFERENCES

1. American Joint Committee on Cancer: AJCC Cancer Staging Manual. 7th ed. New York: Springer. 117-26, 2010
2. Catalano V et al: Gastric cancer. Crit Rev Oncol Hematol. 71(2):127-64, 2009
3. Kim YH et al: Staging of T3 and T4 gastric carcinoma with multidetector CT: added value of multiplanar reformations for prediction of adjacent organ invasion. Radiology. 250(3):767-75, 2009
4. Kunisaki C et al: Risk factors for lymph node metastasis in histologically poorly differentiated type early gastric cancer. Endoscopy. 41(6):498-503, 2009
5. Namikawa T et al: Clinicopathological features of early gastric cancer with duodenal invasion. World J Gastroenterol. 15(19):2309-13, 2009
6. Sim SH et al: The role of PET/CT in detection of gastric cancer recurrence. BMC Cancer. 9:73, 2009
7. Yan C et al: Value of multidetector-row computed tomography in the preoperative T and N staging of gastric carcinoma: A large-scale Chinese study. J Surg Oncol. Epub ahead of print, 2009
8. Sun L et al: Clinical role of 18F-fluorodeoxyglucose positron emission tomography/computed tomography in post-operative follow up of gastric cancer: initial results. World J Gastroenterol. 14(29):4627-32, 2008
9. Chen CY et al: Gastric cancer: preoperative local staging with 3D multi-detector row CT--correlation with surgical and histopathologic results. Radiology. 242(2):472-82, 2007
10. Kwee RM et al: Imaging in local staging of gastric cancer: a systematic review. J Clin Oncol. 25(15):2107-16, 2007
11. Yu JS et al: Value of nonvisualized primary lesions of gastric cancer on preoperative MDCT. AJR Am J Roentgenol. 189(6):W315-9, 2007
12. Lim JS et al: CT and PET in stomach cancer: preoperative staging and monitoring of response to therapy. Radiographics. 26(1):143-56, 2006
13. Shimizu K et al: Diagnosis of gastric cancer with MDCT using the water-filling method and multiplanar reconstruction: CT-histologic correlation. AJR Am J Roentgenol. 185(5):1152-8, 2005
14. D'Angelica M et al: Patterns of initial recurrence in completely resected gastric adenocarcinoma. Ann Surg. 240(5):808-16, 2004
15. Fuchs CS et al: Gastric carcinoma. N Engl J Med. 333(1):32-41, 1995

STOMACH CARCINOMA

Stage IA (T1a N0 M0)

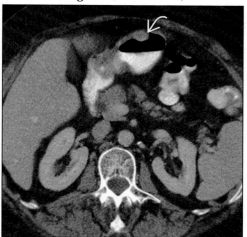

Stage IA (T1a N0 M0)

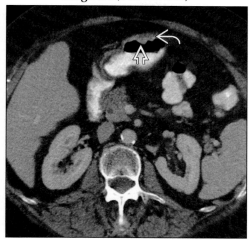

(Left) Axial CECT in a 35-year-old asymptomatic woman, who requested to have a CT of the abdomen because of a strong family history of gastric carcinoma, shows a focal mass ➘ along the anterior wall of the stomach. *(Right)* Axial CECT in the same patient shows focal thickening ➘ of the anterior wall of the stomach with a hypoattenuating stripe ➘ at the base of the mass. A T1a lesion invading the submucosa was found on histological examination.

Stage IIA (T3 N0 M0)

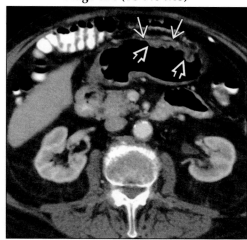

Stage IIA (T3 N0 M0)

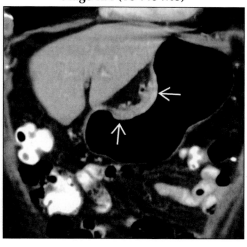

(Left) Axial CECT in an 82-year-old man, who had an abnormal EGD showing an anterior wall gastric mass, reveals an infiltrating polypoid gastric mass ➘ along the anterior wall of the stomach with transmural enhancement. Note the sharp gastric contour at the base of the mass ➘. *(Right)* Coronal CECT in the same patient shows extension of the tumor ➘ along the lesser curvature of the stomach without evidence of invasion beyond the gastric wall.

Stage IIA (T2 N1 M0)

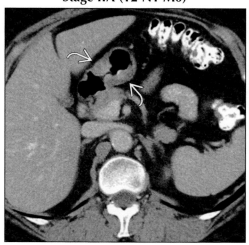

Stage IIA (T2 N1 M0)

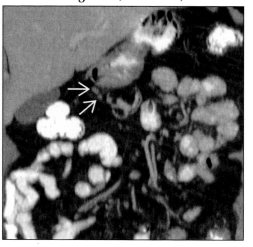

(Left) Axial CECT in a patient who presented with epigastric pain demonstrates circumferential thickening of the antrum ➘. The outer contour of the stomach appears smooth. *(Right)* Coronal CECT in the same patient shows 2 pathologic perigastric lymph nodes ➘. Pathological examination confirmed muscularis propria invasion without involvement of the subserosal connective tissue or T2 category.

STOMACH CARCINOMA

Stage IIB (T2 N2 M0)

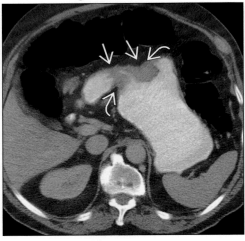

Stage IIB (T2 N2 M0)

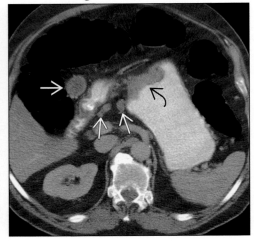

(Left) Axial CECT in a patient who presented with melena shows a circumferential antral mass ➡ causing narrowing of the gastric antrum. The mass exhibits marked scirrhous reaction ➡ with flattening and decreased distensibility of the anterior gastric wall. *(Right)* Axial CECT in the same patient shows the antral mass ➡. Multiple pathologic perigastric nodes are seen ➡. A total of 5 pathologic nodes were found during surgery, making this N2 disease.

Stage IIB (T4a N0 M0)

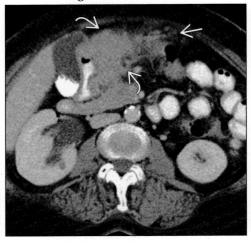

Stage IIB (T4a N0 M0)

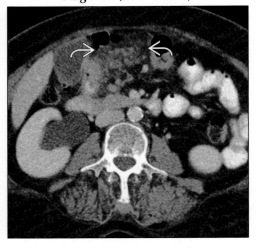

(Left) Axial CECT shows a fungating circumferential mass involving the gastric antrum and pylorus ➡. The mass significantly narrows the stomach at the antrum. Haziness and nodularities ➡ are seen involving the gastrocolic ligament adjacent to the mass. The ligament stretches from the greater curvature of stomach to the transverse colon. *(Right)* Axial CECT in the same patient shows the gastrocolic ligament studded with multiple small nodules ➡.

Stage IIB (T4a N0 M0)

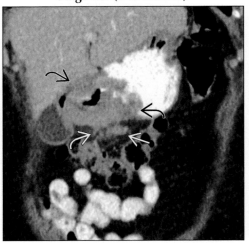

Stage IIB (T4a N0 M0)

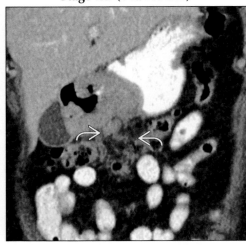

(Left) Coronal CECT in the same patient shows diffuse circumferential thickening of the gastric antrum ➡. Irregularity of the gastric contour ➡ suggests serosal invasion. Haziness and nodularity ➡ of the gastrocolic ligament is again seen. *(Right)* Coronal CECT in the same patient shows nodularity of the gastrocolic ligament ➡. Tumor extending to the gastrocolic ligament without invading the transverse colon is categorized as T4a.

STOMACH CARCINOMA

Stage IIIA (T4a N1 M0)

Stage IIIA (T4a N1 M0)

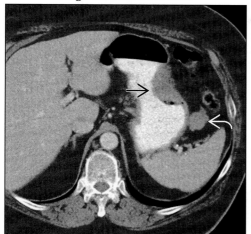

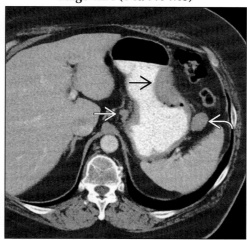

(Left) Axial CECT in a 69-year-old man, who presented with dysphagia and was found to have a gastric mass on EGD, shows a mass ⊡ along the greater curvature with an enlarged greater curvature lymph node ⊡. *(Right)* Axial CECT in the same patient shows a mass ⊡ along the greater curvature, as well as enlarged greater curvature ⊡ and gastrohepatic ⊡ lymph nodes.

Stage IIIA (T4a N1 M0)

Stage IIIA (T4a N1 M0)

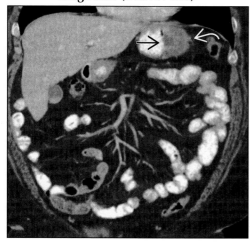

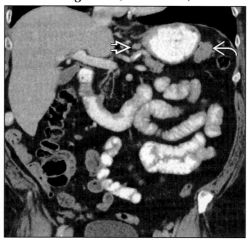

(Left) Coronal CECT in the same patient shows a mass ⊡ along the greater curvature with irregular gastric outer contour ⊡ indicating serosal invasion. *(Right)* Coronal CECT in the same patient shows the greater curvature lymph node ⊡, as well as the enlarged lymph node ⊡ within the gastrohepatic ligament.

Stage IIIA (T4a N1 M0)

Stage IIIA (T4a N1 M0)

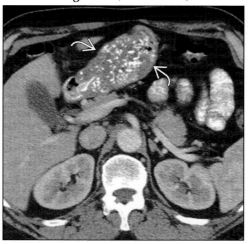

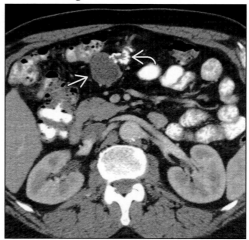

(Left) Axial CECT in a young male who presented with early satiety demonstrates diffuse thickening of the wall of the gastric antrum ⊡. The thick-walled stomach has low attenuation with extensive miliary punctate calcifications. *(Right)* Axial CECT in the same patient shows punctate calcifications ⊡ extending into the gastrocolic ligament indicating serosal violation. Also an enlarged gastroepiploic lymph node ⊡ is seen adjacent to the calcifications.

STOMACH CARCINOMA

Stage IIIA (T4a N1 M0)

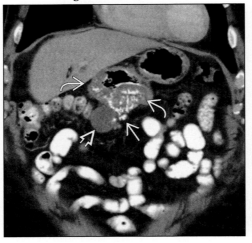

Stage IIIA (T4a N1 M0)

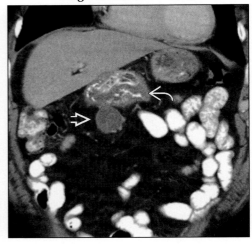

(Left) Coronal CECT in the same patient shows diffuse low-attenuation antral wall thickening ➡ and an enlarged low-attenuation node ⮞, together with tumor extension into the gastrocolic ligament ➡. *(Right)* Coronal CECT in the same patient shows low-attenuation gastric wall thickening ➡ and lymph node ⮞. The presence of low-attenuation gastric wall thickening, calcifications, and low-attenuation node is characteristic of mucinous gastric carcinoma.

Stage IIIB (T4b N1 M0)

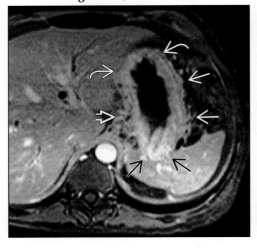

Stage IIIB (T4b N1 M0)

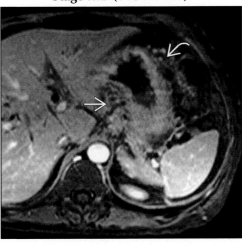

(Left) Axial T1WI C+ FS MR shows marked thickening and transmural enhancement of the gastric wall ➡. Streaks of enhancing tissue extend into the gastrocolic ➡ and gastrohepatic ⮞ ligaments. The stomach abuts the splenic hilum, but the gastric-splenic interface ➡ appears sharp, suggesting the absence of splenic invasion. *(Right)* Axial T1WI C+ FS MR in the same patient shows nodular thickening of the gastrocolic ➡ and gastrohepatic ➡ ligaments.

Stage IIIB (T4b N1 M0)

Stage IIIB (T4b N1 M0)

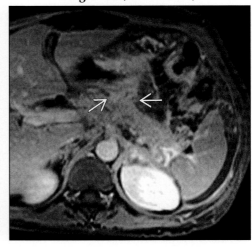

(Left) Axial T1WI C+ FS MR in the same patient shows metastatic nodule within the gastrocolic ligament ➡ and enhancing tumor within the splenorenal ligament ➡. The tumor invades the retroperitoneum ➡ and reaches to the upper pole of the kidney. Low intensity fluid collection ⮞ is a pseudocyst resulting from pancreatitis. *(Right)* Axial T1WI C+ FS MR in the same patient shows tumor extension ➡ through the lesser sac into the body of the pancreas.

STOMACH CARCINOMA

Stage IIIC (T4b N2 M0)

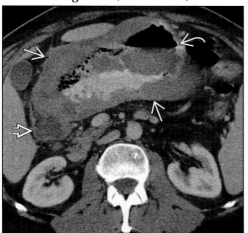

Stage IIIC (T4b N2 M0)

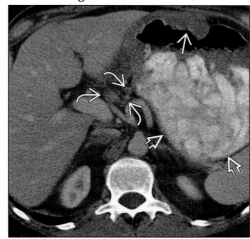

(Left) Axial CECT in a 56-year-old man, who presented with symptoms of gastric outlet obstruction, shows a distended stomach ➡ with diffuse gastric wall thickening ➡ involving the gastric body and antrum. The tumor also involves the proximal duodenum ➡. *(Right)* Axial CECT in the same patient shows gastric wall thickening ➡ and distension ➡. Three enlarged gastrohepatic lymph nodes ➡ are present on this image.

Stage IIIC (T4b N2 M0)

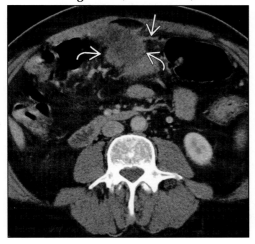

Stage IIIC (T4b N2 M0)

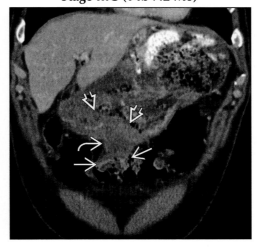

(Left) Axial CECT in the same patient shows tumor ➡ invading the gastrocolic ligament. The landmarks of the ligament are the gastroepiploic vessels ➡. *(Right)* Coronal CECT in the same patient shows tumor along the greater curvature ➡ with invasion through the gastrocolic ligament ➡ into the transverse colon ➡.

Stage IIIC (T4b N2 M0)

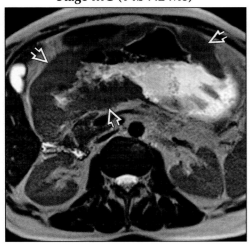

Stage IIIC (T4b N2 M0)

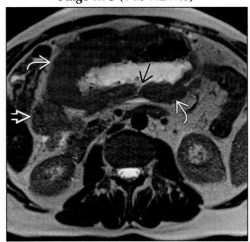

(Left) Axial T2WI MR in the same patient shows circumferential gastric body and antrum wall thickening ➡. The tumor has T2 intermediate signal intensity, similar to the signal intensity of the kidneys. *(Right)* Axial T2WI MR in the same patient shows gastric wall thickening ➡ with malignant ulcer ➡ along the posterior wall. The tumor also causes circumferential thickening of the wall of the duodenum ➡.

STOMACH CARCINOMA

Stage IIIC (T4b N2 M0)

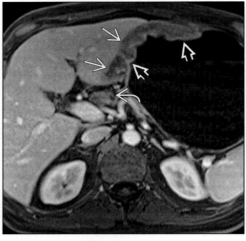

Stage IIIC (T4b N2 M0)

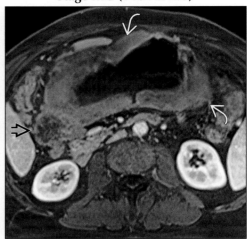

(Left) *Axial T1WI C+ FS MR in the same patient shows enhancing tumor along the anterior wall* ➢ *and gastrohepatic lymph nodes* ➢. *The interface between the tumor and the left lobe of the liver* ➢ *is sharp, indicating absence of hepatic invasion.* *(Right)* *Axial T1WI C+ FS MR in the same patient shows the extensive thickening of the gastric wall (linitis plastica)* ➢ *and invasion of the duodenum* ➢.

Stage IIIC (T4b N2 M0)

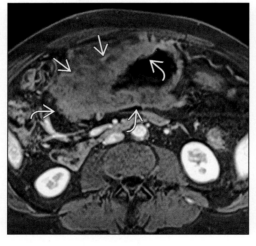

Stage IIIC (T4b N2 M0)

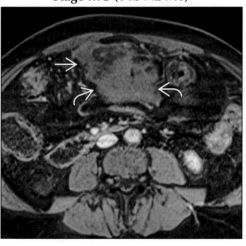

(Left) *Axial T1WI C+ FS MR in the same patient shows gastric wall thickening* ➢ *and invasion of the gastrocolic ligament marked by the gastroepiploic vessels* ➢. *(Right)* *Axial T1WI C+ FS MR in the same patient shows tumor* ➢ *extending inferiorly through the gastrocolic ligament and reaching to the transverse colon* ➢.

Stage IIIC (T4b N2 M0)

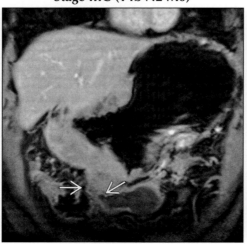

Stage IIIC (T4b N2 M0)

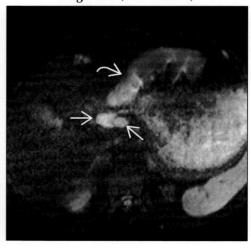

(Left) *Coronal T1WI C+ FS MR in the same patient confirms the invasion of the transverse colon* ➢. *Coronal images are very useful in determining the craniocaudal extension of gastric tumors.* *(Right)* *Axial diffusion-weighted (DWI) MR using b400 shows anterior wall tumor* ➢ *as well as gastrohepatic nodes* ➢. *DWI is very sensitive in detection of nodal metastases.*

STOMACH CARCINOMA

Stage IV (T3 N0 M1)

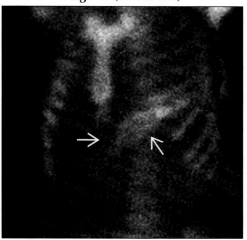

Stage IV (T3 N0 M1)

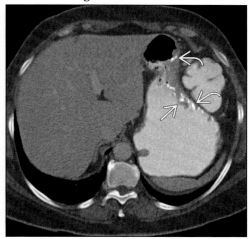

(Left) Oblique projection of a bone scan in a 56-year-old woman, who presented because of right hip pain incidentally, shows tracer accumulation ⮕ in the right upper quadrant. *(Right)* Axial CECT in the same patient shows a scirrhous greater curvature gastric mass ⮕ with punctate calcifications ⮕. The presence of calcification is characteristic of mucinous adenocarcinoma and is probably responsible for tracer accumulation on the bone scan.

Stage IV (T3 N0 M1)

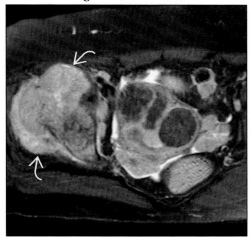

Stage IV (T3 N0 M1)

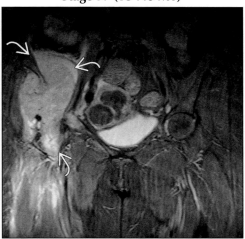

(Left) Axial T2WI FS MR in the same patient shows a large mass ⮕ of high signal intensity replacing the right iliac bone. The uterus is enlarged and contains multiple fibroids. *(Right)* Coronal STIR in the same patient shows the high signal intensity mass ⮕ replacing the right iliac bone.

Stage IV (T3 N0 M1)

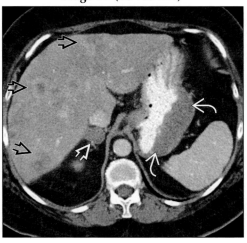

Stage IV (T3 N0 M1)

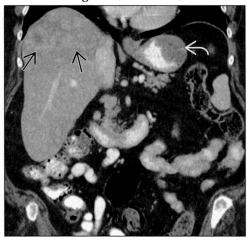

(Left) Axial CECT in a 72-year-old man who presented with right upper quadrant pain shows a mass ⮕ along the greater curvature of the stomach, multiple hepatic metastatic lesions ⮕, and right adrenal mass ⮕. *(Right)* Coronal CECT in the same patient shows the greater curvature gastric mass ⮕ and the enhancing hepatic metastatic lesions ⮕.

STOMACH CARCINOMA

Stage IV (T3 N2 M1)

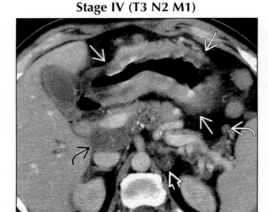

Stage IV (T3 N2 M1)

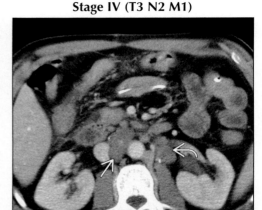

(Left) Axial CECT of a patient with mucinous adenocarcinoma shows diffuse thickening of the stomach wall ➡. Multiple calcified enlarged nodes are seen, including portocaval ➘, paraaortic ➘, and splenic ➘ nodes. *(Right)* Axial CECT in the same patient shows enlarged aortocaval ➡ and paraaortic ➘ lymph nodes. Involvement of intraabdominal lymph nodes, such as hepatoduodenal, mesenteric, and paraaortic, is classified as distant metastasis (M1).

Stage IV (T3 N3a M1)

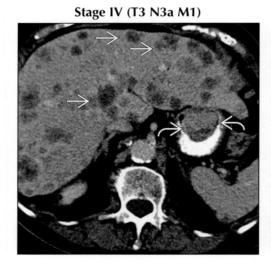

Stage IV (T3 N3a M1)

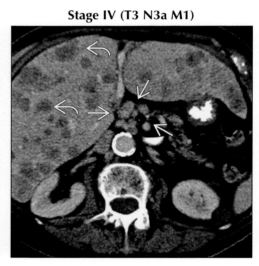

(Left) Axial CECT in a patient who presented with abdominal pain shows a polypoid lesion ➡ arising from the anterior wall of the gastric body. Numerous liver metastatic lesions are also seen ➡. *(Right)* Axial CECT in the same patient shows multiple gastrohepatic lymph nodes ➡, in addition to liver metastases ➡. Pathology confirmed the presence of 8 pathologic nodes.

Stage IV (T4a N1 M1)

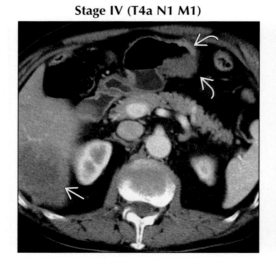

Stage IV (T4a N1 M1)

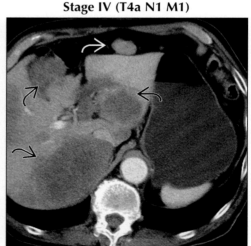

(Left) Axial CECT in a 44-year-old man who presented with hematemesis shows a fungating mass along the greater curvature ➡. There is no evidence of perigastric involvement on this image. Large metastatic lesion ➡ occupies most of segment 6 of the right lobe of the liver. *(Right)* Axial CECT in the same patient shows an enhancing peritoneal mass anterior to the left lobe of the liver ➡. Large hepatic metastatic lesions involve both right and left lobes ➘.

STOMACH CARCINOMA

Stage IV (T4a N1 M1)

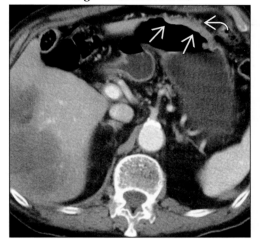

Stage IV (T4a N1 M1)

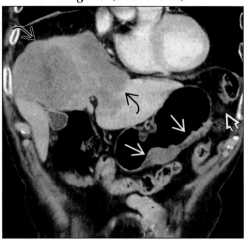

(Left) Axial CECT in the same patient shows thickening of the anterior wall of the stomach ➡. Fine nodularities ➡ along the outer contour of the stomach indicate penetration of serosa. *(Right)* Coronal CECT in the same patient shows tumor along the greater curvature ➡ within the air-filled stomach. Another peritoneal implant is seen ➡, as well as large metastatic liver lesions ➡.

Stage IV (T4a N2 M1)

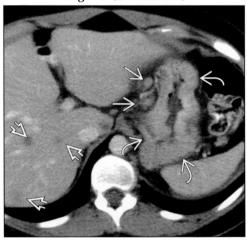

Stage IV (T4a N2 M1)

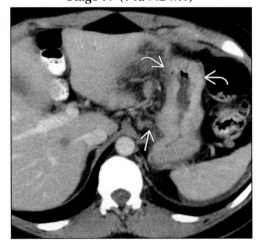

(Left) Axial CECT in a 63-year-old patient who presented with hematemesis shows diffuse thickening of the stomach wall ➡. Multiple gastrohepatic nodes are present ➡. Hypodense lesions ➡ within the liver represent metastatic disease. *(Right)* Axial CECT in the same patient shows gastric wall thickening ➡ with transmural enhancement. Note streaks and nodules of soft tissue density ➡ extending into the fat of the gastrohepatic ligament due to serosal spread.

Stage IV (T4a N2 M1)

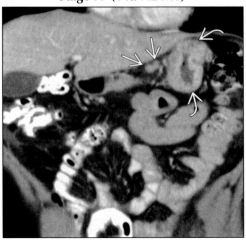

Stage IV (T4a N2 M1)

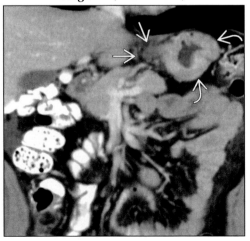

(Left) Coronal CECT in the same patient shows diffuse gastric wall thickening ➡ with transmural enhancement. Multiple lymph nodes ➡ are present within the gastrohepatic ligament. *(Right)* Coronal CECT shows diffuse gastric wall thickening ➡ as well as nodular thickening ➡ of the gastrohepatic ligament resulting from tumor extension into the ligament due to violation of the serosa.

Stage IV (T4a N2 M1)

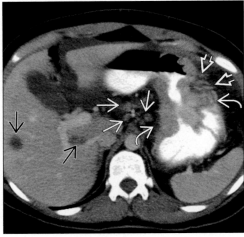

Stage IV (T4a N2 M1)

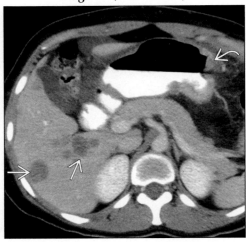

(Left) Axial CECT in a 29-year-old woman who presented with hematemesis shows circumferential thickening of the wall of the gastric body ➡. Nodularity of the outer contour ⮞ indicates serosal invasion. Three gastrohepatic nodes ➡ are present, as are liver metastases ➡. *(Right)* Axial CECT in the same patient shows multiple hepatic metastases ➡ and infiltration of the perigastric fat ➡.

Stage IV (T4a N2 M1)

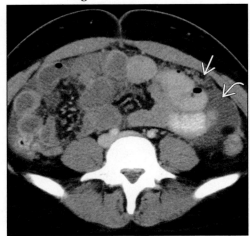

Stage IV (T4a N2 M1)

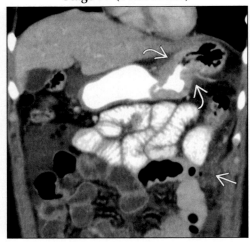

(Left) Axial CECT in the same patient shows subtle omental reticulation ➡ and ascites ➡ due to peritoneal metastatic disease. *(Right)* Coronal CECT in the same patient shows circumferential gastric body wall thickening ➡ and reticular appearance of omentum ➡ due to peritoneal metastases.

Stage IV (T4a N2 M1)

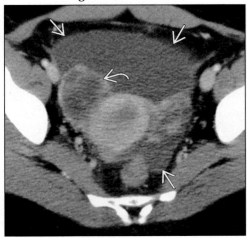

Stage IV (T4a N2 M1)

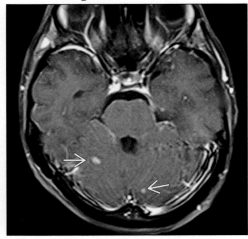

(Left) Axial CECT in the same patient shows enlargement of the right ovary ➡ with a multilocular cystic appearance; on laparoscopy, this proved to be due to metastatic disease (Krukenberg tumor). Ascites ➡ is also present in the pelvis. *(Right)* Axial T1 C+ FS MR in the same patient shows 2 enhancing cerebellar lesions ➡ due to metastatic disease.

STOMACH CARCINOMA

Stage IV (T4a N2 M1)

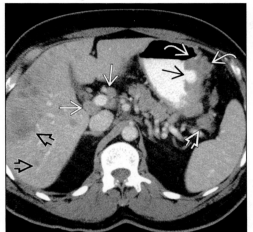

Stage IV (T4a N2 M1)

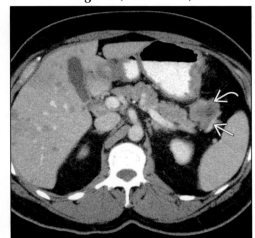

(Left) Axial CECT in a 39-year-old man with history of adenomatous polyposis who underwent colectomy shows a mass along the greater curvature (GC) ➜ with central ulceration ➡ and multiple liver metastases ⇒, as well as tumor masses ⇒ along the gastrosplenic ligament (GSL). Multiple hepatoduodenal nodes ➜, which cannot be explained by the GC tumor, are present. (Right) Axial CECT in the same patient shows tumor ➜ involving the GSL marked by splenic vein ➡.

Stage IV (T4a N2 M1)

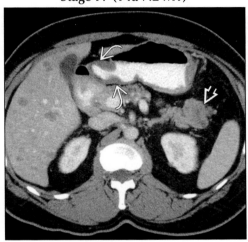

Stage IV (T4a N2 M1)

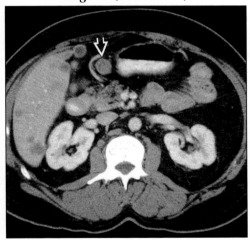

(Left) Axial CECT in the same patient shows mild circumferential thickening of the wall of the antrum ➜. This was found on EGD to represent a 2nd tumor responsible for the enlarged hepatoduodenal lymph nodes. Note also extension of the 1st tumor into the gastrosplenic ligament ➜. (Right) Axial CECT in the same patient shows a round tumor implant or lymph node ➜ within the gastrocolic ligament.

Stage IV (T4a N2 M1)

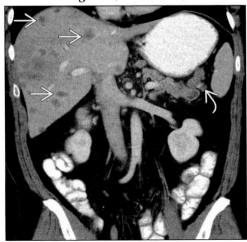

Stage IV (T4a N2 M1)

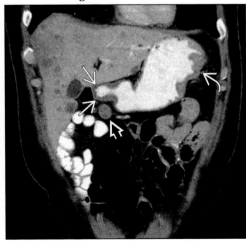

(Left) Coronal CECT in the same patient shows tumor within the gastrosplenic ligament ➜ and multiple hepatic metastases ➡. (Right) Coronal CECT in the same patient shows the 1st tumor along the greater curvature ➜ and the circumferential antral tumor ➡. Note also the peritoneal implant or lymph node ➜ within the gastrocolic ligament.

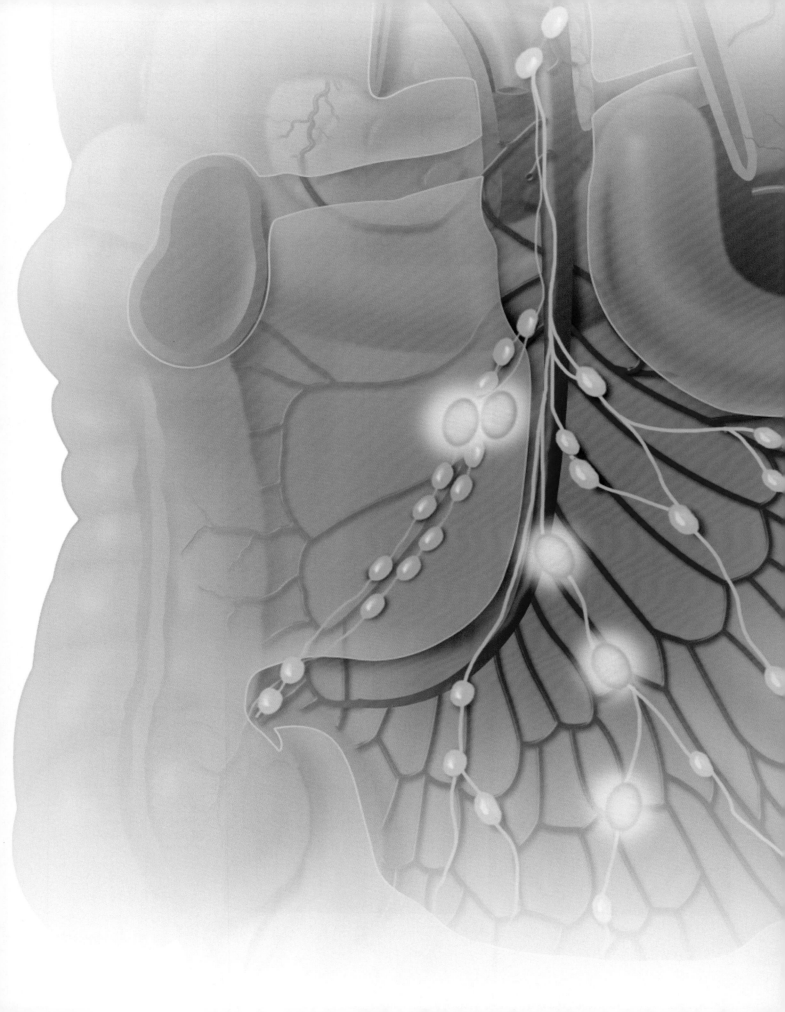

Small Intestine Carcinoma

SMALL INTESTINE CARCINOMA

(T) Primary Tumor

Adapted from 7th edition AJCC Staging Forms.

TNM	Definitions
TX	Primary tumor cannot be assessed
T0	No evidence of primary tumor
Tis	Carcinoma in situ
T1a	Tumor invades lamina propria
T1b	Tumor invades submucosa
T2	Tumor invades muscularis propria
T3	Tumor invades through the muscularis propria into the subserosa or into the nonperitonealized perimuscular tissue (mesentery or retroperitoneum) with extension ≤ 2 cm*
T4	Tumor perforates the visceral peritoneum or directly invades other organs or structures (includes other loops of small intestine, mesentery, or retroperitoneum > 2 cm, and abdominal wall by way of serosa; for duodenum only, invasion of pancreas or bile duct)

(N) Regional Lymph Nodes

NX	Regional lymph nodes cannot be assessed
N0	No regional lymph node metastasis
N1	Metastasis in 1-3 regional lymph nodes
N2	Metastasis in ≥ 4 regional lymph nodes

(M) Distant Metastasis

M0	No distant metastasis
M1	Distant metastasis

The nonperitonealized perimuscular tissue is, for jejunum and ileum, part of the mesentery and, for duodenum in areas where serosa is lacking, part of the interface with the pancreas.

AJCC Stages/Prognostic Groups

Adapted from 7th edition AJCC Staging Forms.

Stage	T	N	M
0	Tis	N0	M0
I	T1	N0	M0
	T2	N0	M0
IIA	T3	N0	M0
IIB	T4	N0	M0
IIIA	Any T	N1	M0
IIIB	Any T	N2	M0
IV	Any T	Any N	M1

SMALL INTESTINE CARCINOMA

Tis

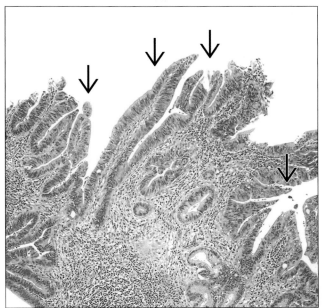

H&E stained section shows small bowel mucosa with numerous villi lined by dysplastic epithelium ➔. The neoplastic cells do not invade the basement membrane or into the lamina propria. (Original magnification 100x.)

Tis

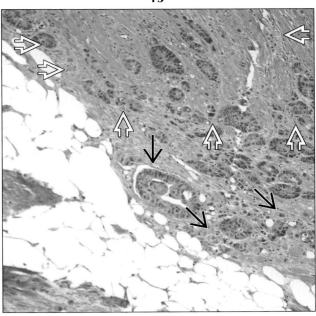

Higher power magnification shows the neoplastic cells extending to the surface/top of the villi with high-grade dysplasia. The dysplastic cells have large nuclei with open/vesicular chromatin and prominent nucleoli. Note the fuzzy border focally ➔, indicating the ciliated epithelium of small bowel. (Original magnification 500x.)

T1a

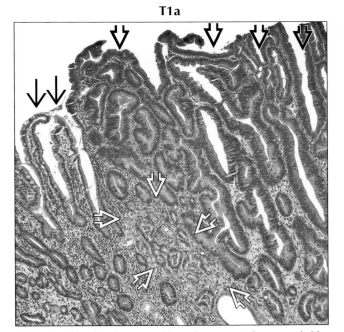

H&E stained section shows small bowel mucosa with unremarkable villi on the left aspect of the slide ➔ and high-grade dysplasia involving the rest of the epithelium on the right side ➔. Note the intramucosal adenocarcinoma ➔ with small and irregular gland buds invading the lamina propria. (Original magnification 100x.)

T3

The adenocarcinoma is arranged in glands and single cells ➔ with extension through the muscularis propria in the upper aspect of the slide. Neoplastic glands ➔ infiltrate through the muscle bundles. The adenocarcinoma extends into the perimuscular/subserosal fibrofatty tissue. (Original magnification 100x.)

SMALL INTESTINE CARCINOMA

T1a

- Epithelium
- Lamina propria

Muscularis mucosae

] Submucosa

Muscularis propria

Subserosa
Serosa

Mucosa

Graphic depicts tumor invading to the level of the lamina propria. The primary tumor is staged according to its depth of penetration of the small bowel wall and invasion of adjacent structures. Lateral spread is not a consideration in the T staging.

T1b

- Epithelium
- Lamina propria

Muscularis mucosae

] Submucosa

Muscularis propria

Subserosa
Serosa

Mucosa

Graphic depicts tumor invading to the level of the submucosa.

T2

- Epithelium
- Lamina propria

Muscularis mucosae

] Submucosa

Muscularis propria

Subserosa
Serosa

Mucosa

Graphic depicts tumor invading to the level of the muscularis propria.

T3

- Epithelium
- Lamina propria

Muscularis mucosae

] Submucosa

Muscularis propria

Subserosa
Serosa

Mucosa

Graphic depicts tumor invading through the muscularis propria into the subserosa.

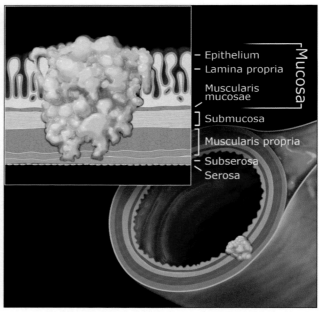

T3

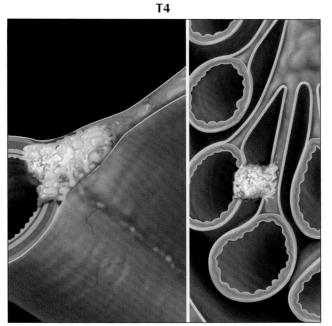

Graphic depicts a tumor invading into the mesenteric attachment of a small bowel loop with extension ≤ 2 cm, consistent with T3 disease. Indeed, by definition, T3 tumors invade such nonperitonealized perimuscular tissue or the retroperitoneal segments of the duodenum with extension ≤ 2 cm.

T4

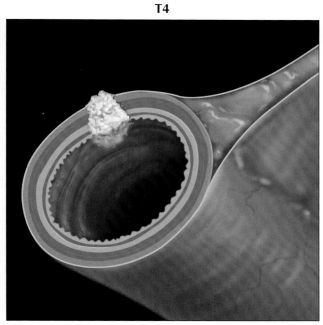

Graphic depicts tumor invading the visceral peritoneal covering of the small bowel. The visceral peritoneum is the serosal layer of the small bowel wall.

T4

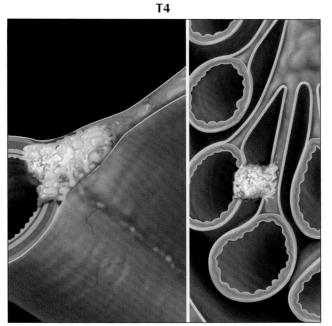

Left graphic depicts tumor invading the nonperitonealized perimuscular tissue at the mesenteric attachment with extension > 2 cm. Duodenal tumor invading the retroperitoneum with extension > 2 cm is also tumor stage T4. Right graphic depicts tumor invading the serosal layer of the bowel wall and adjacent mesentery.

T4

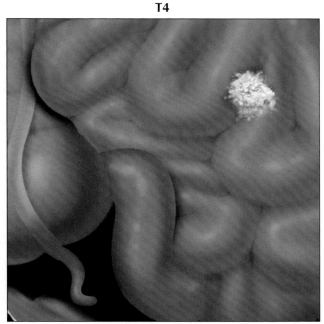

Graphic depicts small bowel tumor invading adjacent loops of small bowel. The primary tumor is staged according to its depth of penetration of the small bowel wall and invasion of adjacent structures. Lateral spread is not a consideration in the T staging.

T4

T4

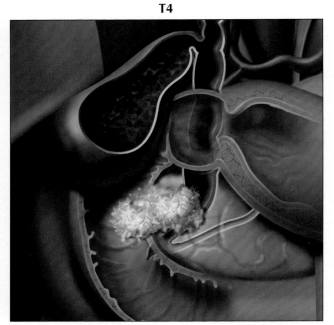

Graphic depicts small bowel tumor invading the abdominal wall.

Graphic depicts tumor arising from the duodenum and invading the pancreatic head and common bile duct. T4 denotes direct invasion of adjacent structures; for tumors originating in the duodenum, the pancreas and bile duct are considered adjacent structures.

Regional Lymph Nodes: Duodenum

Regional Lymph Nodes: Jejunum, Ileum, and Terminal Ileum

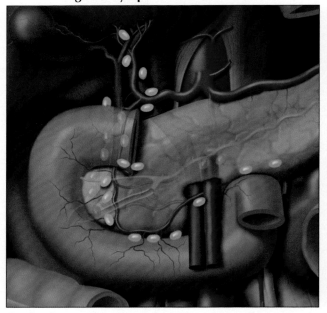

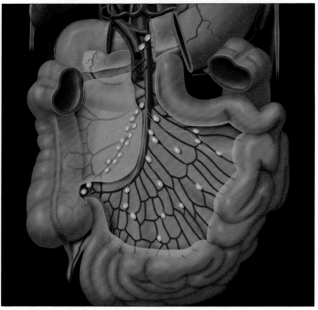

Graphic depicts regional lymph nodes for small bowel carcinoma in the duodenum. Regional lymph nodes include duodenal, hepatic, pancreaticoduodenal, infrapyloric, gastroduodenal, pyloric, superior mesenteric, and pericholedochal.

Graphic depicts regional lymph nodes for small bowel carcinoma in the jejunum and ileum, which include the superior mesenteric and mesenteric nodes (blue). Regional lymph nodes for tumors occurring in the terminal ileum also include cecal and ileocolic chains (orange).

N1

N2

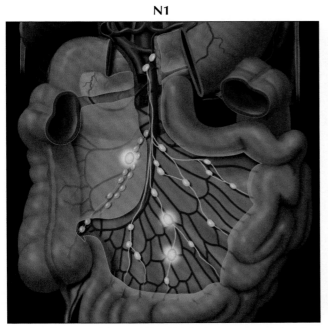

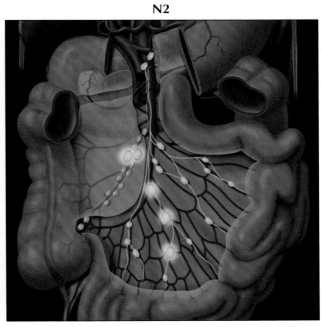

Graphic depicts nodal stage N1, which includes metastasis in 1-3 regional lymph nodes.

Graphic depicts nodal stage N2, which includes metastasis in ≥ 4 regional lymph nodes.

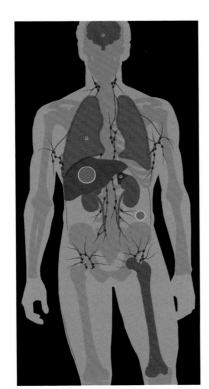

METASTASES, ORGAN FREQUENCY

Liver	59%
Peritoneal cavity	25%
Pulmonary	3%
Adrenal gland	Rare
Extraabdominal lymph nodes	Rare
Brain	Rare

SMALL INTESTINE CARCINOMA

OVERVIEW

General Comments
- Small intestine tumors account for < 2% of GI tract malignancies
- > 50% of primary malignant small intestine tumors are adenocarcinoma

Classification
- Histopathologic types
  - Carcinomas
    - Includes adenocarcinoma and mixed carcinoma/ neuroendocrine
  - Well-differentiated neuroendocrine tumors
    - Staged separately
  - Lymphomas
    - Staged as extranodal lymphomas
  - Gastrointestinal stromal tumors
    - Staged separately
  - Sarcomas
    - Staged separately
    - Includes leiomyosarcoma, angiosarcoma, liposarcoma
- Staging classification does not apply to following tumors
  - Well-differentiated neuroendocrine tumors
  - Lymphoma
  - Carcinoma arising in ileocecal valve
  - Carcinoma arising in Meckel diverticulum
  - Carcinoma of ampulla of Vater

PATHOLOGY

Routes of Spread
- Contiguous spread
  - Important for primary tumor staging
    - Tumor stage determined by depth of penetration in small bowel wall and invasion of adjacent structures
  - Duodenal tumors spread to pancreas, retroperitoneum, and common bile duct
  - Jejunal & ileal tumors tend to spread to nonperitonealized perimuscular tissue or mesentery, other small bowel loops, and abdominal wall
- Lymphatic spread
  - Regional nodes depend on location of primary tumor
    - Duodenum
      - Duodenal
      - Hepatic
      - Pancreaticoduodenal
      - Infrapyloric
      - Gastroduodenal
      - Pyloric
      - Superior mesenteric
      - Pericholedochal
    - Ileum and jejunum
      - Superior mesenteric
      - Cecal (terminal ileum only)
      - Ileocolic (terminal ileum only)
- Hematogenous spread
  - Most commonly to liver
- Peritoneal spread

  - Usually occurs when tumor violates serosal covering

General Features
- Etiology
  - Risk factors
    - Crohn disease
    - Celiac disease
    - Peutz-Jeghers syndrome
    - Hereditary nonpolyposis colorectal cancer
    - Gardner syndrome
    - Lynch syndrome II
    - Familial adenomatous polyposis
    - Congenital bowel duplication
    - Cystic fibrosis
    - Peptic ulcer disease
    - Neurofibromatosis
    - HIV
    - Prior surgery
      - Ileostomy site
      - Surgically bypassed duodenum
      - Jejunal limb of Roux-en-Y esophagojejunostomy
      - Ileal segment of defunctionalized ileocystoplasty
  - Possible dietary risk factors
    - Red meat
    - Smoked & salt-cured foods
    - Bread, pasta, rice
    - Sugar
  - Possible inverse relationship
    - Coffee, fruit, vegetables
- Epidemiology & cancer incidence
  - 6,230 estimated new cases in 2009 in USA
  - 1,110 estimated deaths in 2009 in USA
  - 50x less common than colon cancer
  - 5-year overall survival rate of 26%
- Associated diseases, abnormalities
  - Crohn disease (CD)
    - Most important risk factor
    - Occurs at younger age
    - Male predominance
    - 6-60x increased risk compared to general population
    - 70% occur in ileum
    - Usually at least 10 years from onset of CD to diagnosis of carcinoma, average of 16-21 years
    - Risk factors for adenocarcinoma in patients with CD
      - Male sex
      - Duration of disease
      - Fistulous disease
      - Strictures
      - Surgically excluded loops of bowel
      - Jejunal inflammation

Gross Pathology & Surgical Features
- > 50% of primary small intestine malignancies are adenocarcinomas
- May occur synchronously or metachronously at multiple sites
- Tumor location
  - Duodenum (> 60%)
    - Especially near ampulla
  - Jejunum (20%)
  - Ileum (15%)

SMALL INTESTINE CARCINOMA

- Most common location in patients with Crohn disease
- Proximal tumors
  - Tend to be papillary
- Distal tumors
  - Tend to be annular
  - Tend to cause obstruction
  - Can be polypoid or fungating (20%)

Microscopic Pathology

- H&E
  - Most are moderately to well differentiated
  - May have prominent microvilli
  - Usually have mucin production and CEA reactivity
  - No direct correlation between tumor size and invasiveness
  - Adenoma-carcinoma sequence similar to colorectal cancer
    - Up to 42% of duodenal villous adenomas have malignant cells

IMAGING FINDINGS

Detection

- **Barium examination**
  - 50-60% sensitivity for detection of advanced tumors
  - Techniques
    - Small bowel follow-through
    - Enteroclysis
  - Imaging features of small bowel tumor
    - "Apple core" lesions
      - Annular, circumferential narrowing
      - Involves short segment of small bowel
      - Overhanging borders, both proximally & distally
    - Mucosal ulceration
    - Intussusception
- **CT**
  - Techniques
    - Routine abdominopelvic CT
      - Employs IV contrast & positive enteric contrast
      - Positive enteric contrast may obscure intraluminal and bowel wall abnormalities
      - Adequate for exophytic lesions, bowel complications, such as obstruction or perforation
    - CT enterography
      - Noninvasive exam, requires patient cooperation to drink large volume of enteric contrast
      - Employs IV contrast & neutral enteric contrast
      - Neutral enteric contrast allows visualization of enhancing bowel wall abnormalities
      - Degree of bowel distension less optimal compared with CT enteroclysis
    - CT enteroclysis
      - Invasive procedure requiring nasojejunal intubation
      - Infusion of large volume of enteric contrast for optimal bowel distention
      - Large enteric volume challenge useful to identify subtle bowel wall abnormalities
      - For small bowel neoplasm, best performed with IV contrast and neutral enteric contrast

- Not performed in setting of high-grade obstruction
  - Imaging features of small bowel tumor
    - Focal wall thickening
      - Usually > 1.5 cm
      - Eccentric mucosal fold thickening
      - Asymmetric pattern of valvulae conniventes
    - Annular luminal narrowing
      - "Apple core" lesion
      - Abrupt irregular "overhanging edges"
      - More commonly seen in distal small bowel
      - Usually involves short segment of small bowel
    - Discrete mass
      - Intramural or intraluminal mass
      - Sessile or polypoid
      - CECT: Heterogeneous mass with moderate enhancement
      - Duodenal tumors tend to be polypoid or papillary
      - May cause intussusception
    - Ulcerative lesion
      - Up to 40% of cases
      - Not seen well on CT
  - Bowel inflammation can obscure small lesions
  - May cause partial or complete small bowel obstruction
    - Due to rigid and fibrotic nature of tumors
    - 10% of patients presenting with abdominal pain due to bowel obstruction → etiology is tumor
    - Imaging findings of obstruction
      - Proximal bowel dilation with gradual narrowing
      - Distal bowel collapsed or relatively decompressed
- **MR**
  - Emerging modality for detection of small bowel tumor
    - Studies suggest promising role for tumor detection
    - Efficacy and impact on tumor staging not yet reported
  - Techniques
    - MR enteroclysis
      - Invasive procedure requiring nasojejunal intubation
      - Infusion of large volume of enteric contrast for optimal bowel distention
    - MR enterography
      - Noninvasive exam, requires patient cooperation to drink large volume of enteric contrast
  - Imaging features of small bowel tumor
    - Bowel wall thickening or mass
    - Sessile or pedunculated mass
    - Mean tumor length: 4.8 cm
    - Mean wall thickness: 1.4 cm
    - Adenocarcinoma tends to have intraluminal growth pattern
  - Findings favoring malignant neoplasm
    - Longer tumor length
    - Solitary lesion
    - Nonpedunculated
    - Mesenteric fat infiltration
    - Mesenteric adenopathy
  - Advantages of MR
    - Direct acquisition of multiple planes
    - High intrinsic soft tissue contrast

- No ionizing radiation
- Intravenous contrast not required
- Able to depict extraintestinal involvement

Staging

- Factors affecting tumor stage
  - Depth of tumor penetration in bowel wall
  - Involvement of adjacent structures
  - Spread to distant sites
- Lateral tumor spread within bowel segment does not affect stage
- 30% present with metastatic disease
- **Primary tumor**
  - CT cannot differentiate bowel wall layers or between stage T1 and T2 tumors
  - CT can differentiate early (T1 or T2) from advanced (T3 or T4) tumor
    - Nodular outer contour results from tumor invasion through entire thickness of bowel wall
    - Involvement of surrounding structures represents T4
  - Advantages of CT
    - Determine location of mass in small bowel
    - Define relationship of tumor to lumen
    - Determine invasion of mesentery or adjacent structures
    - Evaluate for concomitant bowel disease
    - Evaluate for complications, such as bowel obstruction & perforation
- **Lymphatic metastasis**
  - Nodal stage determined by number of involved regional nodes
    - N1: Metastasis in 1-3 nodes
    - N2: Metastasis in ≥ 4 nodes
  - Regional lymph nodes depend on tumor location
    - Duodenum
      - Duodenal
      - Hepatic
      - Pancreaticoduodenal
      - Infrapyloric
      - Gastroduodenal
      - Pyloric
      - Superior mesenteric
      - Pericholedochal
    - Jejunum & ileum
      - Superior mesenteric
      - Mesenteric, NOS
    - Terminal ileum
      - Cecal
      - Ileocolic
  - Anatomic imaging (CT & MR)
    - Size ≥ 10 mm short axis
    - Central necrosis
  - Metabolic imaging (PET/CT)
    - Relative ↑ FDG uptake compared to normal lymph nodes
  - Nodal metastases from adenocarcinoma tend to be less bulky than those in lymphoma
  - ↓ 5-year overall survival if positive adenopathy
    - 32% vs. 52%
  - Limitations
    - Micrometastasis (false-negative)
    - Concurrent inflammatory bowel disease (false-positive)
- **Distant metastasis**

- Most common in liver followed by peritoneal cavity
- Other sites of distant metastases
  - Pulmonary
  - Adrenal glands
  - Brain
- Lymph nodes
  - Celiac lymph nodes
  - Extraabdominal lymph nodes

Restaging

- Recurrence
  - Despite cancer-directed surgery, 1 study found
    - Recurrence rate of 39%
    - Median time for recurrence of 25 months
  - Sites of recurrence (in order of frequency)
    - Distant
    - Peritoneal cavity
    - Local
    - Abdominal wall

CLINICAL ISSUES

Presentation

- Age at presentation
  - 50-70 years old
  - ↑ prevalence after age 40
  - Younger if predisposing condition
- Slight male predominance
- Symptoms
  - Abdominal pain
  - Anemia
  - GI bleeding
  - Bowel obstruction
    - More common in distal tumors
  - Bowel perforation
  - Weight loss
- Average delay in diagnosis of 6-8 months from onset of symptoms

Cancer Natural History & Prognosis

- Significant prognostic indicators
  - Extent of tumor (depth of penetration in bowel wall)
    - Strongest indicator of outcome for resectable tumors
  - Regional lymphatic spread
  - Presurgical carcinoembryonic antigen (CEA)
  - Microsatellite instability (MSI)
- Poor prognosis
  - Nonresectable tumor
  - Incomplete resection
  - Regional lymph node metastases
  - Presence of Crohn disease
  - Age > 75 years
    - Relative risk of death 1.8x higher
  - Duodenal adenocarcinoma (compared with distal small intestine)
- Most influential factors for survival
  - Distant metastatic disease
  - Residual disease
- Histologic grade not found to be significant predictor of outcome

SMALL INTESTINE CARCINOMA

Treatment Options

- Major treatment alternatives
  - Surgical resection
    - Chance of cure correlates with ability to completely resect tumor
    - Curative resection possible in 40-65%
    - Overall survival higher with cancer-directed surgery
      - 5-year survival for patients with resected tumors (40-60%)
      - 5-year survival for patients with nonresected tumors (15-30%)
    - Preferred treatment is wide segmental surgical resection
      - Localized duodenal carcinoma → Whipple procedure (pancreaticoduodenectomy)
      - Distal ileum → right hemicolectomy
    - Adequate mesenteric resection may be limited by proximity of tumor or nodes to superior mesenteric artery
  - Radiation therapy
    - Palliation for nonresectable primary tumor
    - Used in conjunction with surgical bypass if obstructing tumor
    - Clinical trials are evaluating utility of radiosensitizers
  - Chemotherapy
    - Adjuvant chemotherapy following resection does not appear to significantly affect survival
    - Clinical trials are evaluating utility in primary unresectable tumor and metastatic disease

REPORTING CHECKLIST

T Staging

- Tumor location
  - Duodenum, jejunum, ileum
- Depth of bowel wall invasion
- Depth of mesenteric/retroperitoneal extension
- Perforation of visceral peritoneum
- Invasion of adjacent structures
  - Duodenum: Pancreas, bile duct
  - Jejunum & ileum: Bowel loops, mesentery/retroperitoneum (> 2 cm), abdominal wall

N Staging

- Regional lymph nodes
  - Depends on tumor location
- Number of regional lymph node metastases
  - N1: 1-3
  - N2: ≥ 4

M Staging

- Liver
- Peritoneal cavity
- Lymph nodes
  - Depends on tumor location

SELECTED REFERENCES

1. American Joint Committee on Cancer: AJCC Cancer Staging Manual. 7th ed. New York: Springer. 127-32, 2010
2. Van Weyenberg SJ et al: MR enteroclysis in the diagnosis of small-bowel neoplasms. Radiology. 254(3):765-73, 2010
3. Kodaira C et al: A case of small bowel adenocarcinoma in a patient with Crohn's disease detected by PET/CT and double-balloon enteroscopy. World J Gastroenterol. 15(14):1774-8, 2009
4. Feldstein RC et al: Small bowel adenocarcinoma in Crohn's disease. Inflamm Bowel Dis. 14(8):1154-7, 2008
5. Ramachandran I et al: Multidetector row CT of small bowel tumours. Clin Radiol. 62(7):607-14, 2007
6. Chan RC et al: Small bowel adenocarcinoma with high levels of microsatellite instability in Crohn's disease. Hum Pathol. 37(5):631-4, 2006
7. Gore RM et al: Diagnosis and staging of small bowel tumours. Cancer Imaging. 6:209-12, 2006
8. Dabaja BS et al: Adenocarcinoma of the small bowel: presentation, prognostic factors, and outcome of 217 patients. Cancer. 101(3):518-26, 2004
9. Horton KM et al: Multidetector-row computed tomography and 3-dimensional computed tomography imaging of small bowel neoplasms: current concept in diagnosis. J Comput Assist Tomogr. 28(1):106-16, 2004
10. Buckley JA et al: CT evaluation of small bowel neoplasms: spectrum of disease. Radiographics. 18(2):379-92, 1998
11. Buckley JA et al: The accuracy of CT staging of small bowel adenocarcinoma: CT/pathologic correlation. J Comput Assist Tomogr. 21(6):986-91, 1997
12. Dudiak KM et al: Primary tumors of the small intestine: CT evaluation. AJR Am J Roentgenol. 152(5):995-8, 1989

SMALL INTESTINE CARCINOMA

Stage I (T2 N0 M0)

Stage I (T2 N0 M0)

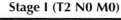

(Left) Axial CECT shows a hypodense intramural mass ➡ in the anterior wall of the 3rd portion of the duodenum. Normal-enhancing bowel wall is seen encasing the mass. *(Right)* Endoscopic image in the same patient shows a submucosal mass ➡ in the 3rd portion of the duodenum.

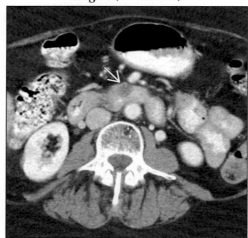

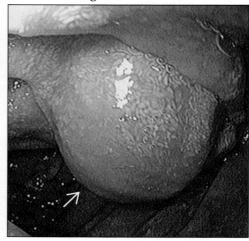

Stage I (T2 N0 M0)

Stage IIA (T3 N0 M0)

(Left) Axial CECT shows a heterogeneously enhancing pedunculated mass ➡ in the ileum. The perienteric fat is preserved, suggesting absence of invasion. The layers of the bowel wall cannot be differentiated on CT; however, surgical pathology showed invasion of the muscularis propria. Mucosal ulceration was present but cannot be appreciated. *(Right)* Axial CECT in a different patient shows segmental mural thickening in the proximal jejunum with irregular overhanging edges ➡.

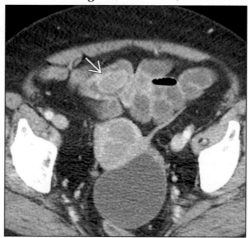

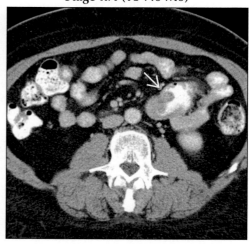

Stage IIA (T3 N0 M0)

Stage IIA (T3 N0 M0)

(Left) Coronal CECT in the same patient shows that the mural thickening is concentric ➡. Positive enteric contrast outlines the abrupt tumor margins and demonstrates luminal narrowing. There is no obstruction to the antegrade passage of contrast. *(Right)* Small bowel follow-through with spot compression in the same patient shows an "apple core" lesion ➡ with a short segment of annular luminal narrowing and irregular overhanging edges.

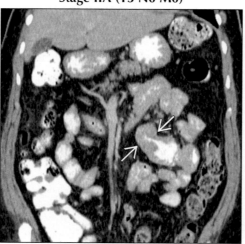

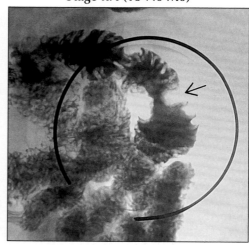

Stage IIA (T3 N0 M0)

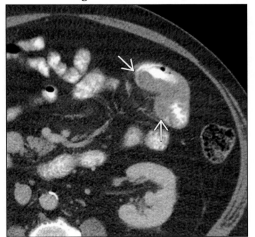

Stage IIA (T3 N0 M0)

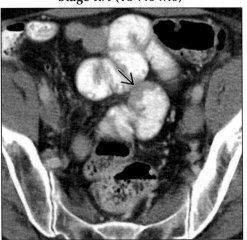

(Left) Axial CECT shows eccentric nodular mural thickening ➔ in the proximal jejunum. Increased density of the perienteric fat is suggestive of a malignant tumor and subperitoneal infiltration. *(Right)* Axial CECT shows focal eccentric mural thickening ➔ of the ileum. Bowel wall layers cannot be differentiated on CT; however, surgical pathology confirmed invasion through the serosa into perienteric fat.

Stage IIB (T4 N0 M0)

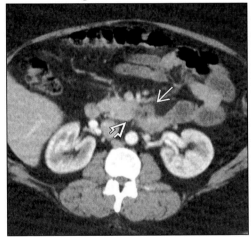

Stage IIB (T4 N0 M0)

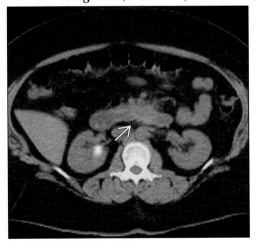

(Left) Axial CECT shows a hypoenhancing mass in the 2nd portion of the duodenum. The mass extends into the retroperitoneal fat ➔. There is invasion of the pancreatic uncinate process ➔, constituting T4 disease for duodenal tumors. *(Right)* Axial fused PET/CT in the same patient shows corresponding avid FDG uptake by the duodenal mass ➔.

Stage IIIA (T4 N1 M0)

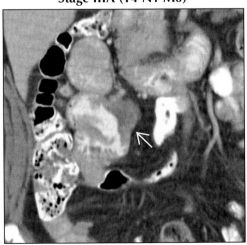

Stage IIIA (T4 N1 M0)

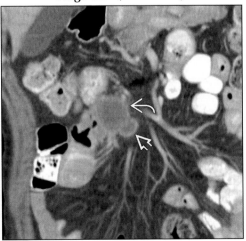

(Left) Coronal CECT shows segmental small bowel wall thickening ➔ with extension into the mesentery. There is an abrupt transition to normal thickness bowel wall. *(Right)* Coronal CECT in the same patient shows the exophytic component ➔ of the small bowel tumor extending into the mesentery more than 2 cm, making this T4 disease. There is an adjacent necrotic mesenteric lymph node ➔, consistent with N1 nodal stage.

SMALL INTESTINE CARCINOMA

Stage IIIA (T3 N1 M0)

(Left) Axial CECT shows hypotonic, mildly dilated small bowel loops ➡, seen particularly well in the left hemiabdomen in this patient with celiac disease. *(Right)* Small bowel follow-through in the same patient shows flocculation of barium ➡ in the left upper quadrant, characteristic of the hypersecretion seen in celiac disease.

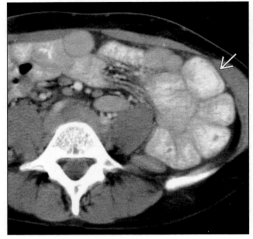

Stage IIIA (T3 N1 M0)

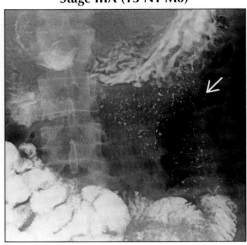

Stage IIIA (T3 N1 M0)

(Left) Axial CECT in the same patient shows distension of the stomach ➡ and proximal duodenum ➡ out of proportion to small and large bowel loops. Stricture ➡ in the 3rd portion of the duodenum is at the point of transition from dilated to collapsed bowel. Pathology revealed adenocarcinoma. *(Right)* Axial CECT in the same patient shows enlarged superior mesenteric nodes ➡. Firm nodes were felt at the base of the superior mesenteric artery at surgery.

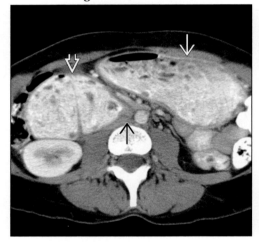

Stage IIIA (T3 N1 M0)

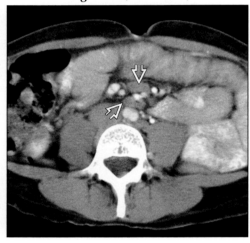

Stage IIIA (T3 N1 M0)

(Left) Upper GI with small bowel follow-through in the same patient shows dilation of the proximal duodenum with abrupt narrowing of the 3rd portion ➡. The stenosis is nonobstructive as demonstrated by distal enteric contrast. *(Right)* Endoscopic image in the same patient taken at the 3rd portion of the duodenum shows nodular friable mucosa ➡ and luminal stenosis ➡, which could not be traversed.

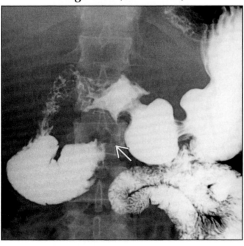

Stage IIIA (T3 N1 M0)

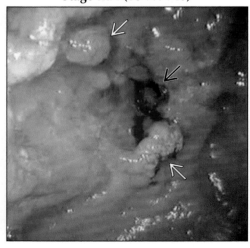

SMALL INTESTINE CARCINOMA

Stage IIIA (T3 N1 M0)

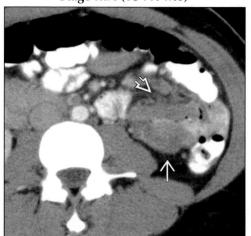

Stage IIIA (T3 N1 M0)

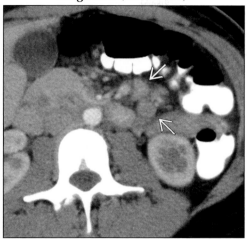

(Left) Axial CECT shows concentric segmental wall thickening of a jejunal loop ➡ *with < 2 cm of extension into the nonperitonealized perimuscular tissue* ➡, *constituting tumor stage T3.* *(Right) Axial CECT in the same patient shows 2 ill-defined enlarged mesenteric lymph nodes* ➡. *If present, fewer than 3 metastatic lymph nodes is nodal stage N1.*

Stage IV (T4 N2 M1)

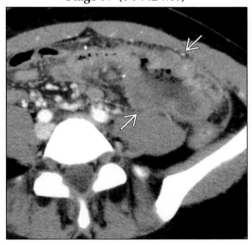

Stage IV (T4 N2 M1)

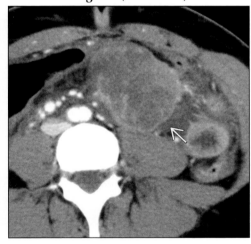

(Left) Axial CECT shows an ileal mass with segmental circumferential nodular wall thickening ➡ *of the involved loop. (Right) Axial CECT in the same patient shows a large exophytic mass* ➡ *arising from the ileum. Although the primary tumor does not invade adjacent structures, > 2 cm of extension into the mesentery is stage T4.*

Stage IV (T4 N2 M1)

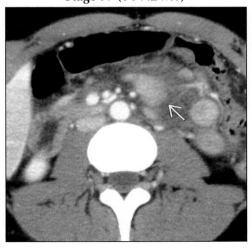

Stage IV (T4 N2 M1)

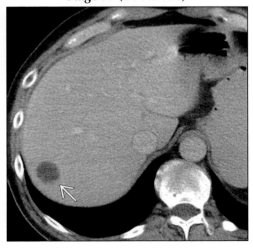

(Left) Axial CECT in the same patient shows an enlarged mesenteric lymph node ➡. *Other images showed additional adenopathy, making the nodal stage N2. (Right) Axial CECT in the same patient shows a hypovascular mass* ➡ *in segment 7 of the liver, consistent with distant metastatic disease. Multiple other liver masses, although present, are not shown. The liver is the most common location for hematogenous metastases.*

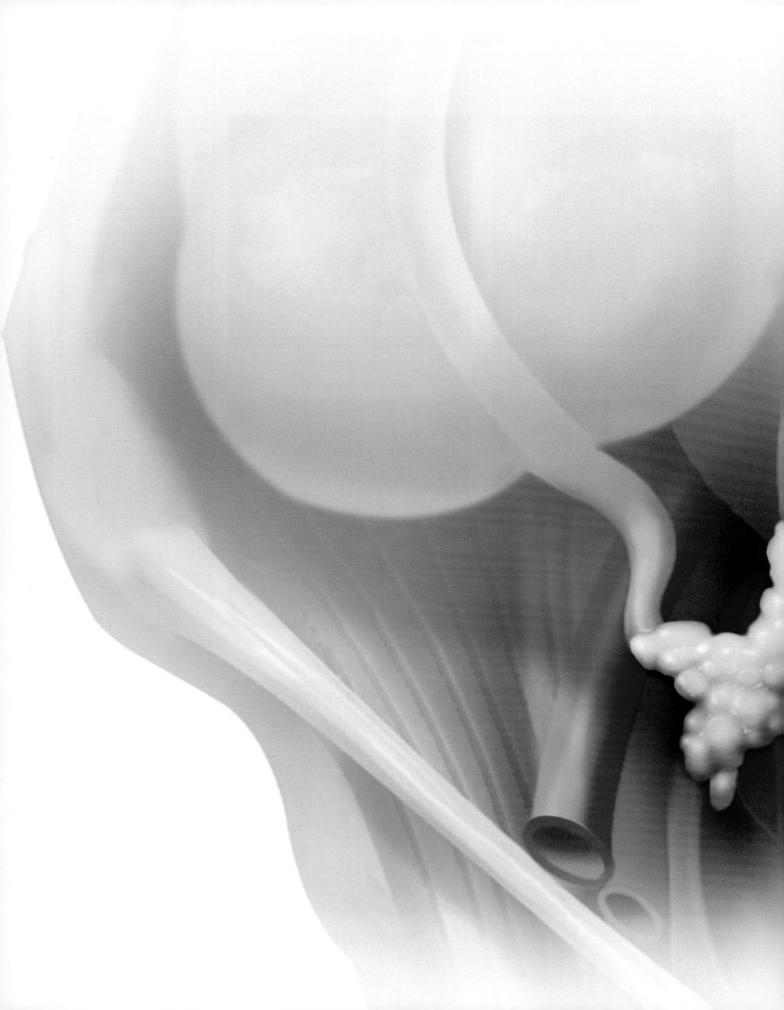

Appendiceal Carcinoma

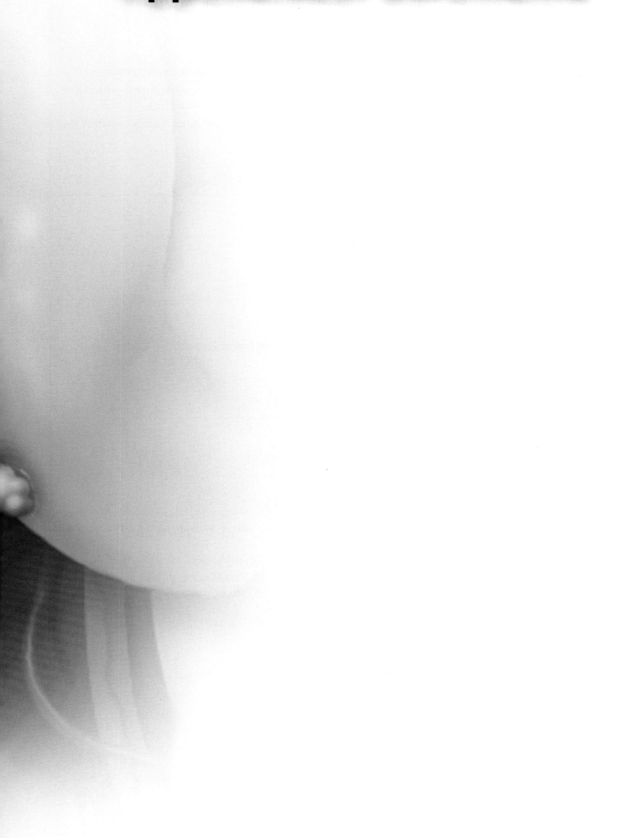

APPENDICEAL CARCINOMA

(T) Primary Tumor

Adapted from 7th edition AJCC Staging Forms.

TNM	Definitions
TX	Primary tumor cannot be assessed
T0	No evidence of primary tumor
Tis	Carcinoma in situ: Intraepithelial or invasion of lamina propria[1]
T1	Tumor invades submucosa
T2	Tumor invades muscularis propria
T3	Tumor invades through muscularis propria into subserosa or into mesoappendix
T4	Tumor penetrates visceral peritoneum, including mucinous peritoneal tumor within the right lower quadrant &/or directly invades other organs or structures[2],[3]
T4a	Tumor penetrates visceral peritoneum, including mucinous peritoneal tumor within the right lower quadrant
T4b	Tumor directly invades other organs or structures

(N) Regional Lymph Nodes

NX	Regional lymph nodes cannot be assessed
N0	No regional lymph node metastasis
N1	Metastasis in 1-3 regional lymph nodes
N2	Metastasis in ≥ 4 regional lymph nodes

(M) Distant Metastasis

M0	No distant metastasis
M1	Distant metastasis
M1a	Intraperitoneal metastasis beyond the right lower quadrant, including pseudomyxoma peritonei
M1b	Nonperitoneal metastasis

(G) Histologic Grade

GX	Grade cannot be assessed
G1	Well differentiated; mucinous low grade
G2	Moderately differentiated; mucinous high grade
G3	Poorly differentiated; mucinous high grade
G4	Undifferentiated

[1]*Tis includes cancer cells confined within the glandular basement membrane (intraepithelial) or lamina propria (intramucosal) with no extension through muscularis mucosae into submucosa.*

[2]*Direct invasion in T4 includes invasion of other segments of the colorectum by way of the serosa, e.g., invasion of ileum.*

[3]*Tumor that is adherent to other organs or structures, grossly, is classified cT4b. However, if no tumor is present in the adhesion, microscopically, the classification should be pT1-3 depending on the anatomical depth of wall invasion.*

APPENDICEAL CARCINOMA

AJCC Stages/Prognostic Groups

Adapted from 7th edition AJCC Staging Forms.

Stage	T	N	M	G
0	Tis	N0	M0	
I	T1	N0	M0	
	T2	N0	M0	
IIA	T3	N0	M0	
IIB	T4a	N0	M0	
IIC	T4b	N0	M0	
IIIA	T1	N1	M0	
	T2	N1	M0	
IIIB	T3	N1	M0	
	T4	N1	M0	
IIIC	Any T	N2	M0	
IVA	Any T	N0	M1a	G1
IVB	Any T	N0	M1a	G2, G3
	Any T	N1	M1a	Any G
	Any T	N2	M1a	Any G
IVC	Any T	Any N	M1b	Any G

(R) Residual Tumor

Adapted from 7th edition AJCC Staging Forms.

TNM	Definitions
R0	Complete resection, margins histologically negative; no residual tumor left after resection
R1	Incomplete resection, margins histologically involved, microscopic tumor remains after resection of gross disease (relevant to resection margins that are microscopically involved by tumor)
R2	Incomplete resection, margins involved or gross disease remains

APPENDICEAL CARCINOMA

T1

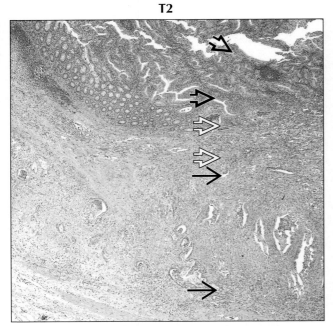

Low-power view of H&E stained section of an appendix shows mucosal epithelium ➡ lining the appendiceal lumen ⇉ with invasive adenocarcinoma ⊡ involving the lamina propria and submucosa but not the muscularis propria ➡. (Original magnification 40x.)

T1

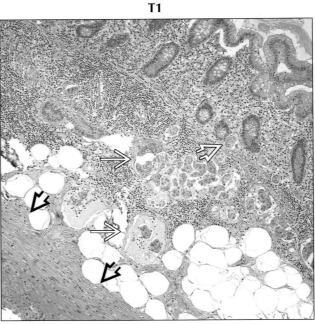

High-power view of H&E stained section shows appendiceal mucosa on the right upper corner with invasive glands in the lamina propria ⊡ as well as in the submucosa ➡. The muscle bundles of the muscularis propria ⊡ are not involved by the neoplastic glands. (Original magnification 100x.)

T2

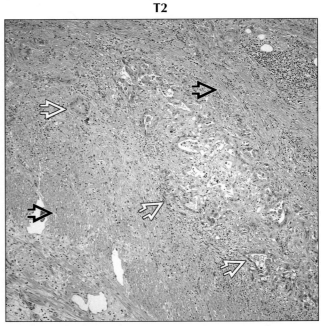

H&E stained section shows the full thickness of an appendix. Tumor involves appendiceal mucosa ⊡ and extends through the submucosa ⇉ to involve the muscularis propria ➡. (Original magnification 20x.)

T2

Higher power magnification shows the neoplastic glands ⇉ infiltrating into the smooth muscle bundles ⊡ of the muscularis propria. (Original magnification 100x.)

T3

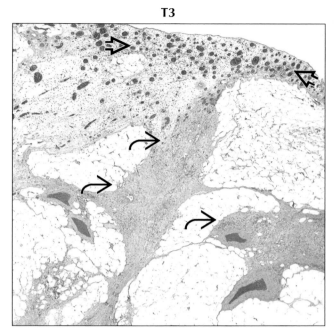

H&E stain shows a section of appendiceal carcinoma that extends beyond the wall of the appendix to involve the fatty tissue of the mesoappendix. The tumor ➔ extends from the left lower corner and invades periappendiceal fat cells (white spaces) but does not involve the serosal surface ➔. (Original magnification 40x.)

T3

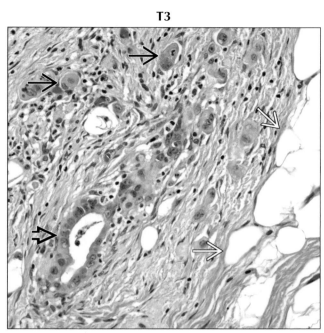

High-power view of H&E stained section shows the neoplastic cells arranged in glands ➔ or singly ➔ surrounded by a desmoplastic reaction (pink areas) that is elicited by the neoplastic cells. Note the fat cells ➔. (Original magnification 400x.)

T4a

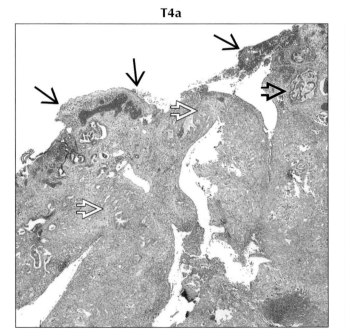

H&E stained section shows invasive appendiceal mucinous carcinoma that extensively involves the periappendiceal tissue. Sheets of the tumor cells ➔ replace the subserosal fatty tissue with numerous glands filled with mucin ➔. The neoplastic cells extend to involve the serosal surface ➔. (Original magnification 20x.)

T4a

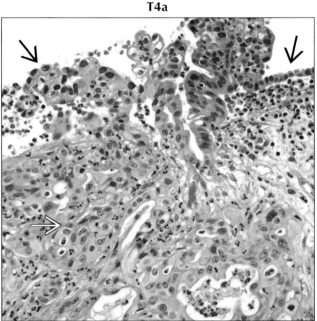

High-power magnification highlights the neoplastic cells ➔ that extend to the upper aspect of the figure and penetrate through serosal surface ➔. (Original magnification 400x.)

APPENDICEAL CARCINOMA

T1

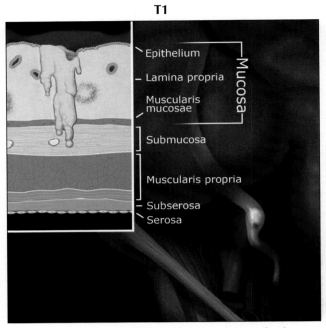

Graphic illustrates T1 tumor, defined as tumor that invades the submucosa.

T2

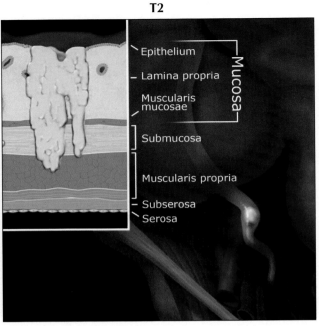

Graphic illustrates T2 tumor, which invades the muscularis propria.

T3

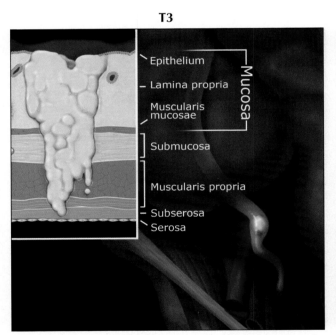

Graphic illustrates T3 tumor, defined as tumor that invades through the muscularis propria into subserosa or into mesoappendix.

T4a

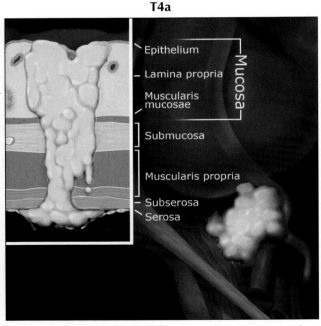

Graphic illustrates T4a tumor, defined as tumor that penetrates the visceral peritoneum. Mucinous peritoneal tumor within the right lower quadrant is also included under T4a.

APPENDICEAL CARCINOMA

T4b

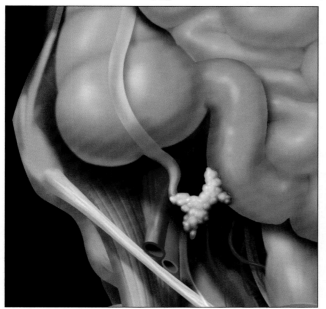

Graphic illustrates T4b tumor invading the terminal ileum. Any direct invasion of other organs or structures is considered T4b.

Nodal Drainage

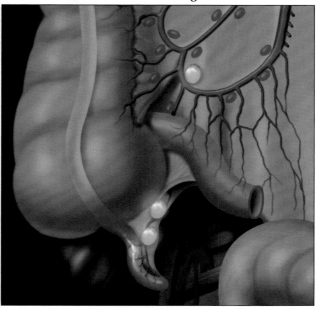

Graphic illustrates nodal drainage of the appendix to the ileocolic lymph nodes.

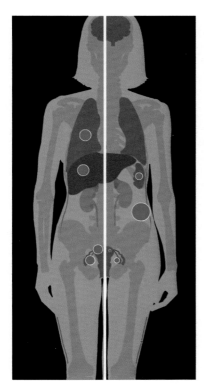

METASTASES, ORGAN FREQUENCY

NONMUCINOUS

Liver	43%
Lung	43%
Ovary	29%
Uterus	29%

MUCINOUS

Peritoneum	70%
Spleen	22%
Ovary	13%
Uterus	4%
Skin	4%

Site of metastases varies based on histology.

APPENDICEAL CARCINOMA

OVERVIEW

General Comments
- Carcinoma constitutes 10-20% of appendiceal tumors
  - Majority of appendiceal tumors are carcinoids

Classification
- Histologic types of appendiceal carcinoma
  - Mucinous carcinoma, colloid type (37%)
    - > 50% of mucinous carcinoma is of colloid type
  - Nonmucinous
    - Adenocarcinoma in situ
    - Adenocarcinoma
      - Referred to as "colonic-type" adenocarcinoma of appendix
    - Medullary carcinoma
    - Signet ring cell carcinoma (> 50% signet ring cells)
    - Squamous cell carcinoma
    - Adenosquamous carcinoma
    - Small cell carcinoma
    - Undifferentiated carcinoma
    - Carcinoma, NOS

PATHOLOGY

Routes of Spread
- Local spread
  - Mucinous carcinoma
    - Peritoneal dissemination
      - Major route of spread of appendiceal mucinous tumors
      - Results from mucocele rupture and dissemination of malignant cells into peritoneal cavity
      - Distribution in peritoneal cavity follows expected peritoneal fluid hemodynamics and gravity
      - But tends to spare bowel due to peristalsis
  - Nonmucinous carcinoma
    - Tends to spread by direct invasion of surrounding structures
- Nodal metastasis
  - Mucinous carcinoma
    - Only 2% of patients have metastatic regional lymph nodes
    - Regional lymph nodes: Ileocolic nodes
  - Nonmucinous carcinoma
    - Behaves more like colorectal carcinoma, metastasizing early to regional lymph nodes
- Hematogenous metastasis
  - Mucinous carcinoma
    - Rare in contrast to colorectal carcinoma
    - Only 2% of patients have liver metastasis
  - Nonmucinous carcinoma
    - Behaves more like colorectal carcinoma, with high propensity to metastasize to liver

General Features
- Etiology
  - Adenoma–carcinoma sequence exists in appendix, similar to colorectal carcinoma
    - Occasional appendiceal carcinomas in patients with familial adenomatous polyposis syndrome

- About 10% of patients with appendiceal epithelial lesion will develop pseudomyxoma peritonei (PMP)
  - Median evolution time from appendiceal neoplasm to PMP is approximately 2 years but can be > 10 years
- Epidemiology & cancer incidence
  - Exceedingly rare
    - Age-adjusted incidence of 0.12 cases per 1,000,000 people per year
  - Malignant appendiceal neoplasms are found in 0.9-1.4% of appendectomy specimens
- Associated diseases, abnormalities
  - Incidence of synchronous colorectal carcinoma is 4-12%

Gross Pathology & Surgical Features
- **Mucocele**
  - Dilated mucus-filled appendix
  - Results from obstruction of appendiceal orifice or overproduction of mucus
  - 0.2-0.3% of appendectomy specimens
  - 8% of appendiceal tumors
- **Pseudomyxoma peritonei (jelly belly)**
  - Description
    - Presence of copious, thick mucinous or gelatinous material covering peritoneal surface and mucinous ascites
    - Deposits most often have gelatinous consistency, also known as gelatinous ascites
  - Incidence
    - Rare condition with reported incidence of 1 case per 1,000,000 population per year
    - Mean age of patients at diagnosis is 49 years (range: 23–83 years)
    - More common in women than men
  - Extensive fibroblastic organization may yield firmer, white appearance
  - Recent studies suggest that majority of cases of pseudomyxoma peritonei are caused by appendiceal mucinous tumors
    - Most develop from low-grade mucinous carcinomas that penetrate or rupture into peritoneal cavity
- **Colonic-type (nonmucinous) adenocarcinoma**
  - Usually detected in setting of suspected appendicitis in older individuals
  - Appears as appendiceal soft tissue mass with propensity to infiltrate surrounding structures

Microscopic Pathology
- **Mucocele**
  - Mucinous cystadenocarcinoma is 1 cause of appendiceal mucocele
    - 10-12% of cases of mucocele caused by mucinous cystadenocarcinoma
    - High risk of perforation with tumor seeding → peritoneal mucinous carcinomatosis
  - Other causes of mucocele
    - Simple mucocele or retention cyst
      - 20% of cases
      - Mild appendiceal dilatation, rarely > 2 cm in diameter
      - Degenerative changes of appendiceal epithelium with no epithelial atypia

APPENDICEAL CARCINOMA

- – Results from appendicolith, postoperative or postinflammatory scarring following appendicitis, appendiceal or cecal carcinoma, or appendiceal volvulus
  - ■ Focal or diffuse mucosal hyperplasia
    - – 20% of cases
    - – Mild appendiceal dilatation
  - ■ Mucinous cystadenoma
    - – Most common type of mucocele (about 50% of cases)
    - – May perforate with mucus seeding → disseminated peritoneal adenomucinosis
  - ○ Distinction between adenoma and carcinoma may be difficult on cytologic examination
    - ■ Mucinous tumors with either mural invasion or peritoneal spread are considered appendiceal carcinoma
- **Pseudomyxoma peritonei (jelly belly)**
  - ○ 3 pathological categories
    - ■ Disseminated peritoneal adenomucinosis (DPAM)
      - – Peritoneal lesions composed of abundant extracellular mucin
      - – Contains scant simple to focally proliferative mucinous epithelium with little cytological atypia or mitotic activity
      - – Does not invade stroma and appears to spread along peritoneal surfaces
      - – Arises from well-differentiated (low-grade) mucinous carcinomas
      - – Amenable to surgical debulking
      - – Tends to have relatively indolent or protracted clinical course, especially if debulking is successful
    - ■ Peritoneal mucinous carcinomatosis (PMCA)
      - – Peritoneal lesions composed of more abundant mucinous epithelium with architectural and cytological features of carcinoma
      - – Originates from high-grade mucinous carcinomas
      - – Large soft tissue and fibrotic component and may be adherent to all peritoneal surfaces
      - – Clinical course is fatal
    - ■ Peritoneal mucinous carcinomatosis with intermediate or discordant features (PMCA-I/D)
      - – Intermediate form between DPAM and PMCA
- **Colonic-type (nonmucinous) adenocarcinoma**
  - ○ Rare
  - ○ Malignant tumor in which < 50% of lesion composed of mucin
  - ○ Cuboidal or columnar neoplastic cells that form infiltrating glands resembling typical colorectal adenocarcinomas
  - ○ Tend not to form mucoceles
- **Goblet cell carcinoids**
  - ○ Referred to as adenocarcinoid
    - ■ Share histological features of both adenocarcinoma and carcinoid tumor
    - ■ 6% of appendiceal carcinoids
  - ○ Composed of small glandular acini and individual cells with eosinophilic and focally granular cytoplasm
  - ○ Staged with adenocarcinoma because biological behavior is closer to carcinomas than to carcinoids

IMAGING FINDINGS

Detection
- **Mucocele**
  - ○ Common presentation of mucinous neoplasms
  - ○ Imaging features
    - ■ Abdominal radiograph
      - – Right lower quadrant soft tissue mass, frequently with curvilinear mural calcification
    - ■ Contrast enema
      - – Smooth impression on medial aspect of cecum
    - ■ US
      - – Anechoic or hypoechogenic tubular structure in right lower quadrant
      - – Low level internal echoes
      - – Acoustic shadowing from mural calcifications
    - ■ CT
      - – Well-circumscribed, homogeneous, low-attenuation, spheric or tubular mass contiguous with base of cecum
      - – Curvilinear mural calcification in less than 50% of cases
      - – Intraluminal gas bubbles or air–fluid level within mucocele suggests superinfection
    - ■ MR
      - – Hyperintense on T2-weighted images
      - – Variably hypointense to isointense on T1-weighted images, depending on mucin concentration
  - ○ Complications of mucocele that can be detected on imaging
    - ■ Acute appendicitis
      - – Stranding of surrounding fat
      - – Presence of air within mucocele
      - – Features suggestive of coexisting mucocele in patients presenting with appendicitis include cystic dilatation of appendix, mural calcification, and luminal diameter > 1.3 cm
    - ■ Intussusception
      - – Well-defined, fluid-filled mucocele surrounded by contrast or fecal material within cecum
    - ■ Torsion
      - – Whorled appearance of supplying mesenteric fat and vessels
      - – Stranding of periappendiceal fat
- **Colonic-type (nonmucinous) adenocarcinomas**
  - ○ Soft tissue mass that involves appendix
  - ○ Usually no mucocele formation
    - ■ Unless appendiceal lumen is obstructed (simple mucocele)
- Morphologic changes of concern for neoplasm in patients presenting clinically with appendicitis
  - ○ Cystic dilatation of appendix (mucocele)
  - ○ Presence of soft tissue mass without appendiceal dilatation
  - ○ Appendiceal diameter > 15 mm

Staging
- **Local staging**
  - ○ Not possible to differentiate among T1, T2, and T3 tumors by imaging
  - ○ T4 disease manifests as soft tissue mass infiltrating surrounding structures
- **Pseudomyxoma peritonei**

APPENDICEAL CARCINOMA

- ○ General features
  - ▪ Disseminated peritoneal adenomucinosis (DPAM)
    - - Tends to spare peritoneal surfaces of bowel
    - - Accumulates beneath right hemidiaphragm; along omental surfaces, cul-de-sac, right retrohepatic and subhepatic spaces, and left paracolic gutter
  - ▪ Peritoneal mucinous carcinomatosis (PMCA)
    - - May be adherent to all peritoneal surfaces including intestinal serosal surfaces
- ○ Sonography
  - ▪ Echogenic ascitic fluid
    - - In contrast to echoes resulting from proteinaceous, bloody, or fibrinous exudates or infection, echoes within PMP are not mobile
    - - Echogenic septations within gelatinous ascites are frequent
    - - Focal or sheet-like echogenic masses that represent involvement of omentum and parietal peritoneum may be present
    - - Scalloping of hepatic and splenic margins may be present
- ○ CT
  - ▪ Mucin is low in CT attenuation (fluid density)
    - - Areas of soft tissue attenuation may be present, representing solid tumor elements, fibrosis, or compression of mesentery
  - ▪ Widespread heterogeneous peritoneal loculi that displace and distort hollow viscera or produce scalloping effect on solid organs
  - ▪ Linear or punctate septal calcification may be apparent
- ○ PET/CT
  - ▪ Patients with DPAM usually have negative scan whereas patients with PMCA or PMCA-I/D usually have positive scan
  - ▪ Preoperative PET/CT predicted type of PMP with sensitivity of 90%, specificity of 77%, accuracy of 85%, PPV of 86%, NPV of 83%
- ○ MR
  - ▪ T1WI: Low signal intensity of both peritoneal implants and mucinous ascites
  - ▪ T2WI: High signal intensity of both tumor implants and mucinous ascites
    - - Mucinous ascites shows higher signal intensity than implants, approaching signal intensities of water
  - ▪ Gadolinium-enhanced MR: Thick and heterogeneously enhancing peritoneal tumor masses
    - - Heterogeneous appearance reflects combination of nonenhancing mucinous material and enhancing cellular tumor
- **Nodal metastasis**
  - ○ Usually to ileocolic lymph nodes
  - ○ Common with colonic-type adenocarcinoma and less common with cystadenocarcinoma
- **Distal metastases**
  - ○ Liver is most common site of distal metastases
    - ▪ Rare in cases of mucinous adenocarcinoma
    - ▪ Common in cases of colonic-type adenocarcinoma
  - ○ Thoracic metastases are rare

- ▪ Direct extension into pleural and pericardial spaces possibly through diaphragm in PMP
- ▪ Pulmonary parenchymal metastases are extremely rare
  - - Can develop years after initial presentation
  - - Usually low-attenuation lesions on CT ± peripheral calcifications

Restaging

- CT is modality of choice for follow-up after curative surgery
- Long-term follow-up in patients with mucinous tumors is required
  - ○ PMP can develop up to 20 years following tumor resection

CLINICAL ISSUES

Presentation

- Most present as acute appendicitis (37%), frequently with appendiceal abscess
  - ○ In about 40% of cases, diagnosis is made after appendectomy
- Mucocele
  - ○ Asymptomatic and incidentally discovered in majority of patients
  - ○ Abdominal pain
  - ○ Palpable right lower quadrant abdominal mass
  - ○ Acute appendicitis if secondarily infected
  - ○ Acute right lower quadrant pain can also result from torsion of mucocele
- Pseudomyxoma peritonei
  - ○ Progressive abdominal pain
  - ○ Increasing abdominal girth
  - ○ Weight loss

Cancer Natural History & Prognosis

- Mucinous carcinoma has better prognosis than nonmucinous adenocarcinoma and is less likely to demonstrate lymphatic or hematogenous spread
- Overall 5-year survival rate by stage
  - ○ Stage I (81%)
  - ○ Stage II (53%)
  - ○ Stage III (33%)
  - ○ Stage IV (23%)

Treatment Options

- Major treatment alternatives
  - ○ Standard surgery
    - ▪ Right hemicolectomy + ileocolic anastomosis + lymph node dissection
    - ▪ Some authors recommend concomitant palliative oophorectomy, especially in postmenopausal women
  - ○ Peritoneal metastases and pseudomyxoma peritonei
    - ▪ Cytoreductive surgery + perioperative intraperitoneal chemotherapy composed of hyperthermic intraperitoneal chemotherapy (HIPEC) ± postoperative intraperitoneal chemotherapy (EPIC)
      - - 5-year survival ranges from 52-96% from time of cytoreductive surgery

- Right hemicolectomy does not confer survival advantage in patients with mucinous appendiceal tumor with peritoneal seeding
  - Appendectomy alone can be performed in this group of patients
- Right hemicolectomy should be performed if
  - Necessary to achieve complete cytoreduction
  - Lymph node involvement is demonstrated by histopathological examination
  - Nonmucinous histological type is identified by histopathological examination

REPORTING CHECKLIST

T Staging
- Not possible to differentiate T1 from T2 from T3 by imaging
- Tumor invading visceral peritoneum and presenting as mass is T4a
- Mucinous tumor limited to right lower quadrant is T4a
- Tumor invading adjacent organs (e.g., small intestine or colon) is T4b

N Staging
- Rare with mucinous tumors
- More common with colonic-type tumors
- Involves ileocolic lymph nodes
  - 1-3 nodes is N1
  - ≥ 4 nodes is N2

M Staging
- Pseudomyxoma peritonei and peritoneal metastases beyond right lower quadrant is M1a
- Nonperitoneal metastases (e.g., to liver) is M1b

SELECTED REFERENCES

1. American Joint Committee on Cancer: AJCC Cancer Staging Manual. 7th ed. New York: Springer. 133-41, 2010
2. Passot G et al: Pseudomyxoma peritonei: role of 18F-FDG PET in preoperative evaluation of pathological grade and potential for complete cytoreduction. Eur J Surg Oncol. 36(3):315-23, 2010
3. Bennett GL et al: CT diagnosis of mucocele of the appendix in patients with acute appendicitis. AJR Am J Roentgenol. 192(3):W103-10, 2009
4. Chua TC et al: Pseudomyxoma peritonei: a need to establish evidence-based standard of care--is this the right trial? Ann Surg Oncol. 16(10):2675-7, 2009
5. Levy AD et al: Secondary tumors and tumorlike lesions of the peritoneal cavity: imaging features with pathologic correlation. Radiographics. 29(2):347-73, 2009
6. Wei-Ming L et al: Intussusception secondary to a giant appendical mucocele: preoperative diagnosis by multi-slice computed tomography. Abdom Imaging. Epub ahead of print, 2009
7. Low RN et al: Mucinous appendiceal neoplasms: preoperative MR staging and classification compared with surgical and histopathologic findings. AJR Am J Roentgenol. 190(3):656-65, 2008
8. Moran B et al: Consensus statement on the loco-regional treatment of appendiceal mucinous neoplasms with peritoneal dissemination (pseudomyxoma peritonei). J Surg Oncol. 98(4):277-82, 2008
9. Smeenk RM et al: Appendiceal neoplasms and pseudomyxoma peritonei: a population based study. Eur J Surg Oncol. 34(2):196-201, 2008
10. Blondiaux E et al: Appendiceal intussusception caused by a mucocele of the appendix: imaging findings. Dig Liver Dis. 39(12):1087, 2007
11. Hebert JJ et al: MDCT diagnosis of an appendiceal mucocele with acute torsion. AJR Am J Roentgenol. 189(1):W4-6, 2007
12. Khan AA et al: Prolonged survival in a patient with recurrent pulmonary metastases secondary to mucinous cystadenocarcinoma of the appendix with pseudomyxomatous peritonei. Ann Thorac Surg. 83(5):1893-4, 2007
13. Sugarbaker PH: New standard of care for appendiceal epithelial neoplasms and pseudomyxoma peritonei syndrome? Lancet Oncol. 7(1):69-76, 2006
14. Pickhardt PJ et al: Primary neoplasms of the appendix: radiologic spectrum of disease with pathologic correlation. Radiographics. 2003 May-Jun;23(3):645-62. Review. Erratum in: Radiographics. 23(5):1340, 2003
15. Stocchi L et al: Surgical treatment of appendiceal mucocele. Arch Surg. 138(6):585-9; discussion 589-90, 2003
16. Kabbani W et al: Mucinous and nonmucinous appendiceal adenocarcinomas: different clinicopathological features but similar genetic alterations. Mod Pathol. 15(6):599-605, 2002
17. Pickhardt PJ et al: Primary neoplasms of the appendix manifesting as acute appendicitis: CT findings with pathologic comparison. Radiology. 224(3):775-81, 2002
18. Sulkin TV et al: CT in pseudomyxoma peritonei: a review of 17 cases. Clin Radiol. 57(7):608-13, 2002
19. Bechtold RE et al: CT appearance of disseminated peritoneal adenomucinosis. Abdom Imaging. 26(4):406-10, 2001
20. Krebs TL et al: General case of the day. Mucinous cystadenocarcinoma of the appendix. Radiographics. 18(4):1049-50, 1998
21. Mortman KD et al: Pulmonary metastases in pseudomyxoma peritonei syndrome. Ann Thorac Surg. 64(5):1434-6, 1997
22. Buy JN et al: Magnetic resonance imaging of pseudomyxoma peritonei. Eur J Radiol. 9(2):115-8, 1989

APPENDICEAL CARCINOMA

Stage I (T2 N0 M0)

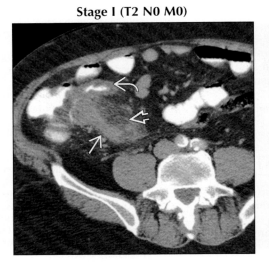

Stage I (T2 N0 M0)

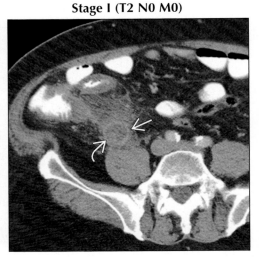

(Left) Axial CECT in a 65-year-old man who presented with acute right lower quadrant pain shows dilated appendix ➡ with extensive periappendiceal stranding ➡ due to acute appendicitis. There is also mild thickening of the wall of the terminal ileum ➡. *(Right)* Axial CECT in the same patient shows dilatation of the tip of the appendix (mucocele) ➡ with a nodular intraluminal soft tissue component ➡.

Stage I (T2 N0 M0)

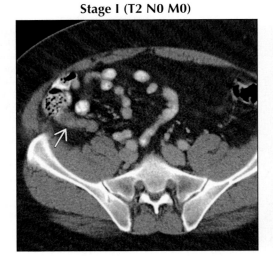

Stage I (T2 N0 M0)

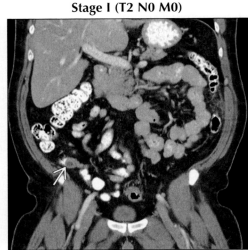

(Left) Axial CECT in a 42-year-old man shows thickened appendix ➡ without periappendiceal stranding or adenopathy. *(Right)* Coronal CECT in the same patient shows dilated appendix with a small cystic component ➡. Pathology revealed tumor invading into the muscularis propria, consistent with T2 disease.

Stage IIA (T3 N0 M0)

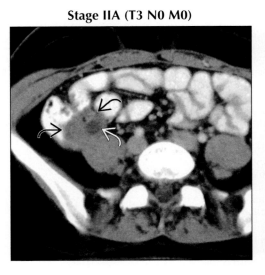

Stage IIA (T3 N0 M0)

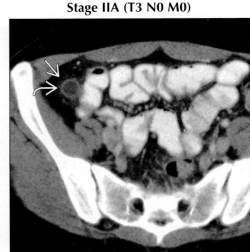

(Left) Axial CECT in a 46-year-old man who presented with signs and symptoms of acute appendicitis shows an appendiceal mucocele ➡ surrounded by a rim of soft tissue ➡. *(Right)* Axial CECT in the same patient shows mild fat stranding ➡ surrounding the distal end of the mucocele ➡. Acute appendicitis was confirmed during surgery, together with a colonic-type appendiceal adenocarcinoma invading into the mesoappendix.

APPENDICEAL CARCINOMA

Stage IIC (T4b N0 M0)

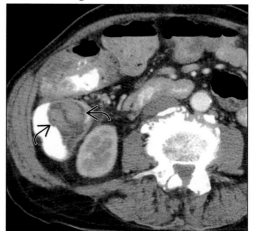

Stage IIC (T4b N0 M0)

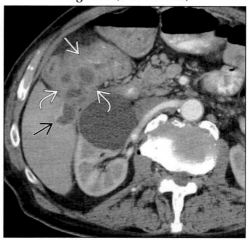

(Left) Axial CECT in a 75-year-old man who presented with right upper quadrant pain shows a large appendiceal mass ⧎ protruding into the cecal lumen. (Right) Axial CECT in the same patient shows a mixed solid and cystic subhepatic mass ⧎ invading into the right lobe of the liver ⧎ and into the transverse colon ⧎.

Stage IIC (T4b N0 M0)

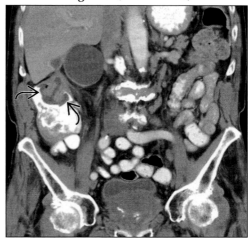

Stage IIC (T4b N0 M0)

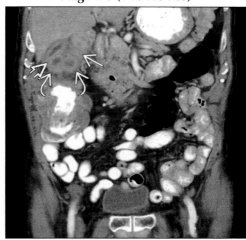

(Left) Coronal CECT in the same patient shows the thickened wall of the appendix ⧎ protruding into the cecum. The patient has cecal bascule, which occurs when the cecum folds anteriorly without torsion so that the appendix lies above the ileocecal valve. (Right) Coronal CECT in the same patient shows tumor ⧎ that invades the wall of the transverse colon ⧎ and is inseparable from the gallbladder ⧎.

Stage IIC (T4b N0 M0)

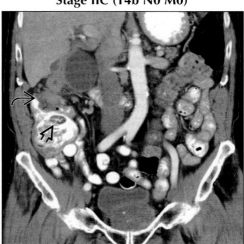

Stage IIC (T4b N0 M0)

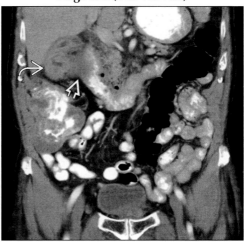

(Left) Coronal CECT in the same patient shows the appendiceal tumor ⧎ protruding into the cecum above the ileocecal valve ⧎. (Right) Coronal CECT in the same patient shows the appendiceal tumor ⧎ in the subhepatic region infiltrating ⧎ into the transverse colon. Appendiceal tumors invading surrounding organs or structures are considered T4b disease.

APPENDICEAL CARCINOMA

Stage IIIA (T2 N1 M0)

Stage IIIA (T2 N1 M0)

(Left) Axial CECT with rectal contrast in a 79-year-old woman who presented with acute right lower quadrant pain shows a fluid-filled tubular right lower quadrant mass ⬇. (Right) Axial CECT in the same patient shows the distal end of the fluid-filled appendix (mucocele) ➡.

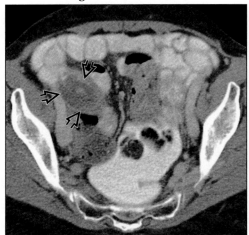

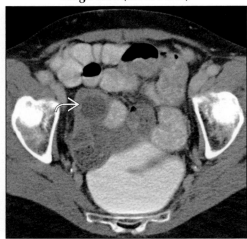

Stage IIIA (T2 N1 M0)

Stage IIIA (T2 N1 M0)

(Left) Sagittal CECT in the same patient shows an appendiceal mucocele ⬇ with peripheral mural calcifications ➡. (Right) Coronal CECT in the same patient shows the appendiceal mucocele ➡ as well as a 9 mm ileocolic lymph node ➡, which was found to be metastatic during surgery. Biopsy showed appendiceal mucinous adenocarcinoma invading into muscularis propria but not into subserosa, consistent with T2 disease.

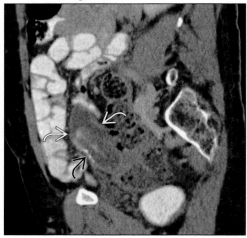

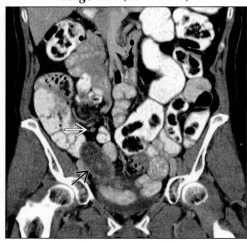

Stage IIIB (T3 N1 M0)

Stage IIIB (T3 N1 M0)

(Left) Axial CECT in a 54-year-old man who presented with vague chronic right lower quadrant pain shows a dilated thick-walled appendix ➡ without periappendiceal stranding. Multiple lymph nodes ➡ are seen along the ileocolic vessels. (Right) Axial CECT in the same patient shows thickening of the wall of the base of the appendix ➡ and distension of its tip ⬇.

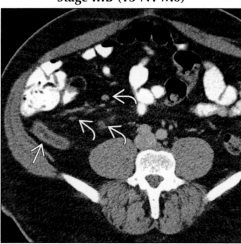

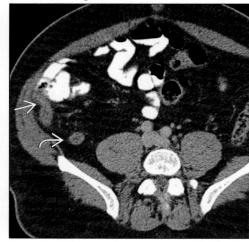

Stage IIIB (T3 N1 M0)

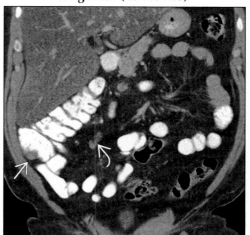

Stage IIIB (T3 N1 M0)

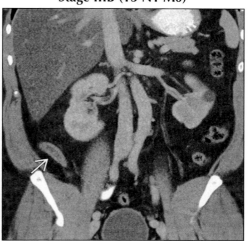

(Left) Coronal CECT in the same patient shows thickening of the base of the appendix ➡ and ileocolic nodes ➡. *(Right)* Coronal CECT in the same patient shows the thick-walled appendiceal mucocele ➡. Surgery revealed T3 tumor reaching to the subserosa without penetration of the serosa and 3 metastatic lymph nodes.

Stage IIIB (T4a N1 M0)

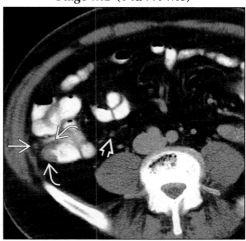

Stage IIIB (T4a N1 M0)

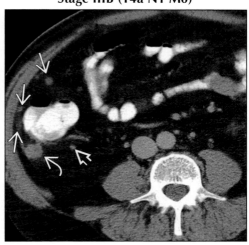

(Left) Axial CECT in a 61-year-old man with a long history of postprandial pain shows thickening of the wall of the appendiceal orifice ➡ with multiple peritoneal nodules ➡ and an ileocolic node ➡. *(Right)* Axial CECT in the same patient shows an appendiceal mass ➡ with a spiculated outer margin, peritoneal nodules ➡, and an ileocolic node ➡.

Stage IIIB (T4a N1 M0)

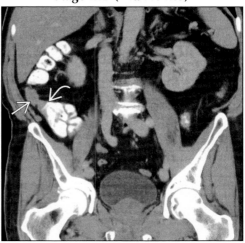

Stage IIIB (T4a N1 M0)

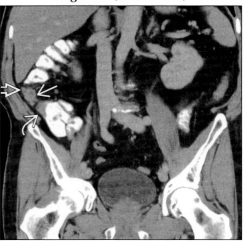

(Left) Coronal CECT in the same patient shows appendiceal tumor ➡ invading into the cecum ➡. *(Right)* Coronal CECT in the same patient shows appendiceal tumor ➡, tumor invasion of the cecum ➡, and peritoneal nodules ➡.

Stage IIIB (T4a N1 M0)

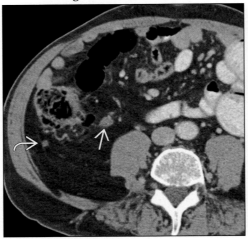

Stage IIIB (T4a N1 M0)

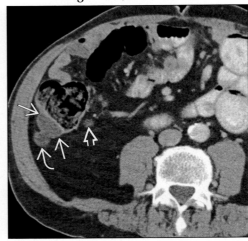

(Left) Axial CECT in a 65-year-old man shows normal appearance of the proximal appendix ➡ and an enlarged node ➡ along the ileocolic vessels. *(Right)* Axial CECT in the same patient shows dilatation of the distal appendix (mucocele) ➡ that has ruptured with mucinous tumor implant on the surface of the cecum ➡. Another ileocolic node ⮞ is present.

Stage IIIB (T4a N1 M0)

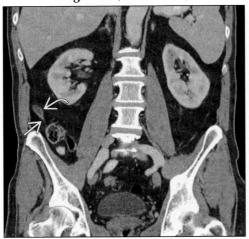

Stage IIIB (T4a N1 M0)

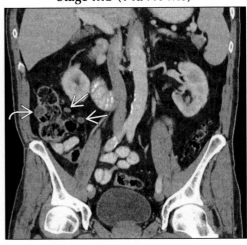

(Left) Coronal CECT in the same patient shows the transition from the normal proximal appendix ➡ to the dilated appendiceal mucocele ➡. *(Right)* Coronal CECT in the same patient shows the mucinous implant ➡ on the surface of the cecum and 2 enlarged ileocolic nodes ➡. Mucinous peritoneal tumor in the right lower quadrant constitutes T4a disease, while peritoneal implants beyond the right lower quadrant constitute M1a disease.

Stage IVA (T4a N0 M1a G1)

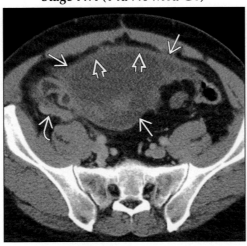

Stage IVA (T4a N0 M1a G1)

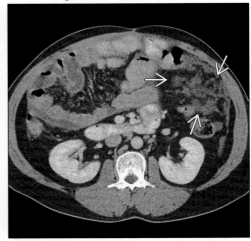

(Left) Axial CECT in a 63-year-old man who presented with worsening abdominal distension shows pelvic fluid collection ➡ with surrounding thick soft tissue rind ➡. The appendix is enlarged ➡ without surrounding inflammatory changes. *(Right)* Axial CECT in the same patient shows extensive peritoneal metastases in the left upper quadrant ➡. Peritoneal implants in pseudomyxoma peritonei tend to spare the bowel peritoneal surfaces.

APPENDICEAL CARCINOMA

Stage IVA (T4a N0 M1a G1)

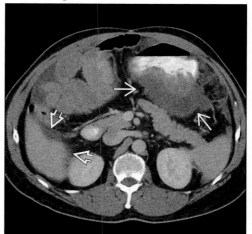

Stage IVA (T4a N0 M1a G1)

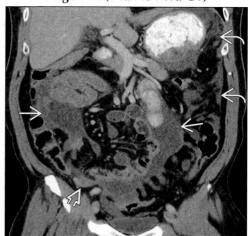

(Left) Axial CECT in the same patient shows accumulation of mucinous ascites within the lesser sac ➡ and along the surface of the liver ➡. *(Right)* Coronal CECT in the same patient shows the mucinous ascites ➡ and peritoneal implants ➡, in addition to the large appendix ➡. M1a disease with G1 histology is staged as IVA, while M1a disease with G2 or G3 histology is staged as IVB.

Stage IVC (T3 N0 M1b)

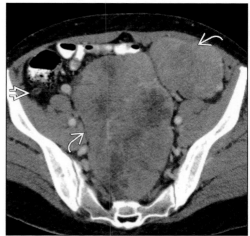

Stage IVC (T3 N0 M1b)

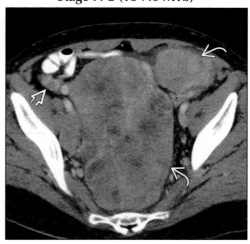

(Left) Axial CECT shows bilateral solid ovarian masses ➡ in a 35-year-old woman who presented with vague pelvic pain and was found to have pelvic mass on physical examination. A normal proximal part of the appendix is seen ➡. *(Right)* Axial CECT in the same patient shows the bilateral ovarian masses ➡ and an enhancing soft tissue mass of the distal end of the appendix ➡. Pathology revealed primary appendiceal adenocarcinoma with ovarian metastases.

Stage IVC (T3 N0 M1b)

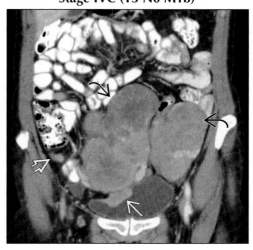

Stage IVC (T3 N0 M1b)

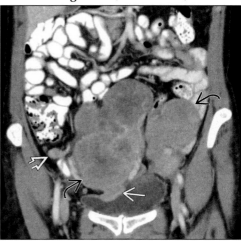

(Left) Coronal CECT in the same patient shows the bilateral solid ovarian masses ➡ and a small enhancing appendiceal mass ➡. There is a peritoneal metastatic lesion ➡ that invades into the wall of the urinary bladder dome. *(Right)* Coronal CECT in the same patient again shows not only the ovarian metastases ➡ and the primary appendiceal tumor ➡ but also a peritoneal metastatic lesion ➡ that invades into the wall of the urinary bladder.

APPENDICEAL CARCINOMA

Stage IVC (T4a N0 M1b)

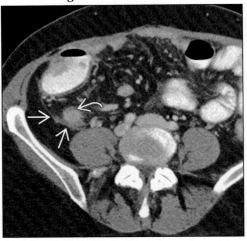

Stage IVC (T4a N0 M1b)

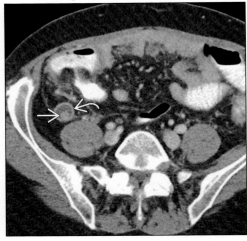

(Left) Axial CECT in a 64-year-old woman who presented with right lower quadrant pain of 2 months duration shows an enhancing large appendix ➔ with surrounding soft tissue/ fluid density ➔. *(Right)* Axial CECT in the same patient shows a dilated fluid-filled appendix (mucocele) ➔ containing an enhancing mural solid component ➔. The presence of a solid component within a mucocele makes the diagnosis almost certainly mucinous cystadenocarcinoma.

Stage IVC (T4a N0 M1b)

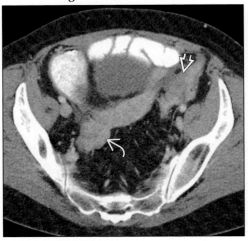

Stage IVC (T4a N0 M1b)

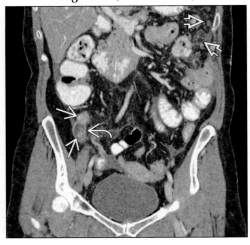

(Left) Axial CECT in the same patient shows an enlarged, solid-appearing right ovary ➔ that was found at surgery to be metastatic carcinoma. Low-density tissue is seen in the region of the left adnexa ➔, which proved to be peritoneal metastasis. *(Right)* Coronal CECT in the same patient shows appendiceal mucocele ➔ with enhancing mural components ➔. Scattered soft tissue nodules ➔ are seen throughout the peritoneum due to peritoneal metastatic disease.

Stage IVC (T4a N0 M1b)

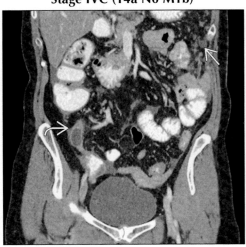

Stage IVC (T4a N0 M1b)

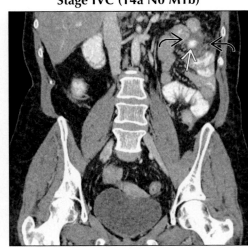

(Left) Coronal CECT in the same patient shows appendiceal mucocele ➔ and nodular peritoneal implants ➔. *(Right)* Coronal CECT in the same patient shows abnormal low-density material ➔ surrounding a jejunal loop ➔ and representing peritoneal mucinous carcinomatosis, which may involve all peritoneal surfaces including the serosal surfaces of the intestine. Pseudomyxoma peritonei, on the other hand, tends to spare the peritoneal surfaces of the bowel.

APPENDICEAL CARCINOMA

Stage IVC (T4a N0 M1b)

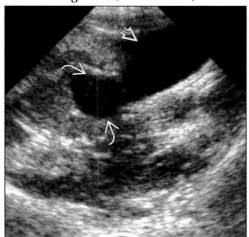

Stage IVC (T4a N0 M1b)

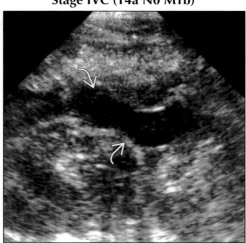

(Left) Transverse transabdominal ultrasound in a 65-year-old man who presented with increasing abdominal girth shows a rounded structure (appendiceal mucocele) ➡ with low level echoes within the right lower quadrant. The anechoic structure adjacent to the mucocele is the urinary bladder ➡. (Right) Longitudinal transabdominal ultrasound in the same patient shows a tubular structure (appendiceal mucocele) ➡ containing low level echoes.

Stage IVC (T4a N0 M1b)

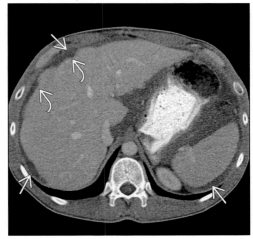

Stage IVC (T4a N0 M1b)

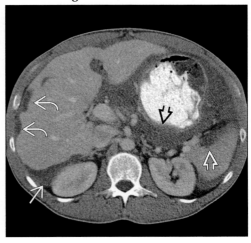

(Left) Axial CECT in the same patient shows low-density material ➡ surrounding the liver and spleen. Note the mass effect on the liver ➡, which manifests as scalloping of the liver contour, characteristic of pseudomyxoma peritonei. (Right) Axial CECT in the same patient shows mucinous ascites causing scalloping of the liver ➡ and splenic ➡ contours. Mucinous material is also present within the lesser sac ➡ and Morrison pouch ➡.

Stage IVC (T4a N0 M1b)

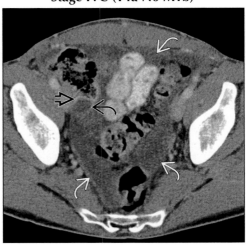

Stage IVC (T4a N0 M1b)

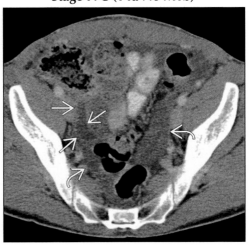

(Left) Axial CECT in the same patient shows pelvic filling with the low-density mucinous material ➡. In addition the basal part of the causative mucocele ➡ is seen at the base of the cecum ➡. The fluid in the mucocele is slightly less dense than the mucinous ascites, allowing its visualization. (Right) Axial CECT in the same patient shows pelvic mucinous ascites ➡ and a long portion of the fluid-filled mucocele ➡.

APPENDICEAL CARCINOMA

Stage IVC (T4a N0 M1b)

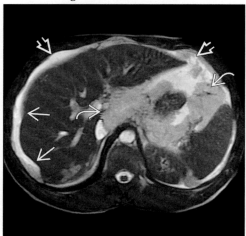

Stage IVC (T4a N0 M1b)

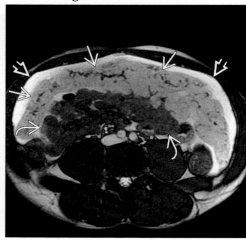

(Left) Axial T2WI MR in the same patient shows scalloping of the liver contour ➡, mucinous ascites ⇉, and slightly lower intensity tumor masses ➡ within the upper abdomen. *(Right)* Axial T2WI MR in the same patient shows mucinous ascites ⇉ and tumor masses involving the omentum ➡. Pseudomyxoma peritonei tends to spare small bowel loops ⇉ because of peristalsis.

Stage IVC (T4a N0 M1b)

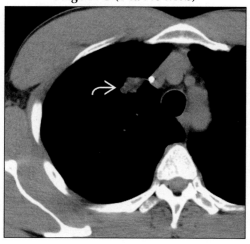

Stage IVC (T4a N0 M1b)

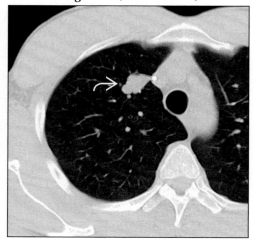

(Left) Axial NECT of the chest, mediastinal window, in the same patient shows a right upper lobe nodule ➡ with low attenuation coefficient (-5 to 10 HU). The low attenuation of the nodule is due to its gelatinous mucinous content. *(Right)* Axial NECT of the chest, lung window, in the same patient shows the lobulated outer contour of the right upper lobe lung nodule ➡. Parenchymal lung nodules, presumed to be due to hematogenous spread, are extremely rare.

Stage IVC (T4a N0 M1b)

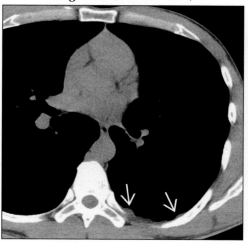

Stage IVC (T4a N0 M1b)

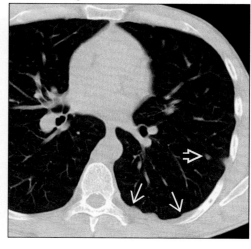

(Left) Axial NECT of the chest, mediastinal window, in the same patient shows nodular thickening ➡ of the left pleura. *(Right)* Axial CECT of the chest, lung window, in the same patient shows nodular thickening ➡ of the pleura with nodules involving the left interlobar fissure ⇉. Pleural metastases, although rare, are more common than parenchymal lung metastases and are presumed to result from extension through the diaphragm.

Stage IVC (T4b N0 M1b)

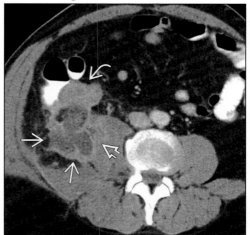

Stage IVC (T4b N0 M1b)

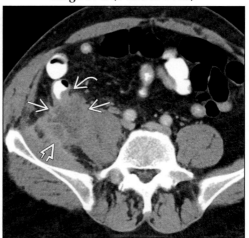

(Left) Axial CECT in a 45-year-old man who presented with right lower quadrant pain of 2 weeks duration shows an appendiceal soft tissue mass ⮞ and a peripherally enhancing, multilocular, fluid density lesion ⮞ involving the right psoas muscle ⮞.
(Right) Axial CECT in the same patient shows the peripheral, enhancing, fluid density lesion ⮞ involving the terminal ileum ⮞ as well as the right iliacus muscle ⮞.

Stage IVC (T4b N0 M1b)

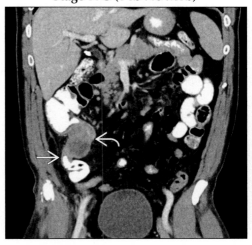

Stage IVC (T4b N0 M1b)

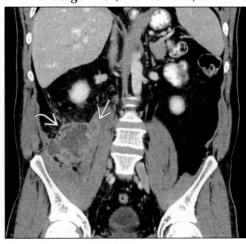

(Left) Coronal CECT in the same patient shows the tubular appendiceal soft tissue mass ⮞. The mass has mixed solid and cystic components, and it invades into the terminal ileum ⮞.
(Right) Coronal CECT in the same patient shows tumor ⮞ invading the psoas muscle ⮞. This was thought to represent an abscess resulting from appendicitis and appendiceal perforation; however, fluid obtained during percutaneous drainage showed necrotic tumor with malignant cells.

Stage IVC (T4b N0 M1b)

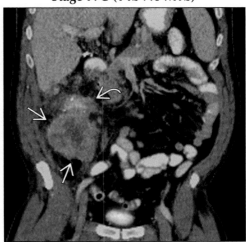

Stage IVC (T4b N0 M1b)

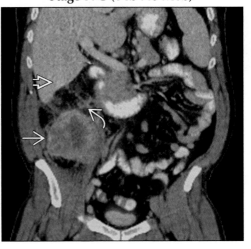

(Left) Coronal PET/CT in the same patient shows increased metabolic activity of the enlarged appendix ⮞ as well as increased activity at the periphery of the cystic component ⮞.
(Right) Coronal PET/CT in the same patient shows increased metabolic activity at the periphery of the cystic component ⮞. In addition, increased activity is present within the mesoappendix ⮞ and within the liver ⮞. Nonperitoneal metastasis constitutes M1b disease.

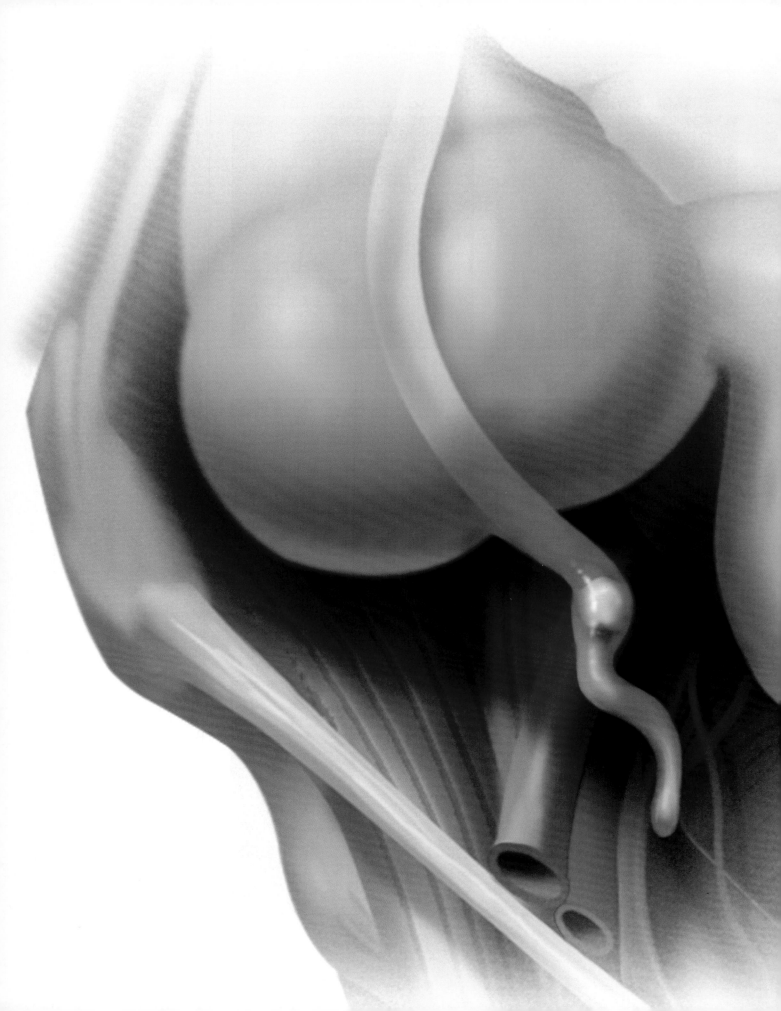

Appendiceal Carcinoid

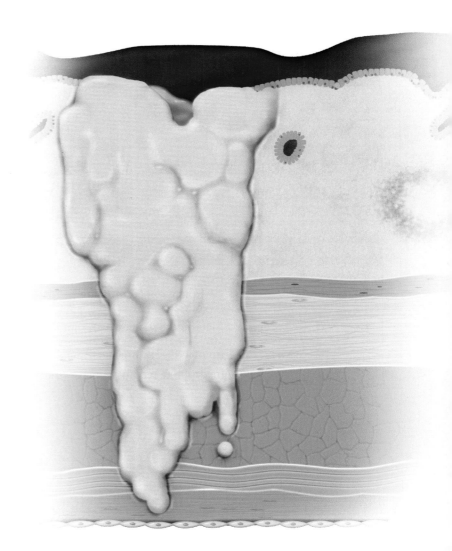

APPENDICEAL CARCINOID

(T) Primary Tumor

Adapted from 7th edition AJCC Staging Forms.

TNM	Definitions
TX	Primary tumor cannot be assessed
T0	No evidence of primary tumor
T1	Tumor ≤ 2 cm in greatest dimensions
T1a	Tumor ≤ 1 cm in greatest dimensions
T1b	Tumor > 1 cm but ≤ 2 cm in greatest dimensions
T2	Tumor > 2 cm but ≤ 4 cm or with extension to the cecum
T3	Tumor > 4 cm or with extension to the ileum
T4	Tumor directly invades other adjacent organs or structures, e.g., abdominal wall and skeletal muscles*

(N) Regional Lymph Nodes

NX	Regional lymph nodes cannot be assessed
N0	No regional lymph node metastasis
N1	Regional lymph node metastasis

(M) Distant Metastasis

M0	No distant metastasis
M1	Distant metastasis

Tumor that is adherent to other organs or structures, grossly, is classified cT4. However, if no tumor is present in the adhesion, microscopically, the classification should be pT1-3 depending on the anatomical depth of wall invasion.

*Penetration of the mesoappendix does not seem to be as important a prognostic factor as the size of the primary tumor and is not separately categorized.

AJCC Stages/Prognostic Groups

Adapted from 7th edition AJCC Staging Forms.

Stage	T	N	M
I	T1	N0	M0
II	T2	N0	M0
	T3	N0	M0
III	T4	N0	M0
	Any T	N1	M0
IV	Any T	Any N	M1

(R) Residual Tumor

Adapted from 7th edition AJCC Staging Forms.

TNM	Definitions
R0	Complete resection, margins histologically negative; no residual tumor left after resection
R1	Incomplete resection, margins histologically involved, microscopic tumor remains after resection of gross disease (relevant to resection margins that are microscopically involved by tumor)
R2	Incomplete resection, margins involved or gross disease remains

APPENDICEAL CARCINOID

T1a

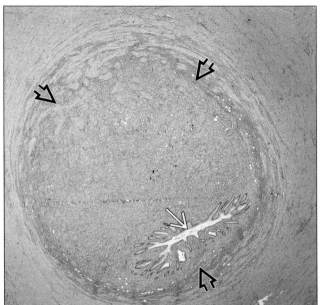

Low-power view of H&E stained section of an appendix shows a 7 mm carcinoid tumor ⇨ involving the lamina propria and submucosa but not the muscularis propria (outer circular pink area). Note the lumen ➡. (Original magnification 20x.)

T1a

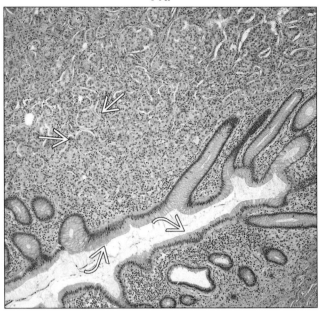

Higher magnification of the previous image shows normal mucosal epithelium ➡ with submucosal carcinoid. Tumor cells ➡ are arranged in nests and clusters composed of uniform cells with round regular nuclei and faint indistinct cell borders. (Original magnification 400x.)

T2

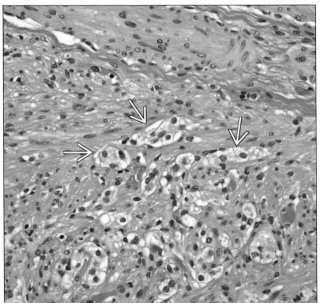

H&E stained section shows portion of the muscularis propria of the cecum with nests of carcinoid tumor cells ➡ invading through the spindle muscle bundles. (Original magnification 500x.)

T2

Immunohistochemical stain for chromogranin antibody, performed on a deeper section than that presented in the previous figure, shows the carcinoid cells staining brown ➡ and infiltrating into the spindle cells of the cecal muscularis propria. (Original magnification 500x.)

APPENDICEAL CARCINOID

T1a

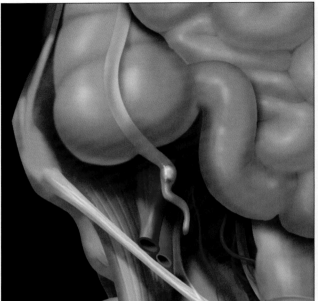

Graphic illustrates an appendiceal tumor that is ≤ 1 cm in greatest dimension, consistent with T1a disease.

T1b

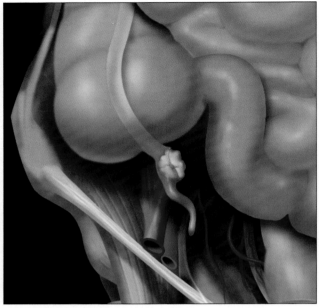

Graphic illustrates an appendiceal tumor that is > 1 cm but ≤ 2 cm in greatest dimension, consistent with T1b disease.

T2

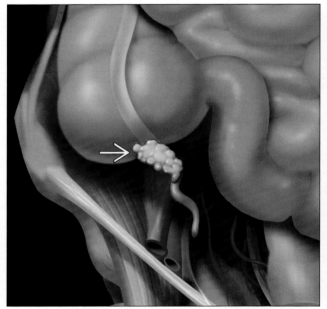

Graphic illustrates an appendiceal tumor infiltrating the cecum ➜, consistent with T2 disease. T2 designates tumor > 2 cm but ≤ 4 cm in greatest dimension or with extension to the cecum.

T3

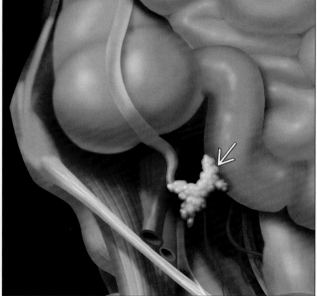

Graphic illustrates an appendiceal tumor infiltrating the ileum ➜, consistent with T3 disease. T3 indicates tumor > 4 cm in greatest dimension or with extension to the ileum.

APPENDICEAL CARCINOID

T1a

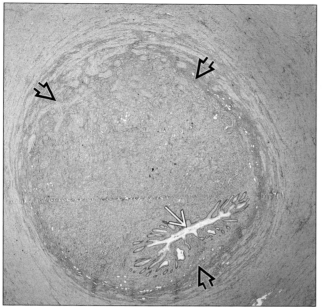

Low-power view of H&E stained section of an appendix shows a 7 mm carcinoid tumor ⧐ involving the lamina propria and submucosa but not the muscularis propria (outer circular pink area). Note the lumen ➡. (Original magnification 20x.)

T1a

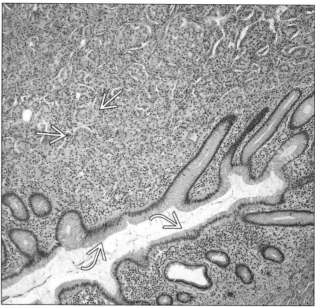

Higher magnification of the previous image shows normal mucosal epithelium ➡ with submucosal carcinoid. Tumor cells ➡ are arranged in nests and clusters composed of uniform cells with round regular nuclei and faint indistinct cell borders. (Original magnification 400x.)

T2

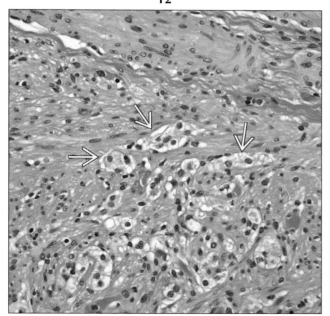

H&E stained section shows portion of the muscularis propria of the cecum with nests of carcinoid tumor cells ➡ invading through the spindle muscle bundles. (Original magnification 500x.)

T2

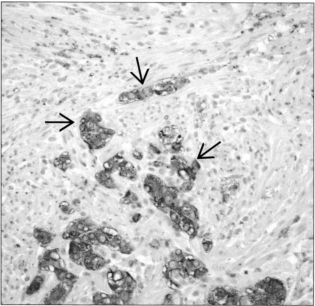

Immunohistochemical stain for chromogranin antibody, performed on a deeper section than that presented in the previous figure, shows the carcinoid cells staining brown ➡ and infiltrating into the spindle cells of the cecal muscularis propria. (Original magnification 500x.)

APPENDICEAL CARCINOID

T1a

T1b

Graphic illustrates an appendiceal tumor that is ≤ 1 cm in greatest dimension, consistent with T1a disease.

Graphic illustrates an appendiceal tumor that is > 1 cm but ≤ 2 cm in greatest dimension, consistent with T1b disease.

T2

T3

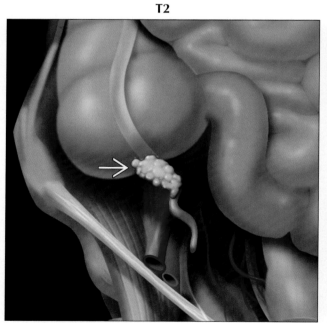

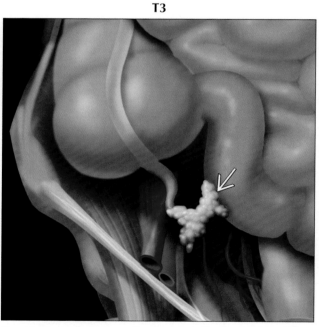

Graphic illustrates an appendiceal tumor infiltrating the cecum ➡, consistent with T2 disease. T2 designates tumor > 2 cm but ≤ 4 cm in greatest dimension or with extension to the cecum.

Graphic illustrates an appendiceal tumor infiltrating the ileum ➡, consistent with T3 disease. T3 indicates tumor > 4 cm in greatest dimension or with extension to the ileum.

APPENDICEAL CARCINOID

T4

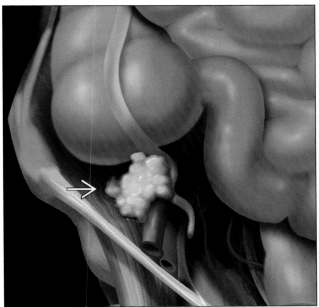

Graphic illustrates tumor directly invading iliacus muscle ➡. *T4 denotes tumor with direct invasion into other adjacent structures or organs such as the abdominal wall and skeletal muscles.*

Nodal Drainage

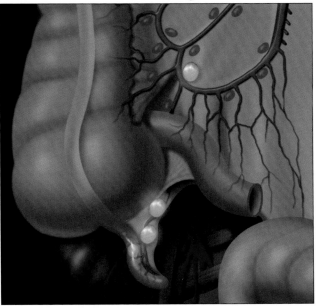

Graphic illustrates nodal drainage of the appendix to the ileocolic lymph nodes.

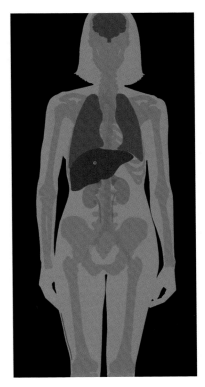

METASTASES, ORGAN FREQUENCY

Distant metastases from appendiceal carcinoid are very rare, occurring in only 0.7% of cases, almost exclusively to the liver.

APPENDICEAL CARCINOID

OVERVIEW

General Comments
- Most common appendiceal neoplasm (80-90%)

Classification
- Histologic types of appendiceal carcinoid
  - Carcinoid tumor
  - Well-differentiated neuroendocrine tumor
  - Tubular carcinoid
  - Goblet cell carcinoid
    - Classified according to staging scheme for appendiceal carcinoma
    - Also called adenocarcinoid
  - Atypical carcinoid

PATHOLOGY

Routes of Spread
- Local spread
  - Rare in tumors < 2 cm
  - Can invade cecum, terminal ileum, abdominal wall, and pelvic side wall
- Nodal metastases
  - Lymph node metastases are rare in small tumors
    - Found in up to 30% of tumors > 2 cm
  - Appendix drains into retrocecal and ileocolic nodes and, eventually, to superior mesenteric nodes
- Distant metastases
  - Rare, occurring in only 0.7% of cases
  - More common when lesions are > 2 cm in diameter
  - Liver is primary site of metastatic disease

General Features
- Epidemiology & cancer incidence
  - Carcinoid is most common appendiceal tumor
    - Found in 0.2-0.7% of all appendectomy specimens
  - Appendix is most common site of carcinoid tumors
  - M:F = 2:3
  - Mean age at diagnosis: ~ 47.1 years
    - Median age: 47 years
    - Age range: 9-89 years
- Associated diseases, abnormalities
  - Multicentric tumors can be seen in 5% of patients
    - Involvement of other portions of GI tract with other primary carcinoid tumors
  - Increased incidence of carcinoid tumors in patients with Crohn disease

Gross Pathology & Surgical Features
- Arise from subepithelial argentaffin cells in lamina propria and submucosa
- Majority are serotonin-producing enterochromaffin cell (EC-cell) tumors similar to those that occur in jejunum and ileum
- Small yellow nodules
- Usually in distal 1/3 of appendix (60-70%)
- When acute appendicitis and appendiceal carcinoid coexist, appendicitis is frequently not caused by carcinoid
  - Carcinoids are frequently located in distal part of appendix
  - Carcinoid causes obstruction in only 25% of cases

Microscopic Pathology
- H&E
  - Composed of small cells with uniform round nuclei that contain stippled chromatin but are without prominent nucleoli
  - Usually no significant mitotic activity, cytologic atypia, or nuclear pleomorphism
  - 4 histologic subtypes
    - Enterochromaffin cell
    - Goblet cell
      - Classified with adenocarcinoma because their biological behavior is closer to carcinomas than to carcinoids
    - Composite cell
    - Atypical cell
  - Recognized growth patterns
    - Insular
    - Trabecular
    - Glandular
    - Diffuse
- Special stains
  - Silver stains and immunohistochemical studies improve specificity of diagnosis

IMAGING FINDINGS

Detection
- Rarely detected on imaging
- Imaging features
  - Ultrasound
    - May present as acute appendicitis
      - Distended noncompressible fluid-filled appendix
    - Rarely appears as hypoechoic nodule within appendix
  - CECT
    - Most commonly appears as acute appendicitis without discernible mass
    - Rarely presents as focal enhancing soft tissue appendiceal mass
    - Tumor obstructing appendiceal lumen may present as mucocele
      - Fluid-filled distended appendix
    - Diffuse circumferential enhancing mural thickening

Staging
- Local spread
  - To adjacent organs: Cecum, terminal ileum, and abdominal wall
  - Appears as soft tissue mass invading these structures
- Nodal spread
  - Enlarged retrocecal, ileocolic, and mesenteric nodes
- Distant metastases
  - Primarily to liver
    - Tumors usually enhancing during arterial phase of contrast-enhanced studies

Restaging
- Follow-up only needed after resection of tumor > 2 cm

APPENDICEAL CARCINOID

CLINICAL ISSUES

Presentation
- Most present as acute appendicitis
  - In about 40% of cases, diagnosis is made after appendectomy
- Incidental finding during surgery performed for other reasons
- Carcinoid syndrome with appendiceal primary site is exceedingly rare

Cancer Natural History & Prognosis
- Most favorable prognosis of all gastrointestinal neuroendocrine tumors
- Tumor size is most important prognostic factor
  - Prognosis for tumors < 2 cm in size is excellent
    - Rarely metastasize
  - Worsened survival as tumor size increases
- Frequency of metastasis is rare
  - 21% with primary lesions 2-3 cm in diameter
  - 44% with primary lesions > 3 cm in diameter
- Well-differentiated tumors have significantly better prognosis than moderately or poorly differentiated tumors
- Overall 5-year survival rate (71-97.5%)
  - Local disease (94%)
  - Regional metastases (85%)
  - Distant metastases (34%)

Treatment Options
- Major treatment alternatives
  - Appendectomy
    - Most carcinoids are diagnosed during histological examination following simple appendectomy
    - Indications for re-intervention (right hemicolectomy + lymphadenectomy) include
      - Lesions > 2 cm in diameter
      - Cecal involvement
      - Lymph node involvement
      - Histological evidence of lymphatic invasion
      - Tumor-positive resection margins
      - High-grade malignant carcinoids and goblet cell adenocarcinoids
      - Cellular pleomorphism with high mitotic index
- Treatment options by stage
  - Stage I
    - Appendectomy is adequate treatment with cure rates of essentially 100%
    - No follow-up management is required if tumor is confined within appendix
    - Mesoappendiceal involvement alone does not affect staging
      - Does not appear to be important prognostic factor
      - Does not warrant right hemicolectomy
  - Stage II
    - Right hemicolectomy + lymphadenectomy
  - Stage III
    - Right hemicolectomy + lymphadenectomy
    - Right hemicolectomy + distal ileectomy + lymphadenectomy
      - If tumor invades terminal ileum
  - Stage IV
    - Surgical resection or debulking of primary tumor for palliation or relief of obstruction
    - Multiple wedge resections, cryosurgery, or radiofrequency ablation of hepatic lesions in patients with carcinoid syndrome

REPORTING CHECKLIST

T Staging
- Appendiceal tumors are rarely detected on imaging
- Aggressive tumors may invade cecum, terminal ileum, and abdominal wall

N Staging
- Usual sites are retrocecal, ileocolic, and mesenteric lymph nodes

M Staging
- Very rare
- Liver is primary site of distant metastases

SELECTED REFERENCES

1. American Joint Committee on Cancer: AJCC Cancer Staging Manual. 7th ed. New York: Springer. 133-41, 2010
2. Butte JM et al: [Long-term survival in carcinoid tumour of the appendix. An analysis of 8903 appendectomies.] Gastroenterol Hepatol. 32(8):537-41, 2009
3. Pasieka JL: Carcinoid tumors. Surg Clin North Am. 89(5):1123-37, 2009
4. In't Hof KH et al: Carcinoid tumour of the appendix: an analysis of 1,485 consecutive emergency appendectomies. J Gastrointest Surg. 12(8):1436-8, 2008
5. Landry CS et al: Analysis of 900 appendiceal carcinoid tumors for a proposed predictive staging system. Arch Surg. 143(7):664-70; discussion 670, 2008
6. Pinchot SN et al: Carcinoid tumors. Oncologist. 13(12):1255-69, 2008
7. Fornaro R et al: Appendectomy or right hemicolectomy in the treatment of appendiceal carcinoid tumors? Tumori. 93(6):587-90, 2007
8. Levy AD et al: From the archives of the AFIP: Gastrointestinal carcinoids: imaging features with clinicopathologic comparison. Radiographics. 27(1):237-57, 2007
9. West NE et al: Carcinoid tumors are 15 times more common in patients with Crohn's disease. Inflamm Bowel Dis. 13(9):1129-34, 2007
10. Deeg KH et al: Sonographic diagnosis of a carcinoid tumour of the appendix in a 14-year-old boy. Ultraschall Med. 24(2):120-2, 2003
11. Goede AC et al: Carcinoid tumour of the appendix. Br J Surg. 90(11):1317-22, 2003
12. Pickhardt PJ et al: Primary neoplasms of the appendix: radiologic spectrum of disease with pathologic correlation. Radiographics. 2003 May-Jun;23(3):645-62. Review. Erratum in: Radiographics. 23(5):1340, 2003
13. Pickhardt PJ et al: Primary neoplasms of the appendix manifesting as acute appendicitis: CT findings with pathologic comparison. Radiology. 224(3):775-81, 2002

APPENDICEAL CARCINOID

Stage I (T1a N0 M0)

Stage I (T1a N0 M0)

(Left) Axial CECT in a 27-year-old man who presented with vague right lower quadrant abdominal pain shows a slightly distended proximal appendix ➡ containing air ➡. *(Right)* Axial CECT in the same patient shows soft tissue thickening of the distal appendix ➡ without surrounding inflammatory changes. Appendectomy and histological examination revealed an 8 mm carcinoid and acute appendicitis.

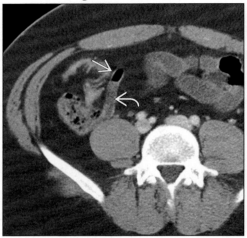

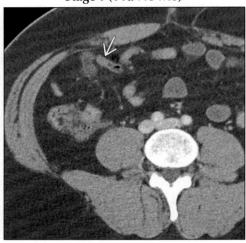

Stage I (T1a N0 M0)

Stage I (T1a N0 M0)

(Left) Axial CECT in a 70-year-old woman who presented with acute right upper quadrant abdominal pain shows a distended fluid-filled appendix ➡ with periappendiceal fat stranding ➡. This was diagnosed as acute appendicitis. Pathological examination revealed carcinoid of the appendiceal tip, which in retrospect can be seen in the same location ➡. *(Right)* Axial CECT in the same patient shows regional lymph nodes ➡. These were found to be inflammatory in nature.

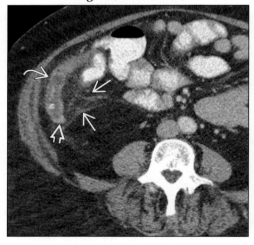

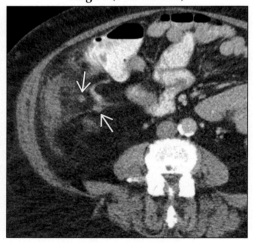

Stage II (T2 N0 M0)

Stage II (T2 N0 M0)

(Left) Axial CECT in a 58-year-old man who presented with a 6-month history of abdominal pain shows a distended fluid-filled appendix (appendiceal mucocele) ➡ and an infiltrative soft tissue mass ➡ at the base of the appendix infiltrating into the cecum ➡. *(Right)* Axial CECT in the same patient shows the appendiceal base soft tissue mass ➡ and the appendiceal mucocele ➡.

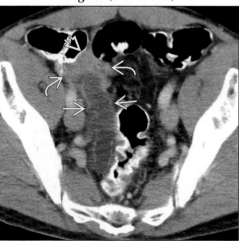

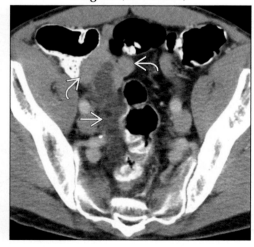

APPENDICEAL CARCINOID

Stage II (T2 N0 M0)

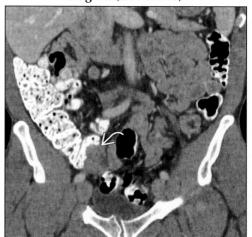

Stage II (T2 N0 M0)

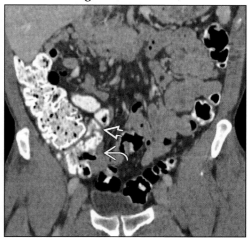

(Left) Coronal CECT in the same patient shows tumor invading the cecum ➘. *(Right)* Coronal CECT in the same patient shows tumor involving the cecum ➘ without involvement of the terminal ileum ➘.

Stage III (T1a N1 M0)

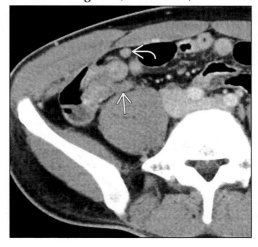

Stage III (T1a N1 M0)

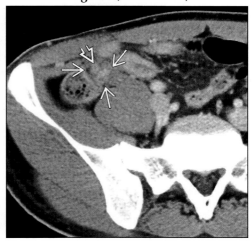

(Left) Axial CECT in a 31-year-old man who presented with acute right lower quadrant abdominal pain shows mild mucosal enhancement of the proximal appendix ➘. An enhancing 9 mm pericecal node ➘ is present. *(Right)* Axial CECT in the same patient shows fat stranding ➘ around the tip of the appendix, indicating acute appendicitis. A small enhancing 9 mm nodule ➘ is seen. Histology confirmed typical carcinoid tumor.

Stage III (T1a N1 M0)

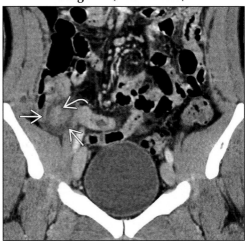

Stage III (T1a N1 M0)

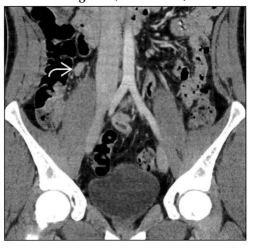

(Left) Coronal CECT in the same patient shows inflammatory changes ➘ around the appendix as well as the enhancing appendiceal nodule ➘. *(Right)* Coronal CECT in the same patient shows a slightly enlarged ileocolic lymph node ➘. The patient underwent right hemicolectomy and adenectomy. Metastatic nodal disease was found on pathological examination.

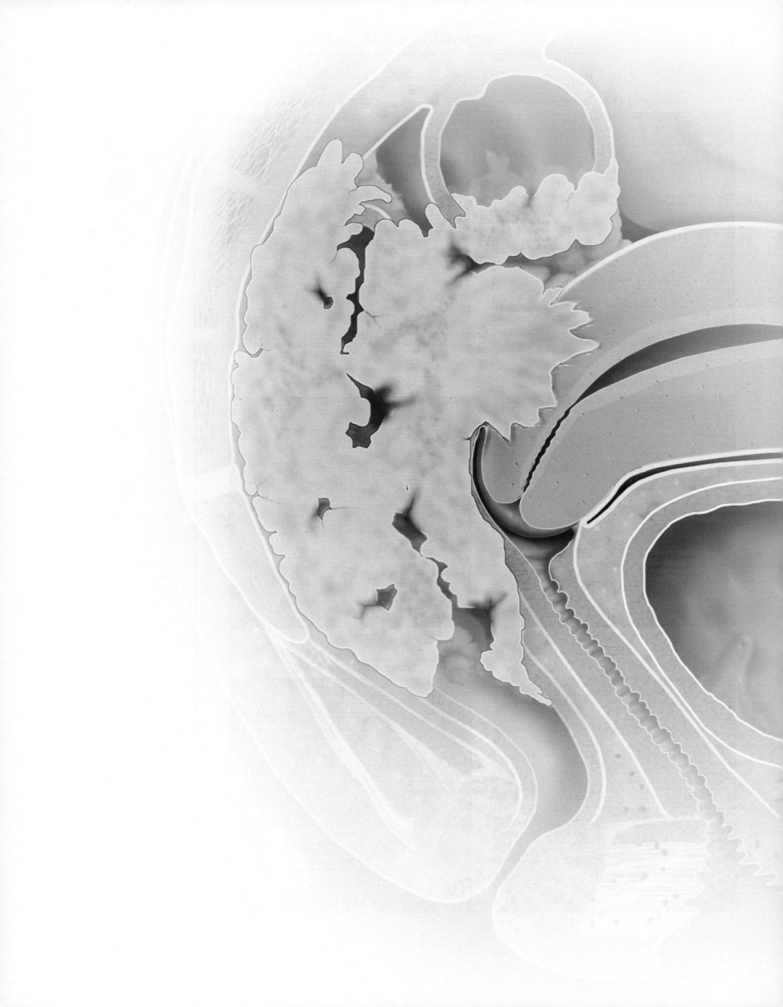

Colorectal Carcinoma

COLORECTAL CARCINOMA

(T) Primary Tumor

Adapted from 7th edition AJCC Staging Forms.

TNM	Definitions
TX	Primary tumor cannot be assessed
T0	No evidence of primary tumor
Tis	Carcinoma in situ: Intraepithelial or invasion of lamina propria[1]
T1	Tumor invades submucosa
T2	Tumor invades muscularis propria
T3	Tumor invades through muscularis propria into perirectal tissues
T4a	Tumor penetrates to surface of visceral peritoneum[2]
T4b	Tumor directly invades or is adherent to other organs or structures[2,3]

(N) Regional Lymph Nodes

NX	Regional lymph nodes cannot be assessed
N0	No regional lymph node metastasis
N1	Metastasis in 1-3 regional lymph nodes
N1a	Metastasis in 1 regional lymph node
N1b	Metastasis in 2-3 regional lymph nodes
N1c	Tumor deposit(s) in subserosa, mesentery, or nonperitonealized pericolic or perirectal tissues without regional nodal metastasis
N2	Metastasis in ≥ 4 regional lymph nodes
N2a	Metastasis in 4-6 regional lymph nodes
N2b	Metastasis in ≥ 7 lymph nodes

(M) Distant Metastasis

M0	No distant metastasis
M1	Distant metastasis
M1a	Metastasis confined to 1 organ or site (e.g., liver, lung, ovary, nonregional node)
M1b	Metastases in > 1 organ/site or the peritoneum

[1]*Tis includes cancer cells confined within the glandular basement membrane (intraepithelial) or mucosal lamina propria (intramucosal) with no extension through the muscularis mucosae into the submucosa.*

[2]*Direct invasion in T4 includes invasion of other organs or other segments of the colorectum as a result of direct extension through the serosa, as confirmed on microscopic examination (for example, invasion of the sigmoid colon by a carcinoma of the cecum) or, for cancers in a retroperitoneal or subperitoneal location, direct invasion of other organs or structures by virtue of extension beyond the muscularis propria (i.e., respectively, a tumor on the posterior wall of the descending colon invading the left kidney or lateral abdominal wall; or a mid or distal rectal cancer with invasion of prostate, seminal vesicles, cervix, or vagina).*

[3]*Tumor that is adherent to other organs or structures, grossly, is classified cT4b. However, if no tumor is present in the adhesion, microscopically, the classification should be pT1-4a depending on the anatomical depth of wall invasion. The V and L classifications should be used to identify the presence or absence of vascular or lymphatic invasion, whereas the PN site-specific factor should be used for perineural invasion.*

COLORECTAL CARCINOMA

(G) Histologic Grade*

Adapted from 7th edition AJCC Staging Forms.

TNM	Definitions
GX	Grade cannot be assessed
G1	Well differentiated
G2	Moderately differentiated
G3	Poorly differentiated
G4	Undifferentiated

*G1-G2 can be designated low grade. G3-G4 as high grade may contribute to overall outcome independent of TNM staging.

AJCC, Dukes, and MAC Stages/ Prognostic Groups

Adapted from 7th edition AJCC Staging Forms.

AJCC	T	N	M	Dukes[1]	MAC[2]
0	Tis	N0	M0	-	-
I	T1	N0	M0	A	A
	T2	N0	M0	A	B1
IIA	T3	N0	M0	B	B2
IIB	T4a	N0	M0	B	B2
IIC	T4b	N0	M0	B	B3
IIIA	T1-T2	N1/N1c	M0	C	C1
	T1	N2a	M0	C	C1
IIIB	T3-T4a	N1/N1c	M0	C	C2
	T2-T3	N2a	M0	C	C1/C2
	T1-T2	N2b	M0	C	C1
IIIC	T4a	N2a	M0	C	C2
	T3-T4a	N2b	M0	C	C2
	T4b	N1-N2	M0	C	C3
IVA	Any T	Any N	M1a	D	D
IVB	Any T	Any N	M1b	D	D

[1]*Dukes B is a composite of better (T3 N0 M0) and worse (T4 N0 M0) prognostic groups, as is Dukes C (Any T N1 M0 and Any T N2 M0).*

[2]*MAC is the modified Astler-Coller classification. Description of MAC: B1 is defined as invasion into the muscularis propria without nodal disease; B2 is invasion into the perirectal or pericolic fat without nodal disease; B3 represents involvement of adjacent structures; C1 is B1 with nodal disease; C2 is B2 with nodal disease; and C3 is B3 with nodal metastasis.*

COLORECTAL CARCINOMA

Tis

Tis

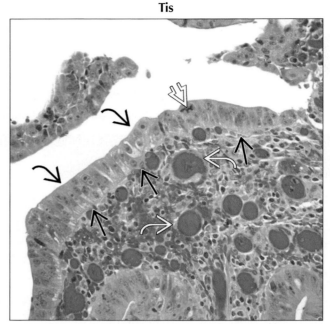

Low magnification of H&E stained section of colonic mucosa shows a dysplasia of the surface epithelium ➡ (intraepithelial tumor without invasion into the lamina propria). The dysplastic changes involve the left aspect of the mucosa, and the normal epithelium is on the right ➡. (Original magnification 40x.)

Higher magnification discloses neoplastic cells with crowded and stratified nuclei with prominent nucleoli ➡ and a mitotic figure ➡. The neoplastic cells are limited to the basement membrane ➡. Numerous dilated/congested blood vessels are noted in the lamina propria ➡. (Original magnification 400x.)

T1

T2

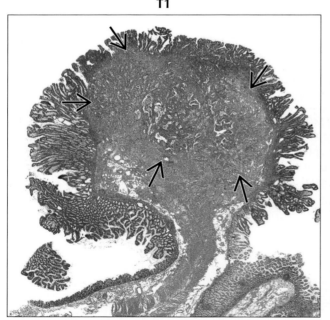

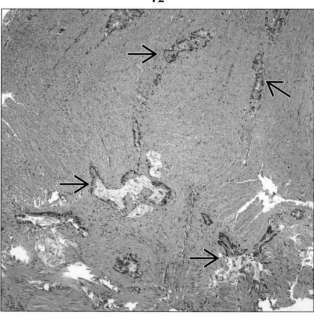

H&E stained section of an adenomatous polyp arising from the colonic side of the ileocecal valve in a right hemicolectomy specimen shows an invasive colonic adenocarcinoma ➡ involving the lamina propria and the submucosa. (Original magnification 10x.)

H&E stained section shows invasive colonic carcinoma that involves muscularis propria. The neoplastic cells are arranged in irregular well-formed glands ➡ that dissect through the muscle bundles of the muscularis mucosa. (Original magnification 40x.)

COLORECTAL CARCINOMA

T2

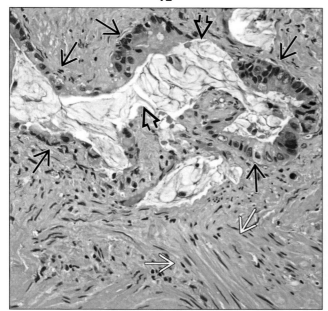

Higher magnification of T2 shows irregular gland composed of neoplastic cells ➡. The lumen of the neoplastic gland ⮞ is filed with mucinous secretions. The neoplastic gland dissects the surrounding bundles (composed of pink cells with spindle nuclei) ➡ of the muscularis propria. (Original magnification 400x.)

T2

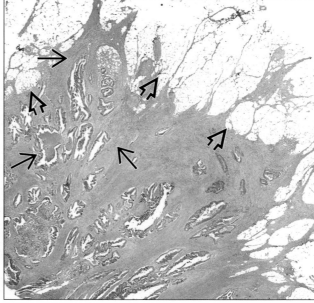

H&E stained section shows adenocarcinoma of the colon that invades through the muscularis propria and extends to involve the pericolonic fatty tissue. The tumor ➡ invades through the pink muscularis propria toward the pericolonic fat ⮞. (Original magnification 40x.)

T2

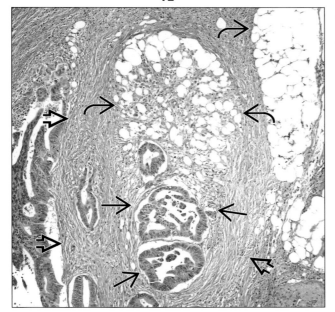

Higher magnification shows colonic adenocarcinoma ➡ invading into the pericolonic fat ➡. Note the desmoplastic reaction (pink areas) ⮞ elicited by the neoplastic cells. (Original magnification 400x.)

T4a

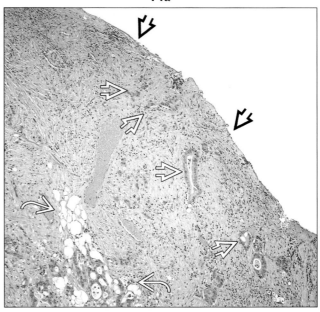

H&E stained section shows invasive colonic adenocarcinoma that extends to the serosal surface ⮞. The neoplastic glands ⮞ invade the pericolonic fat ➡ and extend to involve the serosal surface without extension to adjacent organs. (Original magnification 400x.)

Surgical Treatment for Colorectal Carcinoma

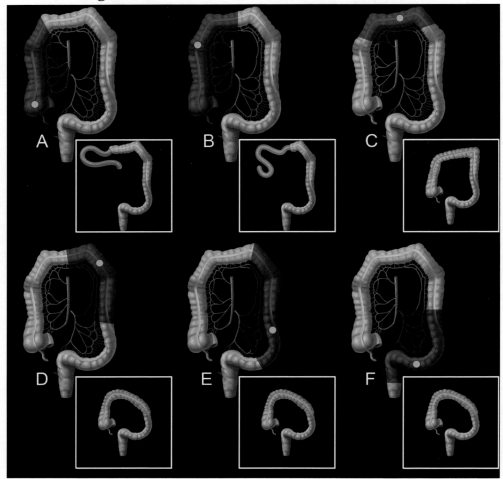

Surgical resection of colonic carcinoma depends on the site of the primary tumor. This composite graphic shows the portion of colon resected in blue, as well as the appearance of the colon after anastomosis. Right hemicolectomy is performed for tumors of the cecum (A) or ascending colon (B). Transverse colectomy is performed for tumors of the transverse colon (C). Left hemicolectomy is performed for tumors of the distal transverse (D) and descending colon (E) and in selected patients with proximal sigmoid colon tumors. Sigmoid colectomy is performed for sigmoid tumors (F).

Adenoma-Carcinoma Sequence

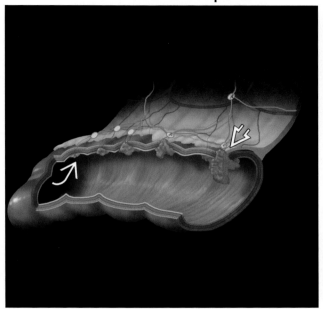

Graphic shows progression of carcinogenesis of adenomatous polyp from in situ dysplasia ➔ through T4 disease ➔.

T1

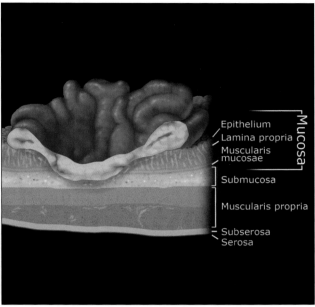

Graphic shows an ulcerating mass invading into the submucosa, classified as T1 disease.

T2

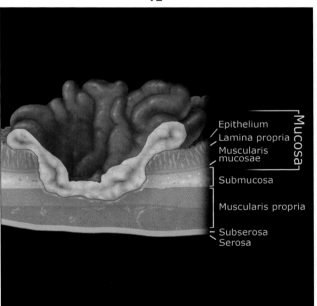

Graphic demonstrates an ulcerating mass invading into the muscularis propria, consistent with T2 disease.

T3

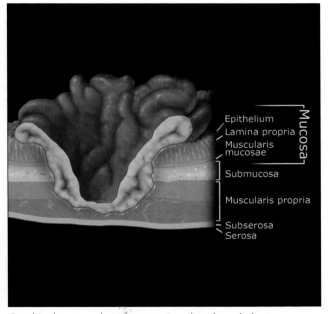

Graphic shows an ulcerating mass invading through the muscularis propria into the subserosa. Tumor that invades into the nonperitonealized pericolic tissue is also considered T3 disease.

COLORECTAL CARCINOMA

T4a

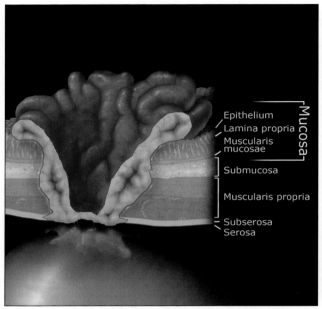

Epithelium
Lamina propria — Mucosa
Muscularis mucosae
Submucosa
Muscularis propria
Subserosa
Serosa

Graphic reveals an ulcerating mass invading through all layers of the colonic wall to penetrate the serosa (visceral peritoneum), indicative of T4a disease.

T4b

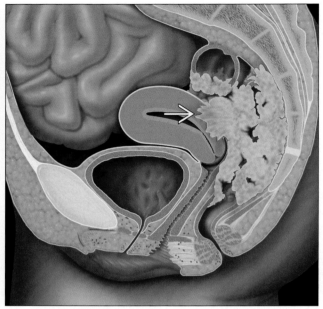

Graphic shows that T4b tumor ➡ that invades or is adherent to adjacent structures.

Nodal Drainage of Cecum, Ascending and Transverse Colon

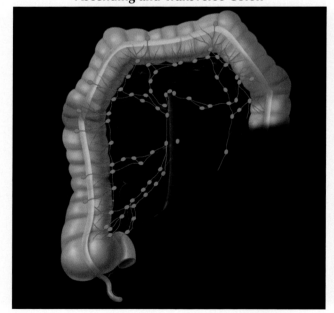

Regional nodes include pericolic nodes (located along the mesocolic border of the colon), nodes along the vascular arcades of the marginal arteries, and nodes along the ileocolic and right colic vessels for the ascending colon and along the middle colic vessels for the transverse colon.

Nodal Drainage of Desending and Sigmoid Colon

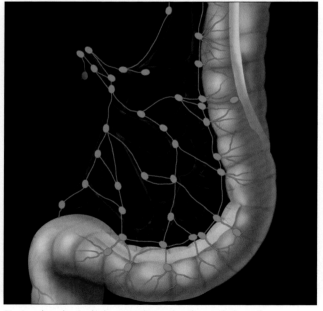

Regional nodes include pericolic nodes (located along the mesocolic border of the colon), nodes along vascular arcades of the marginal arteries, and nodes along the left colic and inferior mesenteric arteries.

COLORECTAL CARCINOMA

N1a and N1b

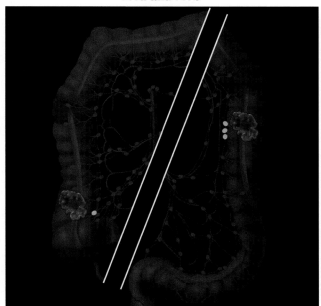

N2

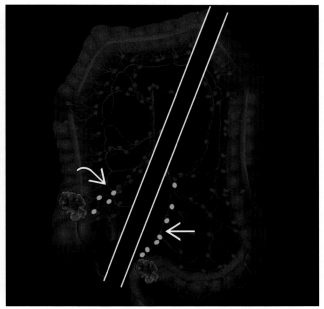

N1 disease involves metastases in 1-3 regional lymph nodes: N1a describes metastasis in a single node (left); N1b describes metastases in 2-3 regional lymph nodes (right); N1c (not shown) is tumor deposit(s) in the subserosa, mesentery, or nonperitonealized pericolic or perirectal tissues without regional nodal metastasis.

N2 disease involves metastases in ≥ 4 regional lymph nodes: N2a applies to metastases in 4-6 regional lymph nodes ⬈; N2b describes metastases in ≥ 7 regional lymph nodes ➡.

METASTASES, ORGAN FREQUENCY

Liver	28%
Lung	12%
Bone	2%
Brain	Rare

COLORECTAL CARCINOMA

OVERVIEW

General Comments
- Colorectal cancer (CRC): Deadly disease
  - Accurate staging has important treatment and outcome implications

Classification
- Applies only to colorectal carcinomas
  - Separate staging system for appendiceal and anal carcinomas
  - Specific staging applies to lymphomas, carcinoid tumors, and sarcomas
- Histological types
  - Adenocarcinoma in situ
    - Synonymous with "high-grade" or "severe dysplasia"
  - Adenocarcinoma (90%)
  - Medullary carcinoma
  - Signet ring cell carcinoma
    - > 50% signet ring cells
  - Mucinous (colloid type)
    - > 50% mucinous carcinoma
  - Others (10%)
    - Squamous cell (epidermoid)
    - Adenosquamous
    - Small (oat cell) carcinoma
    - Undifferentiated
    - Carcinoma, NOS

PATHOLOGY

Routes of Spread
- Local
  - Contiguous invasion of adjacent organs
    - Retroperitoneal invasion
      - Posterior walls of ascending and descending colon are retroperitoneal
      - Upper 1/3 of rectum is covered by peritoneum anteriorly and laterally
      - Middle 1/3 of rectum is covered by peritoneum only anteriorly
      - Lower 1/3 of rectum is not covered by peritoneum
    - Ileum
    - Stomach
    - Bladder
    - Prostate
  - Peritoneal spread
    - Ascending and descending colon are covered by visceral peritoneum anteriorly
    - Transverse colon is suspended by transverse mesocolon
    - Sigmoid and cecum are peritonealized
    - Peritoneal spread to ovaries (Krukenberg tumor)
- Lymphatic
  - 20% of patients have metastatic disease to lymph nodes at presentation
  - Initially epicolic and paracolic lymph nodes, then to regional nodes along mesenteric vasculature
  - Nodes involved by tumor location
    - Cecum
      - Pericolic, anterior and posterior cecal, ileocolic, right colic nodes
    - Ascending colon
      - Pericolic, ileocolic, right colic, middle colic nodes
    - Hepatic flexure
      - Pericolic, right colic, middle colic nodes
    - Transverse colon
      - Pericolic, middle colic nodes
    - Splenic flexure
      - Pericolic, middle colic, left colic, inferior mesenteric nodes
    - Descending colon
      - Pericolic, left colic, inferior mesenteric, sigmoid nodes
    - Sigmoid colon
      - Pericolic, inferior mesenteric, superior rectal, sigmoidal, sigmoid mesenteric nodes
    - Rectosigmoid
      - Pericolic, perirectal, left colic, sigmoid, superior rectal, middle rectal nodes
    - Rectum
      - Initial tumor spread to mesorectal lymph nodes
      - Upper 1/3 → superior rectal nodes → inferior mesenteric nodes
      - Middle and lower 1/3 → middle and inferior rectal nodes → internal iliac nodes
      - Other nodes include obturator, median sacral, and, less commonly, external or common iliac nodes
      - Paraaortic and inguinal nodes are nonregional, and involvement of these nodes constitutes M1 (stage IV) disease
- Hematogenous
  - Common sites include liver, lung, brain, and bone

General Features
- Comments
  - Many inherited and modifiable risk factors with several screening and preventative measures tailored to decrease incidence and improve treatment
  - Adenomatous polyps
    - Dysplasia-adenoma-carcinoma sequence
      - Describes progressive carcinogenesis from dysplastic epithelium, through benign adenoma to frank malignancy
    - Overall chance of developing carcinoma in polyp is estimated at 5%
    - ↑ risk of cancer in
      - Polyps > 1 cm
      - Polyps with high-grade dysplasia
      - Polyps with > 25% villous histology
    - Histologic classification
      - Tubular (80%)
      - Villous (5-15%)
      - Tubulovillous (5-15%)
    - Morphology
      - Sessile
      - Pedunculated
      - Depressed
    - Size and risk of dysplasia/cancer
      - < 1 cm (1-10%)
      - 1-2 cm (10%)
      - > 2 cm (30-50%)
- Genetics

COLORECTAL CARCINOMA

- Majority of CRCs are sporadic
- 10% of colorectal cancer patients have inherited predisposition
  - Familial adenomatous polyposis (FAP)
    - 1% of colorectal cancers
    - Group of syndromes including Gardner syndrome, Turcot syndrome, attenuated adenomatous polyposis coli
    - Adenomas appear in childhood, often symptomatic by teens to 20s
    - 90% of untreated patients will progress to colorectal cancer by 45 years of age
    - Associated with germline mutation involving *APC* gene on chromosome 5
    - Colorectal cancer develops as result of complex process involving oncogenes (*K-ras*) and several tumor suppressor genes (*APC* gene and *P53*)
  - Hereditary nonpolyposis colorectal cancer (Lynch syndrome)
    - Autosomal dominant syndrome more common than FAP
    - 1-5% of CRCs
    - Caused by mutations in 1 of mismatch repair genes, *hMLH1*, *hMSH2*, *hMSH6*, or *PMS2*
    - Early age of presentation
    - Right colon disease predominantly, 70% occur proximal to splenic flexure
    - Synchronous tumors in 10% of patients
    - Associated with endometrial cancer, increased risk for additional malignancies
  - Hyperplastic polyposis syndrome (HPS)
    - > 30 hyperplastic polyps spread throughout colon
    - Or ≥ 5 hyperplastic polyps proximal to sigmoid colon with ≥ 2 being large (> 10 mm)
    - Or any number of hyperplastic polyps in first-degree relative of individual with HPS
  - Up to 25% of patients with CRC have familial predisposition without clear heritable pattern
    - Single affected first-degree relative increases risk by 1.7x above general population
  - *KRAS* mutation has been associated with poor response to treatment with monoclonal antibodies directed toward epidermal growth factor receptors; treatment for patients with metastatic disease
  - 18qLOH is emerging as marker for need for adjuvant therapy in patients with stage II disease
- Etiology
  - Greatest risk factor for colorectal cancer is advanced age
  - Additional modifiable risk factors include
    - Alcohol consumption
    - Obesity
    - Diet low in fiber
- Epidemiology & cancer incidence
  - 3rd most common cancer in both men and women
    - Next to prostate and lung in men, next to breast and lung in women
    - Estimated 146,970 new cases of CRC in USA in 2009
  - 2nd highest cause of cancer-related death
    - Next only to lung cancer
    - Estimated 49,920 deaths from CRC in USA in 2009

- 50% of patients die within 5 years of diagnosis and "curative" surgical resection
- Estimated number of new cases of colorectal cancer cases per year in United States is 108,070 with 29,960 deaths
  - Highest incidence is in people > 50 years of age
  - Incidence rates (1998-2005) per 100,000 were 61.2 for men and 44.8 for women
- Increasing incidence in right-sided cancers in USA and internationally, which may be due to improved diagnostic techniques
- Associated diseases, abnormalities
  - Inflammatory bowel disease
    - Pancolitis increases risk by 5-15% above general population
  - Diabetes mellitus and insulin resistance
  - Familial adenomatous polyposis

Gross Pathology & Surgical Features
- Tumors of right colon are commonly polypoid or fungating masses
  - Women are more likely to have polyps or primary cancers within proximal bowel
- Tumors of distal colon are more frequently circumferential lesions resulting in classic "apple core" appearance
- Circumferential radial margins at resection influence treatment and clinical outcome but have not been validated as distinct staging criteria
- 3-5% of patients have synchronous disease at presentation
  - Synchronous tumors have same prognosis as solitary tumors according to standard staging
- Metachronous tumors develop in 1-3% of patients within 5 years of initial diagnosis
  - Location: Cecum (10%), ascending colon (15%), transverse colon (15%), descending colon (5%), sigmoid colon (25%), rectosigmoid (10%), rectum (20%)

Microscopic Pathology
- H&E
  - Adenocarcinomas are classified according to histologic grade
    - Histologic grade relies on extent of well-formed glandular tissue combined with additional structural or cytologic features
      - High-grade tumors have < 50% gland formation and worse prognosis
      - Low-grade tumors have well or moderately differentiated glandular elements
  - Histologic type has not proven to be independent factor in overall prognosis

IMAGING FINDINGS

Detection
- Conventional endoscopy
  - Current standard technique for evaluating entire colon
  - High sensitivity for mucosal lesions
  - Possibility of performing biopsy and polypectomy during procedure
  - Rate of incomplete colonoscopy ranges from 6-26%

COLORECTAL CARCINOMA

- Because up to 15% of patients present with obstructing lesion, complete bowel evaluation is not possible
  - Entire bowel must be evaluated to exclude synchronous disease
  - Errors of lesion localization can occur
    - No internal landmarks
  - Complications include perforation and major bleeding related to polypectomy
    - Rate: 1 per 1,000 procedures
- Flexible sigmoidoscopy
  - Evaluation up to splenic flexure only
  - Frequently utilized by primary care physicians
  - Studies suggest up to 66% of disease can be missed due to incomplete bowel evaluation
- Capsule endoscopy
  - Ingested capsule provides photographic evaluation of colon
  - Sensitivity 64%, specificity 84% for ≥ 6 mm polyps
- Double contrast barium enema (DCBE)
  - Advantages
    - Less expensive diagnostic method
    - Useful in evaluation of patients referred due to incomplete endoscopy
  - Disadvantages
    - Requires technical experience and trained radiologist
    - Involves inherent radiation exposure
    - Patient will require additional procedure for any intervention
  - DCBE detects only 20% of polyps detected on colonoscopy
    - Rate of detection of adenomas by DCBE is related to their size
      - ≤ 0.5 cm (21%)
      - 0.6-1.0 cm (42%)
      - > 1.0 cm (46%)
    - Location of adenomas affects rate of detection by DCBE
      - Higher rates for left side polyps
  - Imaging findings
    - Early sessile cancer
      - Flat, protruding lesion with broad base and little mucosal elevation in profile view
      - Curvilinear or undulating borders en face
    - Early pedunculated cancer
      - Short thick polyp on stalk with irregular or lobulated margins
    - Advanced polypoid cancer
      - Filling defect vs. etched in barium depending on position
    - Advanced annular cancer
      - Circumferential luminal narrowing, associated with proximal obstruction and thumbprinting of adjacent mucosa
    - Advanced carpet lesion
      - Minimal luminal protrusion, can manifest as nodules surrounded by barium or reticular pattern
- CECT
  - Not useful for early tumor detection
  - Imaging findings
    - Asymmetric mural thickening ± luminal narrowing
      - Wall thickness: 3-6 mm → undetermined
      - Wall thickness: > 6 mm → abnormal
    - Intraluminal polypoid mass
- CT colonography (CTC)
  - Advantages
    - Useful in evaluation of obstructive lesions and in instance of incomplete colonoscopy
    - Can also perform simultaneous evaluation for extracolic disease
    - Noninvasive
    - Valuable in localizing rectal cancer relative to anal canal sphincter and pelvic floor
    - Reported comparable rates of detection with conventional colonoscopy
    - Reported sensitivity of up to 90% in patients with lesions ≥ 10 mm in diameter
  - Disadvantages
    - Requires bowel preparation, stool tagging, image reconstruction
    - Requires training and testing of radiologists
    - Radiation exposure
      - Radiation dose of CTC is about 1/2 that used for standard body CT examination
      - Minimal average dose of approximately 5 mSv
      - Less radiation than barium enema
  - 83-95% accuracy in preoperative T staging, 80-85% accuracy for preoperative N staging

Staging
- No role for endoscopy or DCBE in staging
- CECT or PET/CT are modalities of choice for tumor staging
  - US can be helpful for detection of liver metastases
  - MR is probably as accurate as CT for staging
- **CT**
  - CECT should be obtained in all patients with stage II, III, or IV disease prior to or following resection
    - Preoperative staging with CT showed average savings of $24,000 for patients with higher stages of disease
    - Preoperative CT in patients with CEA 2x upper limit of normal generated average savings of $54,000 in higher stages of disease
  - Key diagnostic tool for noninvasive evaluation of tumor extension, distant metastatic disease, synchronous disease, lymphatic involvement, and tumor-related complications
    - Highly variable reported sensitivity and specificity for tumor recognition based on size of primary lesion
      - Unable to detect T1 or T2 tumors reliably
    - Reported rates of extracolonic findings (24%)
      - Highly variable sensitivity for peritoneal implants dependent on location and size
    - Sensitivity for detecting distant metastasis (75-87%)
      - Higher accuracy for detection of hepatic metastatic disease than nodal metastasis
      - Sensitivity for nodal involvement (45-87%)
- **PET/CT**
  - Important role in initial staging and monitoring of disease recurrence by combining morphologic information of CT with metabolic information of PET

COLORECTAL CARCINOMA

- Fluorine 18-labeled deoxyglucose uptake is 2x higher in tumors relative to nonmalignant lesions
  - Contributes to changes in clinical stage and management in up to 40% of patients
  - Highest diagnostic sensitivity, but dependent on histology
    - Poor sensitivity and reliability in staging patients with mucinous-type cancer
- **MR**
  - Primarily used in staging and surveillance in rectal cancer when utilizing endorectal coil
    - Valuable in recognition of perirectal node involvement
    - Best test to predict circumferential resection margins of rectal cancer
    - Improved field of view compared to transrectal ultrasound (TRUS)
    - Less operator dependent than TRUS
    - Assess feasibility of sphincter sparing treatments
  - Used in patients with hepatic metastasis to evaluate treatment options
- **Transrectal ultrasound (TRUS)**
  - Diagnosis and staging of depth and circumferential margins in rectal cancer
    - Similar reported diagnostic sensitivity of US, CT, and MR for recognition of perirectal nodal involvement
    - Superior diagnostic accuracy compared to all other modalities in description of depth of invasion
      - TRUS: 80-95% sensitivity
      - CT: 65-75% sensitivity
      - MR: 75-85% sensitivity
      - Digital rectal examination: 62% sensitivity
  - Possibility of biopsy at time of evaluation improves nodal staging over conventional methods
- **Local staging**
  - Tis-T2
    - Can be radiographically occult
    - Sessile or pedunculated lesions
    - Well-defined peripheral wall with clear adjacent fat
    - Luminal narrowing without extension through serosa
    - CECT and CTC do not allow reliable differentiation among stages of tumor confined to colonic wall
  - T3
    - Invasion into subserosa of peritonealized organs
    - Poorly defined peripheral wall with nodular margin and pericolonic fat infiltration
    - Extension to nonperitonealized surfaces
      - Retroperitoneal extension from posterior walls of ascending colon and descending colon, as well as rectum distal to peritoneal reflections
  - T4
    - Loss of fat planes between colon and adjacent structures
    - Pericolonic mass
    - Stranding of pericolic fat indicates extension through serosal or peritoneal surfaces
- **Nodal staging**
  - CT, MR, PET/CT, and CT colonography can be used to evaluate nodal disease

- Regional nodal involvement is present in 34% of colon cancer patients and 38% of rectal cancer patients at presentation
  - Nodes often radiographically occult
  - Radiographic features
    - Large nodes ≥ 10 mm
    - Nodes may have hazy outer margins
    - Found along bowel surface and associated vascular pedicle
- **Liver metastases**
  - Occur in 22-77% of patients
  - Presence indicates nonresectable primary disease
  - Any cross-sectional modality can be used in diagnosis
    - PET/CT has best sensitivity in detection of metastatic lesions
  - Tendency to cause intrahepatic bile duct dilatation (more than noncolorectal metastases or hepatocellular carcinoma)
    - Due to intrabiliary growth (much as cholangiocarcinoma)
    - Presence of biliary dilatation in presence of hepatic metastatic disease and unknown primary should raise possibility of CRC
  - CT appearance
    - Calcifications may be seen in hepatic metastases initially or following chemotherapy
      - Occur in 11% of patients
    - Portal venous phase is most reliable in detection of colorectal liver metastases
      - Hypoattenuating relative to liver with occasional faint ring of enhancement
      - Sensitivity (85.1%)
  - MR appearance
    - T1WI: Usually slightly hypointense relative to normal liver
    - T2WI: Slightly hyperintense relative to normal liver
    - Gadolinium-enhanced T1WI
      - Metastases are usually hypovascular, best seen on portal venous phase
      - Thin peripheral ring of strong enhancement that persists through all phases of enhancement
      - Metastases > 3 cm in size show cauliflower appearance
  - US appearance
    - Usually hypoechoic relative to liver parenchyma
    - May be hyperechoic if calcified or hemorrhagic
- Other distant metastatic locations
  - Lung
    - 2nd most common site of metastatic disease
    - Chest x-ray and cross-sectional imaging can be used
  - Bone
    - Infrequent site of metastatic disease
    - Lytic or blastic osseous lesion depending on histologic subtype
  - Brain
    - Very rare, multiple or solitary
    - Not frequently evaluated preoperatively
    - MR is preferred method of diagnosis and characterization

COLORECTAL CARCINOMA

Restaging
- Multiple diagnostic modalities and laboratory parameters can be used to evaluate recurrence and subsequent restaging
- CECT and PET/CT are most commonly utilized to monitor response to therapy
- PET/CT is advocated for use in asymptomatic patients with rising CEA levels to exclude recurrent disease
  - More sensitive than conventional CT in post-treatment surveillance
  - Overall specificity and sensitivity for detection of recurrent cancer is 97% and 76%, respectively

CLINICAL ISSUES

Presentation
- Common symptoms
  - Abdominal pain (44%)
  - Change in bowel habits (43%)
  - GI bleeding (40%)
  - Weakness (20%)
  - Isolated anemia (11%)
  - Weight loss (6%)
- Right colon tumors
  - Bleeding and anemia
- Left colon tumors
  - Constipation, bowel dysfunction, or obstruction
- Rectal tumors
  - Painless bleeding
  - Palpable on exam frequently
  - Locally advanced at diagnosis

Cancer Natural History & Prognosis
- 5-year survival by stage
  - Colon
    - Stage I (93%)
    - Stage IIA (85%)
    - Stage IIB (72%)
    - Stage IIIA (83%)
    - Stage IIIB (64%)
    - Stage IIIC (44%)
    - Stage IV (8%)
    - Stage II and III disease survival highly variable depending on number of lymph nodes analyzed at time of surgical exploration
  - Rectum
    - Stage I (75.7-96.6%)
    - Stage II (44.7-78.7%)
    - Stage IIIA (55.1%)
    - Stage IIIB (35.3%)
    - Stage IIIC (24.5%)
    - Stage IV (4%)
- Prognostic factors
  - Lymphatic and venous invasion are independent adverse prognosticators regardless of T stage
  - Patients with tumors arising around peritoneal reflections, either rectosigmoid or rectal, have worse 5-year survival rate regardless of stage
  - Patients with distal bowel cancers have worse prognosis independent of stage
  - Presenting with obstruction or perforation increases mortality

- 5-year survival rate for patients with symptomatic disease 49% vs. 71% for asymptomatic patients
- Serum CEA levels
  - ≥ 5.0 ng/mL has adverse impact on survival independent of stage
  - Elevated levels serve as marker for recurrent disease after resection
    - Measured preoperatively for baseline
- Tumor deposits
  - Number of satellite tumor deposits separate from leading edge of primary carcinoma
- Tumor regression grade
  - Pathologic features that allow response to adjuvant therapies to be assessed
- Circumferential resection margin
  - Measured in millimeters from tumor edge to nearest margin of surgical resection
- Presentation with obstruction or perforation increases mortality
- *KRAS* gene analysis
- Microsatellite instability
- Perineural invasion

Treatment Options
- Major treatment alternatives
  - Surgical resection of colon primary
    - Right hemicolectomy
      - Tumors of cecum, ascending colon, or proximal transverse colon
      - Ileocolic, right colic, and right branch of middle colic vessels are divided and removed with contiguous mesentery
    - Transverse colectomy
      - Mid transverse colon cancers with satisfactory resection margins
      - Transverse colon is resected along with middle colic vessels and their mesentery
    - Left hemicolectomy
      - Tumors in distal transverse or descending colon, selected patients with proximal sigmoid colon cancer
      - Left branch of middle colic vessels, inferior mesenteric vein, and left colic vessels and their mesenteries are included with specimen
    - Sigmoid colectomy
    - Subtotal or total colectomy
      - For synchronous neoplasms on right and left sides of colon
  - Surgical resection of rectal primary
    - Abdominal perineal resection
      - Includes both abdominal and perineal incisions in treatment of distal rectal tumors
      - Complete proctectomy and creation of permanent colostomy
      - T3 or T4 tumors often treated initially with neoadjuvant chemotherapy to increase likelihood of sphincter sparing procedure
    - Low anterior resection
      - Used for invasive tumors of proximal rectum
      - Generally sphincter sparing depending on distal margins
      - Dissection and anastomosis below peritoneal reflection, with ligation of superior and middle hemorrhoidal arteries

- Additional dissection along prostate gland or plane of anterior rectal wall
  - Coloanal anastomosis
    - Allows sphincter preservation for distal cancers
    - J-pouch is created by folding distal bowel back on itself, creating neorectum
    - Requires temporary diverting ostomy
  - ○ Adjuvant chemotherapy
  - ○ Prophylactic oophorectomy
    - Synchronous and metachronous ovarian tumors occur in 1-8%
  - ○ Resection of hepatic metastatic disease is current recommended treatment
    - 10% of patients meet surgical criteria of > 1 cm surgical margin and absence of portal lymph node involvement
    - 5-year relapse-free survival rates of 24-38% for patients with < 4 hepatic lesions treated with surgical resection
    - Involvement of > 70% of liver precludes resection
    - 5-year survival of patients with resected hepatic metastatic disease averages 40%, 10-year survival 25%
- Major treatment roadblocks
  - ○ Widespread metastatic disease
  - ○ Locally advanced primary tumors
  - ○ Perforation and obstruction upon presentation
  - ○ Lack of adequate resection margins
    - Higher rate of rectal cancer recurrence due to confined anatomy within bony pelvis, proximity to adjacent organs, inadequate lymph node sampling
- Treatment options by stage
  - ○ Carcinoma in situ: Stage I
    - Local excision
    - Transanal endoscopic microsurgery has been increasingly utilized in T1 tumors
  - ○ Stage II-III
    - Wide surgical resection
      - En bloc tumor resection as well as major vascular pedicle and lymphatic drainage basin
      - > 5 cm surgical margins desired
  - ○ Stage IV
    - Wide surgical resection
      - Requires multivisceral en bloc resection with possible radiation therapy
    - Adjuvant chemotherapy
      - T4 rectal disease may be treated with chemotherapy prior to resection
    - Resection of metastatic disease
    - Tumor palliation
      - Radiofrequency ablation or chemoembolization

REPORTING CHECKLIST

T Staging

- Colonoscopy is modality of choice for tumor detection
- CT, PET/CT for tumor staging
- Not possible to differentiate early stage (T1 and T2) tumors on imaging
- Evaluate entire colon for synchronous lesion

N Staging

- Evaluate for regional nodes in peritumoral region and along supplying vessels

M Staging

- Liver metastatic disease most common
- Lung metastases occur with high frequency
- Presence of osseous or brain metastatic disease can be evaluated with target modalities according to symptoms

SELECTED REFERENCES

1. American Joint Committee on Cancer: AJCC Cancer Staging Manual. 7th ed. New York: Springer. 143-64, 2010
2. Jhaveri KS et al: Intrahepatic bile duct dilatation due to liver metastases from colorectal carcinoma. AJR Am J Roentgenol. 193(3):752-6, 2009
3. Johnson CD: CT colonography: coming of age. AJR Am J Roentgenol. 193(5):1239-42, 2009
4. Kim DH et al: CT colonography versus colonoscopy for the detection of advanced neoplasia. N Engl J Med. 357(14):1403-12, 2007
5. Kim JH et al: Incomplete colonoscopy in patients with occlusive colorectal cancer: usefulness of CT colonography according to tumor location. Yonsei Med J. 48(6):934-41, 2007
6. Kung JW et al: Colorectal cancer: screening double-contrast barium enema examination in average-risk adults older than 50 years. Radiology. 240(3):725-35, 2006
7. Kumar V et al: Robbins and Cotran: Pathologic Basis of Disease. 7th ed. Philadelphia, 2005
8. Rockey DC et al: Analysis of air contrast barium enema, computed tomographic colonography, and colonoscopy: prospective comparison. Lancet. 365(9456):305-11, 2005
9. Silva AC et al: CT colonography with intravenous contrast material: varied appearances of colorectal carcinoma. Radiographics. 25(5):1321-34, 2005
10. Ng CS et al: Extracolonic findings in patients undergoing abdomino-pelvic CT for suspected colorectal carcinoma in the frail and disabled patient. Clin Radiol. 59(5):421-30, 2004
11. Rockey DC et al: Prospective comparison of air-contrast barium enema and colonoscopy in patients with fecal occult blood: a pilot study. Gastrointest Endosc. 60(6):953-8, 2004
12. Danet IM et al: Spectrum of MRI appearances of untreated metastases of the liver. AJR Am J Roentgenol. 181(3):809-17, 2003
13. Winawer SJ et al: A comparison of colonoscopy and double-contrast barium enema for surveillance after polypectomy. National Polyp Study Work Group. N Engl J Med. 342(24):1766-72, 2000
14. Zerhouni EA et al: National Cancer Institute partnerships with Academia and Industry in Cancer Diagnosis and Treatment: report of the workshop. Acad Radiol. 5(2):133-40, 1998
15. Easson AM et al: Calcification in colorectal hepatic metastases correlates with longer survival. J Surg Oncol. 63(4):221-5, 1996

COLORECTAL CARCINOMA

Stage 0 (Tis N0 M0)

Stage 0 (Tis N0 M0)

(Left) Endoscopic image shows a sessile polyp ➡. *(Right)* Endoscopic image in another patient shows a sessile tubulovillous polyp ➡. Because colonoscopy allows biopsy and polypectomy of lesions encountered during the procedure, it is the procedure of choice for tumor detection. The major disadvantage of colonoscopy, however, is its inability to accurately stage tumors detected during the procedure.

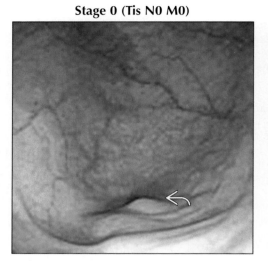

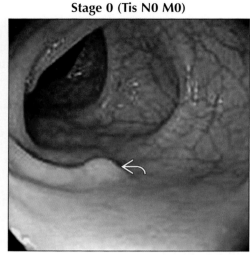

Stage I (T2 N0 M0)

Stage I (T2 N0 M0)

(Left) Axial CECT shows colocolonic intussusception. Intraluminal mesocolic fat ➡ is seen within the dilated sigmoid colon ➡. *(Right)* Coronal CECT in the same patient shows colocolonic intussusception. The intussuscipiens ➡ represents the dilated segment invaginated by the intussusceptum ➡, which is surrounded by the mesocolic fat ➡.

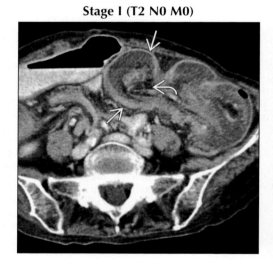

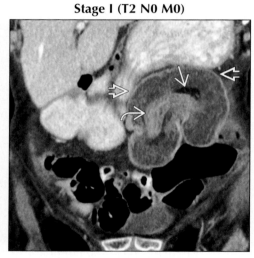

Stage I (T2 N0 M0)

Stage I (T2 N0 M0)

(Left) Coronal CECT in the same patient shows colocolonic intussusception of the sigmoid colon. The intussuscipiens ➡, the mesocolon ➡, and the intussusceptum ➡ are well seen. *(Right)* Axial CECT in the same patient shows intussusceptum ➡ reaching to the level of the rectum ➡. This was found to be secondary to radiographically occult, T2 colonic carcinoma that was found on colonoscopy.

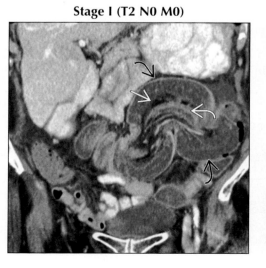

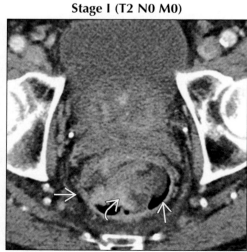

Stage I (T2 N0 M0)

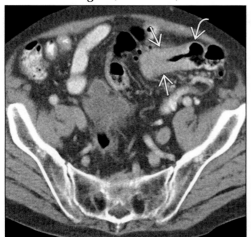

Stage I (T2 N0 M0)

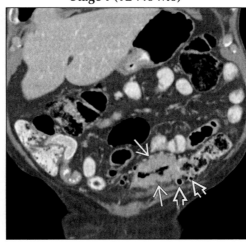

(Left) Axial CECT shows concentric sigmoid colon wall thickening ➡ with abrupt transition from normal to abnormally thick-walled colon ➡. No pericolic tumor stranding or adenopathy is present. (Right) Coronal CECT in the same patient again shows sigmoid colon wall thickening ➡. Multiple diverticula ➡ are also present. Differentiating colonic carcinoma from diverticulitis can be difficult, and repeated imaging after resolution of acute symptoms can be helpful.

Stage IIB (T4a N0 M0)

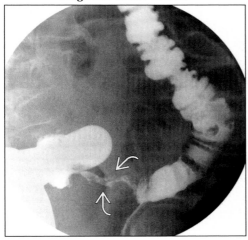

Stage IIB (T4a N0 M0)

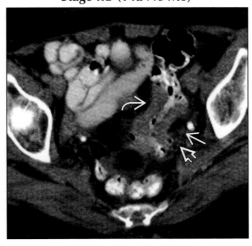

(Left) Contrast enema image shows concentric obstructing lesion ➡ of sigmoid colon found during endoscopy. (Right) Axial CECT in the same patient shows concentric thickening of the sigmoid colon ➡, nodularity of the pericolic fat ➡, and thickening of the peritoneal reflections ➡.

Stage IIB (T4a N0 M0)

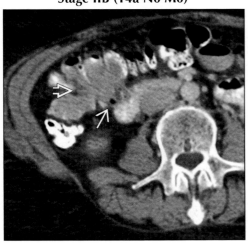

Stage IIB (T4a N0 M0)

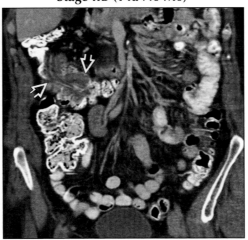

(Left) Axial CECT in the same patient demonstrates a 2nd synchronous tumor ➡ at the hepatic flexure with invasion into the pericolonic tissue ➡. An advantage of CECT over endoscopy is its ability to detect synchronous tumors when the scope cannot be advanced beyond an obstructing lesion. (Right) Coronal CECT in the same patient shows the hepatic flexure mass ➡.

COLORECTAL CARCINOMA

Stage IIB (T4a N0 M0)

(Left) Endoscopic image reveals circumferential carcinoma ➡ of the sigmoid colon. When encountered during endoscopy, the tumor limited additional evaluation of the remaining colon. *(Right)* Axial CECT of sigmoid colon shows massive concentric wall thickening ➡ found during endoscopy. The colonic lumen appears obliterated ⇥. There is significant engorgement of the vessels of the sigmoid mesocolon ➡.

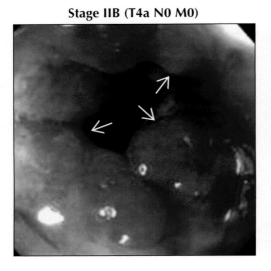

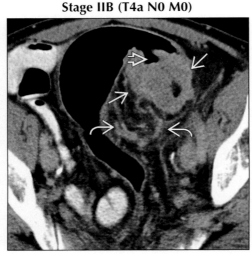

Stage IIC (T4b N0 M0)

(Left) Axial CECT shows concentric thickening of the wall of the cecum ➡ with direct invasion of the terminal ileum ⇥. *(Right)* Axial CECT in the same patient shows concentric thickening of the wall of the cecum ➡ with pericolic tumor extension ➡.

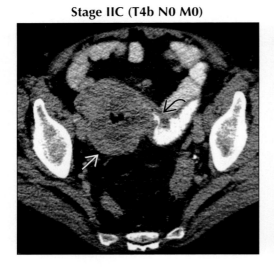

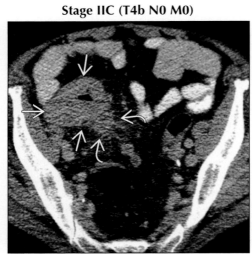

Stage IIC (T4b N0 M0)

(Left) Axial CECT shows tumor of the posterior wall of the descending colon ➡ invading into the retroperitoneum ➡ and reaching to the posterior abdominal wall ⇥. *(Right)* Axial CECT in the same patient shows tumor in the retroperitoneum ➡ with invasion of the transversalis abdominis muscle ⇥.

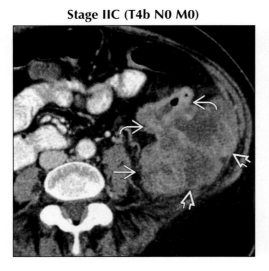

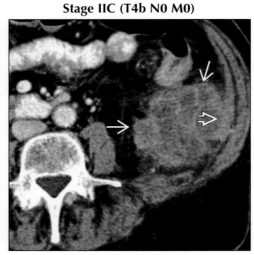

COLORECTAL CARCINOMA

Stage IIIA (T2 N1b M0)

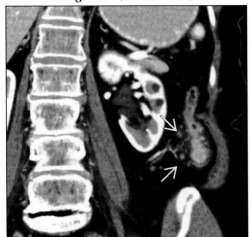

Stage IIIA (T2 N1b M0)

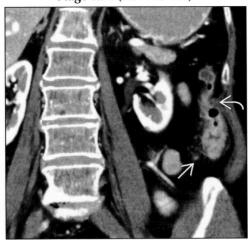

(Left) Coronal CECT in a patient with radiographically occult T2 tumor of descending colon, initially seen on colonoscopy, shows enlarged pericolic lymph nodes ➡. *(Right)* Coronal CECT in the same patient shows a nondistensible portion of descending colon ➡ and metastatic lymph nodes ➡. Pathological examination revealed metastatic deposits in 3 lymph nodes, consistent with N1b disease.

Stage IIIB (T3 N1b M0)

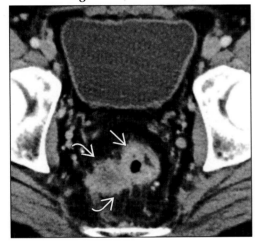

Stage IIIB (T3 N1b M0)

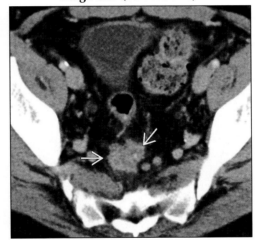

(Left) Axial CECT shows concentric rectal wall thickening ➡ with tumor extending into perirectal tissues ➡ below the peritoneal reflection. *(Right)* Axial CECT in the same patient with rectal primary shows large infiltrative lymph node ➡ along superior rectal vessels. Two adjacent nodes are also present, and all 3 were found to contain metastatic deposits on pathological examination.

Stage IIIB (T4a N1b M0)

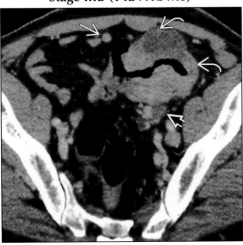

Stage IIIB (T4a N1b M0)

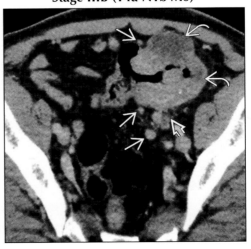

(Left) Axial CECT shows concentric thickening of the wall of the sigmoid colon ➡ with extension into the pericolic tissues ➡ and multiple enlarged pericolic lymph nodes ➡. *(Right)* Axial CECT in the same patient shows concentric thickening of the wall of the sigmoid colon ➡ with tumor extension into the pericolic tissues ➡ and additional enlarged pericolic lymph nodes ➡.

COLORECTAL CARCINOMA

Stage IIIC (T4a N2a M0)

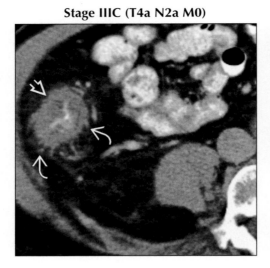

Stage IIIC (T4a N2a M0)

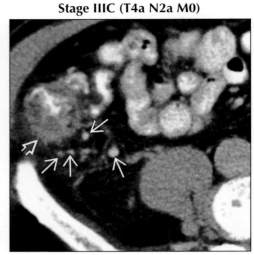

(Left) Axial CECT shows concentric thickening of the wall of the cecum ➡ with tumor strands ➡ invading the visceral peritoneum and extending into the perirectal fat. *(Right)* Axial CECT in the same patient shows cecal wall thickening ➡ and multiple enlarged pericecal lymph nodes ➡. As there are more than 4 metastatic lymph nodes, this constitutes N2 disease.

Stage IIIC (T4a N2a M0)

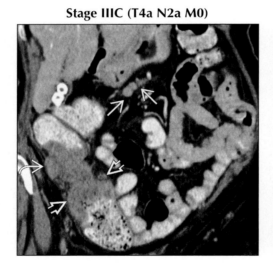

Stage IIIC (T4a N2a M0)

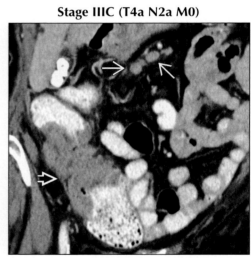

(Left) Coronal CECT shows concentric thickening of the wall of the ascending colon ➡ with extension into the pericolonic tissues ➡ and multiple lymph nodes ➡ along the superior mesenteric vessels. *(Right)* Coronal CECT in the same patient shows ascending colon wall thickening ➡ and additional metastatic lymph nodes ➡ along the superior mesenteric vessels.

Stage IIIC (T4a N2a M0)

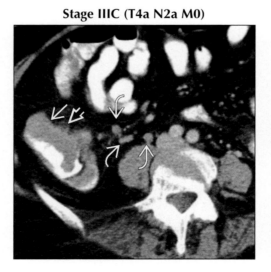

Stage IIIC (T4a N2a M0)

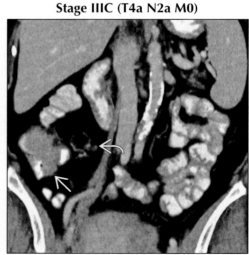

(Left) Axial CECT shows an eccentric cecal mass ➡ infiltrating into the pericecal fat ➡ with 3 enlarged ileocolic lymph nodes ➡. During surgery, metastases were found in 5 regional nodes, compatible with N2a disease. *(Right)* Coronal CECT in the same patient shows the cecal mass ➡ with enlarged regional ileocolic lymph nodes ➡.

COLORECTAL CARCINOMA

Stage IIIC (T4b N2a M0)

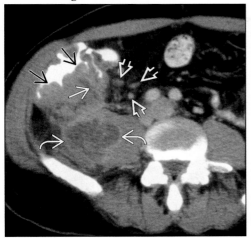

Stage IIIC (T4b N2a M0)

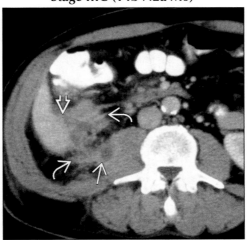

(Left) Axial CECT shows polypoid thickening of the wall of the cecum ⇨ with tumor invading through the retroperitoneum into the psoas muscle ⇨. Tumor also invades the terminal ileum ⇨. Note multiple enlarged lymph nodes ⇨. *(Right)* Axial CECT in the same patient with tumor extending superiorly to invade through the retroperitoneum ⇨ into the psoas muscle ⇨. The tumor also invades the lowermost aspect of the right lobe of the liver ⇨.

Stage IIIC (T4b N2a M0)

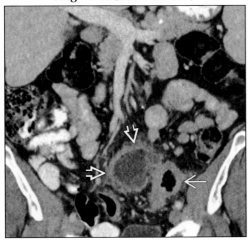

Stage IIIC (T4b N2a M0)

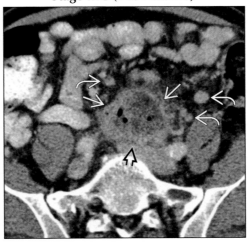

(Left) Coronal CECT shows a fluid collection ⇨ resulting from colonic perforation adjacent to the thick-walled sigmoid colon ⇨. *(Right)* Axial CECT in the same patient shows fluid and air collection ⇨ with a thick soft tissue rind surrounded by fat stranding. The lesion is adherent to the left common iliac vein ⇨. Multiple small lymph nodes ⇨ are present. Viable tumor with necrotic center communicating with colonic lumen was found during surgery.

Stage IIIC (T3 N2b M0)

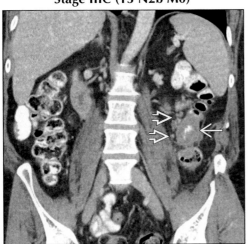

Stage IIIC (T3 N2b M0)

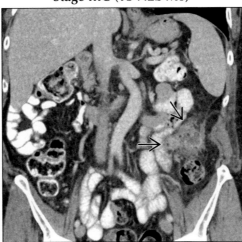

(Left) Coronal CECT shows thickening of the wall of the descending colon ⇨ with 7 enlarged pericolic lymph nodes ⇨. *(Right)* Coronal CECT in the same patient shows the extent of the pericolic tumor invasion ⇨.

COLORECTAL CARCINOMA

Stage IIIC (T3 N2b M0)

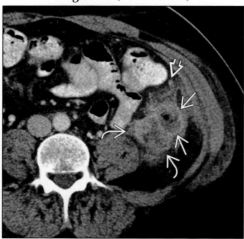

Stage IIIC (T3 N2b M0)

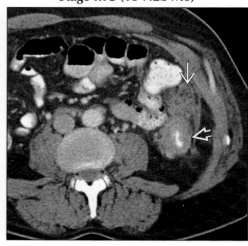

(Left) Axial CECT in a 54-year-old man who presented with acute left lower quadrant abdominal pain shows thickening of the wall of the descending colon ➡ with pericolic stranding due to tumor spread to the retroperitoneum ➡ and omentum ➡. *(Right)* Axial CECT in the same patient shows thickening of the wall of the descending colon ➡ and tumor invading into the omentum ➡.

Stage IIIC (T4a N2b M0)

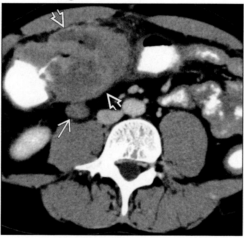

Stage IIIC (T4a N2b M0)

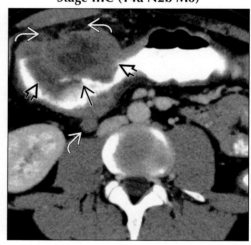

(Left) Axial CECT in a 25-year-old patient with a history of ulcerative colitis demonstrates marked thickening of the wall of the transverse colon ➡ with an enlarged pericolic lymph node ➡. *(Right)* Axial CECT in the same patient shows a large transverse colon mass ➡ with central ulceration ➡. There is stranding in the pericolic fat ➡.

Stage IIIC (T4a N2b M0)

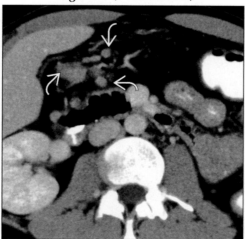

Stage IIIC (T4a N2b M0)

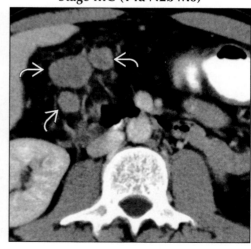

(Left) Axial CECT in the same patient shows multiple enlarged metastatic lymph nodes ➡. *(Right)* Axial CECT in the same patient shows multiple enlarged metastatic lymph nodes ➡. Metastases in 7 or more nodes constitutes N2b disease.

COLORECTAL CARCINOMA

Stage IVA (T4b N2b M1a)

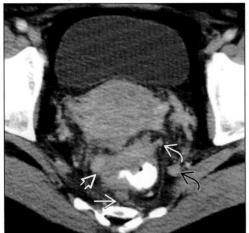

Stage IVA (T4b N2b M1a)

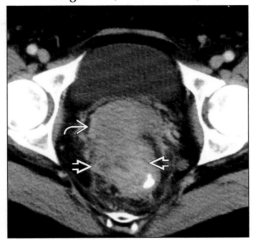

(Left) Axial CECT shows thickening of the wall of the rectum ⮕ with tumor infiltrating into the perirectal fat ⮕ and reaching posteriorly almost to the sacrum ⮕. An enlarged perirectal node ⮕ is also present. *(Right)* Axial CECT in the same patient shows loss of the fat plane between the rectal mass ⮕ and the lower uterus ⮕ due to local tumor invasion.

Stage IVA (T4b N2b M1a)

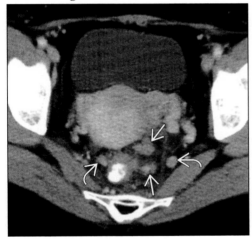

Stage IVA (T4b N2b M1a)

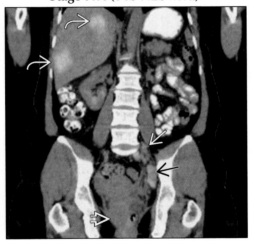

(Left) Axial CECT in the same patient shows multiple enlarged perirectal lymph nodes ⮕ in addition to tumor deposits in the perirectal fat ⮕. *(Right)* Coronal PET/CT in the same patient shows increased metabolic activity in the rectum ⮕, metastatic internal ⮕ and common ⮕ iliac lymph nodes, and liver metastases ⮕.

Stage IVB (T3 N0 M1b)

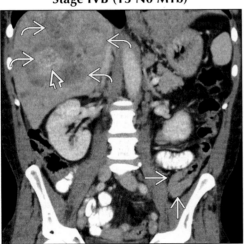

Stage IVB (T3 N0 M1b)

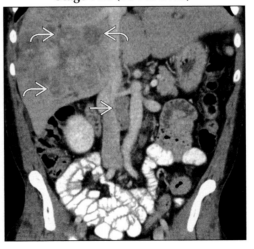

(Left) Coronal CECT shows circumferential thickening of the descending colon ⮕. Multiple liver lesions ⮕ are also present. Some of the liver lesions show high attenuation ⮕ due to calcifications. *(Right)* Coronal CECT in the same patient shows liver metastases ⮕ and an enlarged aortocaval lymph node ⮕. The presence of nodal metastases outside the regional lymph nodes represents distant metastatic disease (M1).

COLORECTAL CARCINOMA

Stage IVB (T3 N0 M1b)

Stage IVB (T3 N0 M1b)

(Left) Axial CECT in the same patient shows multiple liver metastases ➡. Some of the liver metastases show calcifications ➡, which occur in about 11% of colonic metastases to the liver. *(Right)* Axial CECT in the same patient shows multiple liver metastases ➡ almost filling the right lobe. There is biliary dilatation involving mainly the left hepatic duct ➡ and its tributaries ➡.

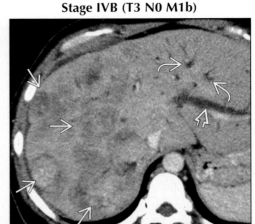
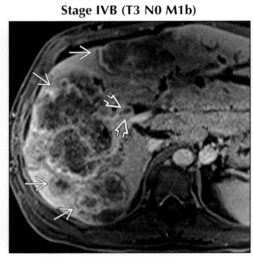

Stage IVB (T3 N0 M1b)

Stage IVB (T3 N0 M1b)

(Left) Coronal T2WI MR (HASTE) shows dilatation of the left lobe bile ducts ➡ with abrupt occlusion of the left hepatic duct due to tumor ➡. *(Right)* Axial T1WI C+ FS MR shows multiple peripherally enhancing hepatic masses ➡ and an intraluminal ductal mass ➡ that is causing biliary obstruction. Metastases from colorectal cancer tend to invade the bile ducts, both centrally and peripherally, and to cause biliary obstruction.

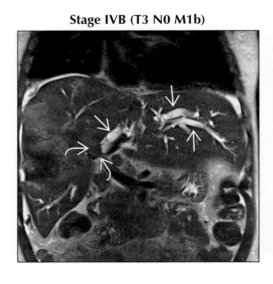

Stage IVB (T3 N0 M1b)

Stage IVB (T3 N0 M1b)

(Left) Axial CECT shows a polypoid cecal mass ➡ without pericolonic stranding or adenopathy. *(Right)* Axial CECT in the same patient shows multiple hypoattenuating liver masses ➡ due to metastatic disease. The portal venous phase is the best phase for detection of hepatic colonic metastases.

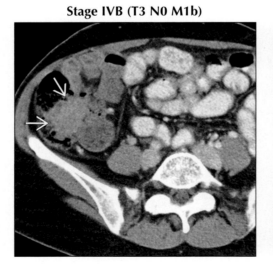
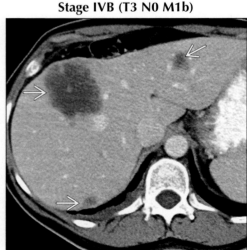

COLORECTAL CARCINOMA

Stage IVB (T3 N0 M1b)

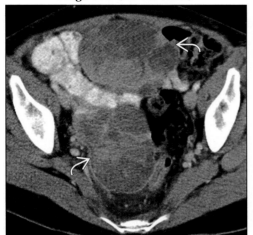

Stage IVB (T3 N0 M1b)

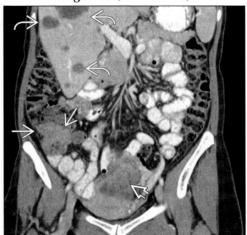

(Left) Axial CECT in the same patient shows bilateral mixed solid-cystic adnexal masses ➡ due to ovarian metastatic lesions (Krukenberg tumors). *(Right)* Coronal CECT in the same patient shows the primary cecal mass ➡, multiple liver metastases ➡, and ovarian metastasis ➡. M1b is defined as metastases in more than 1 organ or in the peritoneum.

Stage IVB (T3 N2b M1b)

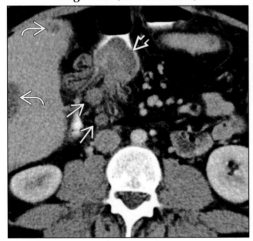

Stage IVB (T3 N2b M1b)

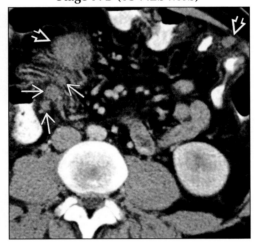

(Left) Axial CECT shows a mass in the transverse colon ➡ with multiple pericolic nodes ➡ as well as hepatic lesions ➡. *(Right)* Axial CECT in the same patient shows multiple peritoneal masses ➡ as well as multiple pericolic enlarged lymph nodes ➡. The presence of hepatic metastases and peritoneal implants represents M1b disease.

Recurrent Metastatic Disease

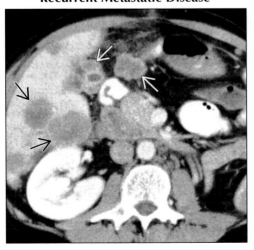

Recurrent Metastatic Disease

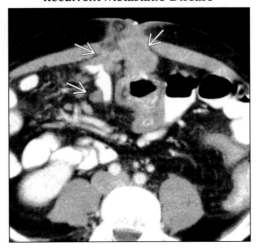

(Left) Axial CECT 5 months following surgical resection of the transverse colon for T4a tumor shows multiple hepatic masses ➡ and multiple peritoneal necrotic masses ➡. *(Right)* Axial CECT in the same patient shows peritoneal masses ➡ extending into the umbilicus. This corresponds to the "Sister Mary Joseph nodule" sign, which refers to a palpable nodule bulging into the umbilicus resulting from abdominal peritoneal metastasis.

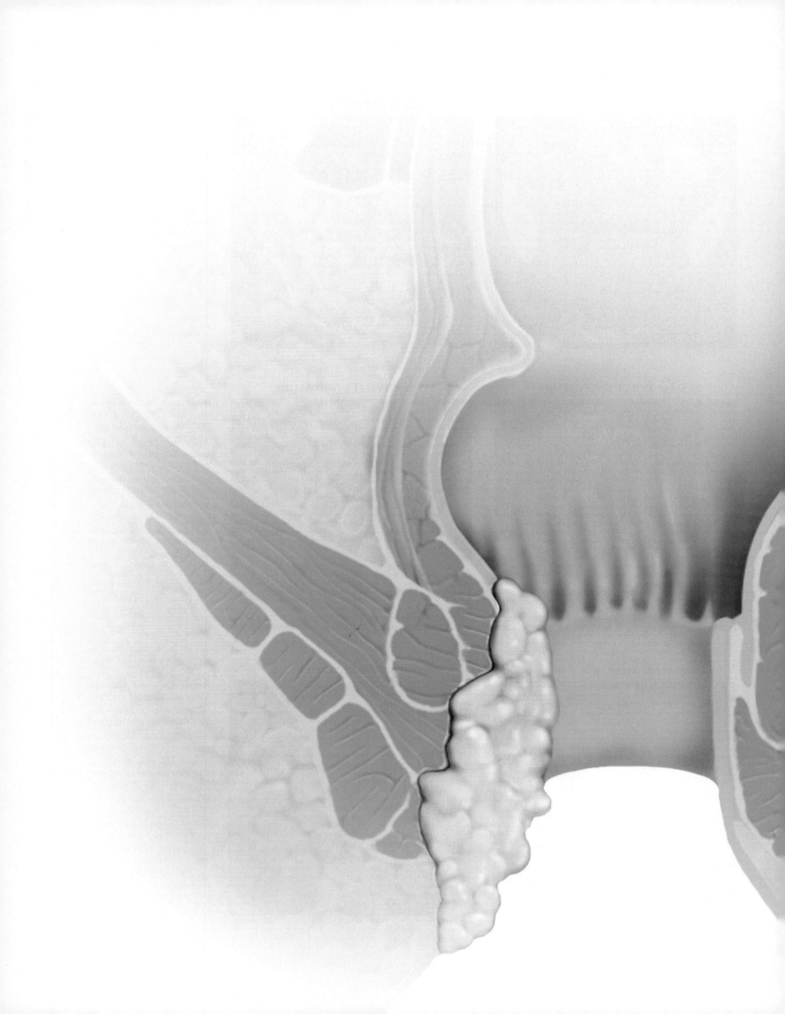

Anal Canal Carcinoma

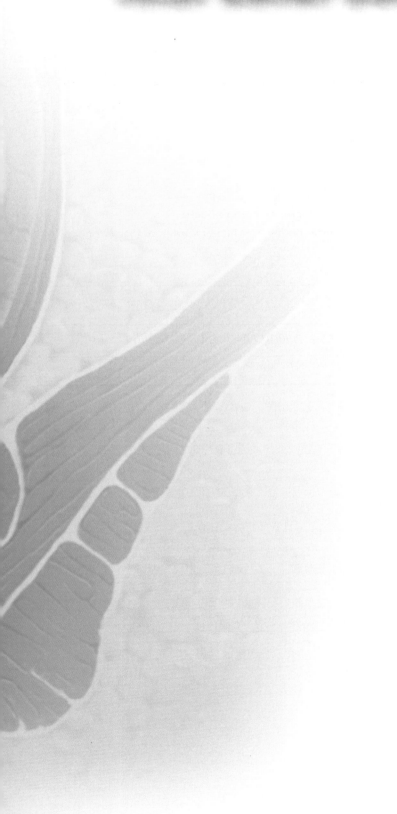

ANAL CANAL CARCINOMA

(T) Primary Tumor

Adapted from 7th edition AJCC Staging Forms.

TNM	Definitions
TX	Primary tumor cannot be assessed
T0	No evidence of primary tumor
Tis	Carcinoma in situ (Bowen disease, high-grade squamous intraepithelial lesion [HSIL], anal intraepithelial neoplasia II-III [AIN II-III])
T1	Tumor ≤ 2 cm in greatest dimension
T2	Tumor > 2 cm but ≤ 5 cm in greatest dimension
T3	Tumor > 5 cm in greatest dimension
T4	Tumor of any size invading adjacent organ(s), e.g., vagina, urethra, bladder*

(N) Regional Lymph Nodes

NX	Regional lymph nodes cannot be assessed
N0	No regional lymph node metastasis
N1	Metastasis in perirectal lymph node(s)
N2	Metastasis in unilateral internal iliac &/or inguinal lymph node(s)
N3	Metastasis in perirectal and inguinal lymph nodes &/or bilateral internal iliac &/or inguinal lymph nodes

(M) Distant Metastasis

M0	No distant metastasis
M1	Distant metastasis

Direct invasion of the rectal wall, perirectal skin, subcutaneous tissue, or the sphincter muscle(s) is not classified as T4.

AJCC Stages/Prognostic Groups

Adapted from 7th edition AJCC Staging Forms.

Stage	T	N	M
0	Tis	N0	M0
I	T1	N0	M0
II	T2	N0	M0
	T3	N0	M0
IIIA	T1	N1	M0
	T2	N1	M0
	T3	N1	M0
	T4	N0	M0
IIIB	T4	N1	M0
	Any T	N2	M0
	Any T	N3	M0
IV	Any T	Any N	M1

ANAL CANAL CARCINOMA

Tis

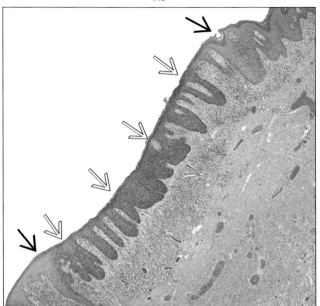

Low-power view of H&E stained section of hemorrhoidectomy specimen shows incidental anal intraepithelial neoplasia (AIN). AIN ➡ involves most of the thickness of the squamous epithelium and has a darker color with abrupt demarcation from the normal squamous epithelium ➨. (Original magnification 20x.)

Tis

Higher magnification of AIN depicted in the previous image shows crowded neoplastic cells (left upper corner) with increased nuclear to cytoplasmic ratio and numerous mitotic figures ➨. The cells respect the basement membrane ➨ with no evidence of invasion. (Original magnification 400x.)

T1

Scanned whole mount of H&E stained section shows invasive squamous cell carcinoma ➡ of the anus arising from the squamous epithelium and invading into the submucosa. The tumor measures 12 mm. Compare with normal glandular mucosa on the left side ➨ and the uninvolved squamous epithelium on the right ➨.

T1

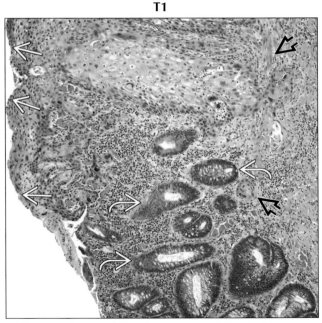

Higher magnification of the right upper part of the prior image shows the invasive squamous cell carcinoma extending from the surface ➡ and invading into the submucosa ➨. Note the adjacent uninvolved glands of the colorectal mucosa ➨. (Original magnification 100x.)

T1

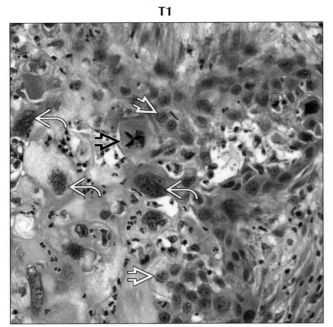

Higher magnification of the previous image shows the pleomorphic atypical cells with numerous large cells ⇒, intermediate to small neoplastic cells ⇒, and a tripolar mitotic figure ⇒. (Original magnification 500x.)

T2

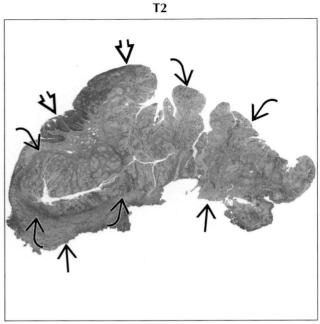

Scanned whole mount of H&E stained section with invasive squamous cell carcinoma of the anus shows a 2.9 cm tumor ⇒. Note the resection margin ⇒ and the surface mucosa ⇒.

T2

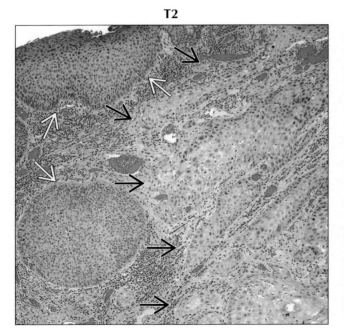

Higher magnification of the previous image shows the invasive squamous carcinoma ⇒ in close proximity to intraepithelial carcinoma ⇒. (Original magnification 100x.)

T2

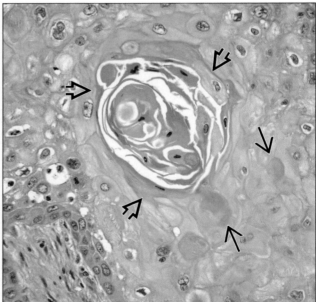

Higher magnification of the invasive squamous cell carcinoma cells shows cytoplasmic eosinophilic pink materials (keratin) ⇒ as well as keratin pearl formation ⇒, indicating a well-differentiated squamous cell carcinoma. (Original magnification 400x.)

ANAL CANAL CARCINOMA

T1

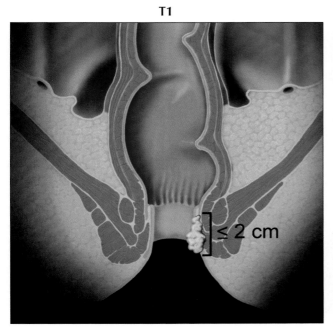

Graphic illustrates an anal canal tumor 2 cm or less in greatest dimension, consistent with T1 disease.

T2

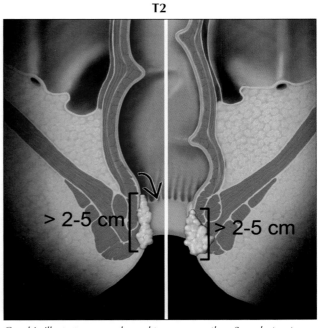

Graphic illustrates an anal canal tumor more than 2 cm but not more than 5 cm in greatest dimension. On the left side of the graphic, tumor extends above the dentate line ⊘.

T3

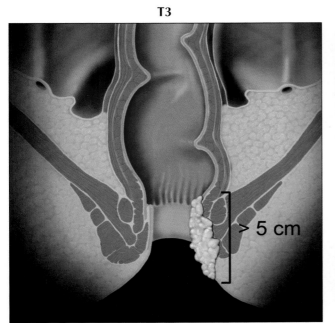

Graphic illustrates an anal canal tumor more than 5 cm in greatest dimension, which is classified as T3 disease.

T4

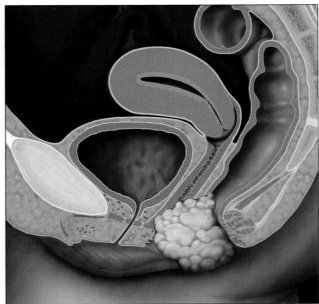

Graphic illustrates an anal canal tumor invading the vagina. T4 tumor is defined as tumor of any size invading adjacent organs or structures, such as vagina, urethra, or urinary bladder.

N1

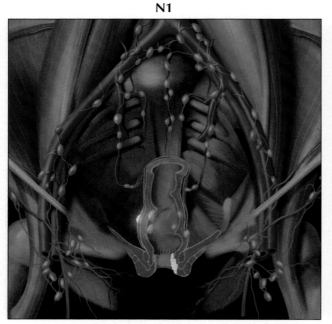

Graphic shows metastasis in a perirectal lymph node, consistent with N1 disease. Even if multiple perirectal lymph nodes were affected, the N classification would still be N1.

N2

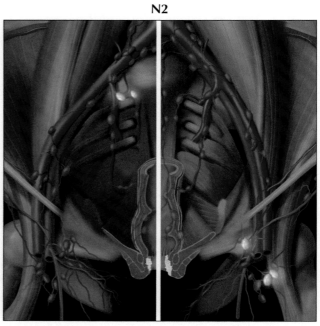

Graphic shows metastases to a single group of nodes, internal iliac (left) or inguinal (right). N2 is defined as metastases in unilateral internal iliac &/or inguinal lymph nodes.

N2

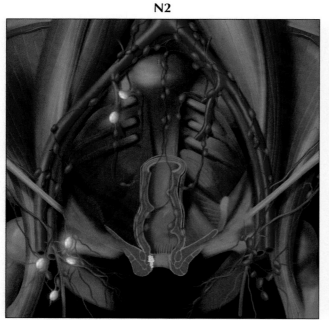

Graphic shows unilateral metastases to both internal iliac and inguinal lymph nodes, another scenario that is considered N2.

N3

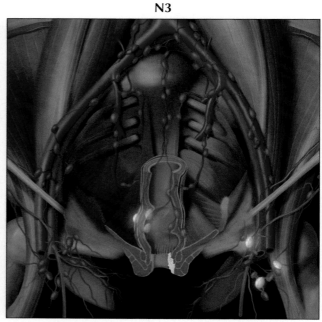

Graphic illustrates metastases to perirectal and inguinal lymph nodes. N3 is defined as metastases in perirectal and inguinal lymph nodes &/or bilateral internal iliac &/or inguinal lymph nodes.

ANAL CANAL CARCINOMA

N3

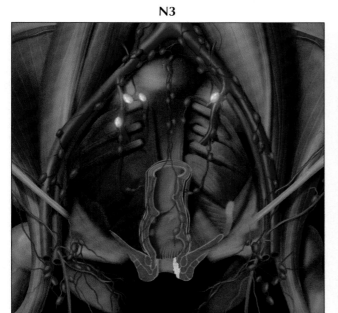

N3

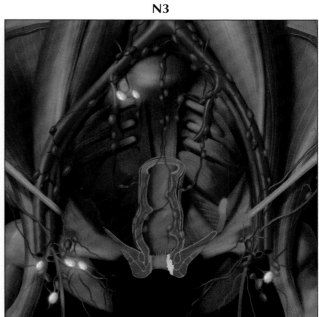

Graphic illustrates metastases to bilateral internal iliac lymph nodes, consistent with N3 disease.

Graphic illustrates metastases to bilateral inguinal and unilateral internal iliac lymph nodes, which is also N3 disease.

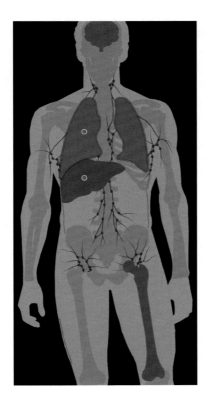

METASTASES, ORGAN FREQUENCY

Liver

Lung

Distant metastases occur in about 10% of cases. No data are available regarding the frequency of metastases. The liver is the most common site, and liver metastases usually occur in patients who have tumor extension to the rectum.

ANAL CANAL CARCINOMA

OVERVIEW

General Comments
- Tumors that arise from anal mucosa are called anal canal carcinomas
  - Include tumors arising from glandular, transitional, and squamous epithelium (from proximal to distal)
- Tumors arising from perianal skin (distal to squamous mucocutaneous junction) are called perianal carcinomas
  - Not included in this staging scheme
    - Staged with skin cancers

Classification
- WHO histological classification
  - Squamous cell carcinomas (SCC) make up majority of all primary anal carcinomas (80% of anal canal tumors)
    - Cloacogenic (basaloid or transitional cell) are considered variants of SCC
      - Exhibit similar natural history, response to treatment, and prognosis
      - All are associated with human papilloma virus (HPV) infection
  - Adenocarcinomas (10%)
    - Rectal type
    - Adenocarcinomas of anal glands
    - Adenocarcinomas within anorectal fistula
  - Mucinous adenocarcinoma
  - Small cell carcinoma
  - Undifferentiated carcinoma

PATHOLOGY

Routes of Spread
- Local spread
  - Local spread can occur to adjacent structures, including vagina, urethra, and urinary bladder
- Nodal spread
  - Metastatic spread to regional lymph nodes represents most common mode of tumor spread
  - Lymphatic drainage depends on location of tumor in relation to dentate line
    - Tumors below dentate line → inguinal and femoral nodes
    - Tumors above dentate line → perirectal and paravertebral nodes
      - Similar to rectal cancers
  - Regional nodes are inguinal, internal iliac, and perirectal (anorectal, perirectal, and lateral sacral) nodes
  - Incidence of nodal metastasis ~ 10% at diagnosis
    - May be as high as 20–60% for T4 lesions
- Distant metastases
  - Occur in ~ 10% of cases of anal carcinoma
  - Mainly to liver and lungs

General Features
- Etiology
  - Risk of anal cancer is rising
  - Known risk factors include
    - History of persistent high-risk genotype HPV infection

- HPV infection is strongly associated with anal cancer development and may be a necessary step in its carcinogenesis
  - Infection with multiple HPV genotypes
  - Cervical dysplasia or cancer
  - HIV seropositivity
  - Low CD4 count
  - Cigarette smoking
  - Anoreceptive intercourse
  - High lifetime number of sexual partners
  - Immunosuppression following solid organ transplant
  - Crohn disease
- Epidemiology & cancer incidence
  - Uncommon malignancy
    - 1.5% of digestive system cancers in USA
    - 4-5% of anorectal malignancies
  - Estimated 5,290 new cases in USA in 2009
  - Estimated 710 deaths in USA in 2009
  - Wide age range; peak incidence during 7th decade of life
  - Marked female predominance
    - M:F = 1:5

Gross Pathology & Surgical Features
- Anal carcinomas are usually nodular and often ulcerated

Microscopic Pathology
- Majority of anal canal carcinomas are squamous cell carcinomas
  - Variants include
    - Large cell keratinizing
    - Large cell nonkeratinizing
    - Basaloid
- Other less common types include adenocarcinoma, melanoma, and small cell carcinoma

IMAGING FINDINGS

Detection
- Because of their location, anal canal cancers are easy to evaluate clinically
  - Examining finger can gauge primary tumor size and degree of fixation
  - All lesions are within easy reach of biopsy
- Endorectal ultrasonography
  - Can give accurate information about size of lesion and possible perirectal lymph node involvement
  - Sensitivity of 100% in primary tumor detection
  - Superior to MR for detection of small superficial tumors
- CT
  - Difficult to detect anal carcinoma due to poor tissue contrast
  - Only large lesions causing significant contour deformity can be seen
  - CT visualized 59% of cases of anal carcinoma in 1 study
- MR
  - Majority of tumors are heterogeneously hyperintense on T2 and STIR images
  - Sensitivity of 89% in primary tumor detection
- PET/CT

ANAL CANAL CARCINOMA

○ PET/CT detects 91-100% of nonexcised primary tumors

Staging

- Endorectal ultrasonography
  - ○ Important tool used to stage patients not undergoing excisional therapy
  - ○ Imaging field of view is limited
    - ▪ Mesorectal lymph nodes located far from endoanal probe may be missed
    - ▪ Inguinal nodes cannot be assessed during endorectal sonographic examination
- CT
  - ○ Not useful for local staging of anal carcinoma due to poor tissue contrast
  - ○ Can detect enlarged perirectal and inguinal lymph nodes
    - ▪ Sensitivity of 62%
  - ○ Useful for detection of metastatic disease to liver and lungs
- MR
  - ○ Local tumor
    - ▪ Good correlation between maximum tumor size as determined by MR imaging and clinical assessment
    - ▪ Good agreement in T staging of tumor by MR imaging and clinical assessment
      - - Clinical examination may actually underestimate degree of local invasion in T4 tumors
- PET/CT
  - ○ PET/CT appears more useful than CT in detection of metastases
    - ▪ Sites of metastases not observed on CT scan were identified in 24% of patients
      - - These included pelvic adenopathy and peritoneal metastases
  - ○ In 1 study, tumor stage group was changed in 23% of patients as result of findings on PET/CT
    - ▪ 15% upstaged, 8% downstaged
  - ○ Sensitivity for nodal regional disease is 89%
    - ▪ Compared to only 62% with conventional imaging

Restaging

- CT
  - ○ Can be used for detection of metastatic disease to liver and lungs
  - ○ Not useful for detection of local recurrence
- MR
  - ○ Can be used for follow-up of patients after chemoradiation
    - ▪ MR criteria for tumor response
      - - Reduction in tumor size
      - - Decreased tumor signal intensity on T2WI
- PET/CT
  - ○ Post-treatment PET scans appear to be of little value in predicting durability of local response
    - ▪ Minimal residual PET activity at primary site on 1 month follow-up PET can be seen in patients without recurrence
    - ▪ Recurrences possible in patients who had negative post-treatment PET studies
  - ○ Useful for detection of distant metastases

CLINICAL ISSUES

Presentation

- 20% of patients have no symptoms at time of diagnosis
- Presentation is very nonspecific
  - ○ Most patients (70-80%) are initially diagnosed as having benign anorectal conditions
- Most patients present with rectal bleeding
  - ○ Occurs in 45% of patients
  - ○ Diagnosis can be delayed because bleeding is often ascribed to hemorrhoids
- Rectal pain &/or mass sensation
  - ○ Occurs in approximately 30% of patients
- History of anorectal warts
  - ○ Present in approximately 50% of homosexual men with anal cancer
  - ○ Present in only 20% of women and heterosexual men with anal cancer

Cancer Natural History & Prognosis

- Stage at diagnosis
  - ○ Stage I (25.3%)
  - ○ Stage II (51.8%)
  - ○ Stage III (17.1%)
  - ○ Stage IV (5.7%)
- 5-year survival by stage
  - ○ Stage I (63-70%)
  - ○ Stage II (57-59%)
  - ○ Stage III (41-48%)
  - ○ Stage IV (19%)
- Tumor size is most important prognostic factor

Treatment Options

- Major treatment alternatives
  - ○ Traditional management is abdominoperineal resection (APR) for tumors of anal region
  - ○ Chemoradiation therapy
    - ▪ Replaced APR as treatment of choice
    - ▪ Chemotherapy with fluorouracil + mitomycin combined with radiation therapy appears to be more effective than radiation therapy alone
    - ▪ Survival and recurrence rates equivalent to those achieved with surgery
    - ▪ Preserves sphincter function
  - ○ Local excision
    - ▪ Can be considered for small well-differentiated carcinomas of anal margin
      - - i.e., tumor ≤ 2 cm in diameter without nodal spread (T1 N0)
- Treatment options by stage
  - ○ Stage 0
    - ▪ Surgical resection is used for treatment of lesions of perianal area not involving anal sphincter
  - ○ Stage I, II, and IIIA
    - ▪ Standard therapy consists of radiotherapy of
      - - Anal canal
      - - Perianal region
      - - Distal rectum
      - - Perirectal, internal iliac, inguinal, and presacral lymph nodes
    - ▪ Selected tumors are also suitable for interstitial radiation therapy
  - ○ Stage IIIB

ANAL CANAL CARCINOMA

- **More extensive therapy**
  - Radiation therapy + chemotherapy (as described above)
  - + surgical resection of residual local disease (local resection or abdominoperineal resection)
  - + unilateral or bilateral superficial and deep inguinal node dissection for residual or recurrent tumor
- ○ **Stage IV**
  - Palliative surgery
  - Palliative radiation therapy
  - Palliative chemotherapy + radiation therapy
- ○ **Recurrent disease**
  - Radical resection for residual or recurrent disease after nonoperative therapy
  - Salvage chemotherapy with fluorouracil and cisplatin + radiation boost
    - May avoid permanent colostomy in selected patients with small amounts of residual tumor following initial nonoperative therapy
  - Interstitial iridium-192 after external beam radiation therapy
    - May convert some patients with residual disease into complete responders

REPORTING CHECKLIST

T Staging

- MR is superior to CT in local staging
- Good correlation between MR and clinical examination in estimation of tumor size
  - ○ Determination of T1-T3
- MR is also useful in evaluation of local extension to urethra, bladder, and vagina

N Staging

- PET/CT is superior to CT and MR in detection of perirectal, inguinal, and pelvic lymphadenopathy

M Staging

- CT, PET/CT, and MR can be used for detection of distant metastases, mainly to liver and lungs

SELECTED REFERENCES

1. American Joint Committee on Cancer: AJCC Cancer Staging Manual. 7th ed. New York: Springer. 165-73, 2010
2. Engledow AH et al: The role of FDG PET/CT in the clinical management of anal squamous cell carcinoma. Colorectal Dis. Epub ahead of print, 2010
3. Goh V et al: Magnetic resonance imaging assessment of squamous cell carcinoma of the anal canal before and after chemoradiation: can MRI predict for eventual clinical outcome? Int J Radiat Oncol Biol Phys. Epub ahead of print, 2010
4. McMahon CJ et al: Lymphatic metastases from pelvic tumors: anatomic classification, characterization, and staging. Radiology. 254(1):31-46, 2010
5. Bilimoria KY et al: Outcomes and prognostic factors for squamous-cell carcinoma of the anal canal: analysis of patients from the National Cancer Data Base. Dis Colon Rectum. 52(4):624-31, 2009
6. Glynne-Jones R et al: Anal cancer: ESMO clinical recommendations for diagnosis, treatment and follow-up. Ann Oncol. 20 Suppl 4:57-60, 2009
7. Otto SD et al: Staging anal cancer: prospective comparison of transanal endoscopic ultrasound and magnetic resonance imaging. J Gastrointest Surg. 13(7):1292-8, 2009
8. Winton E et al: The impact of 18-fluorodeoxyglucose positron emission tomography on the staging, management and outcome of anal cancer. Br J Cancer. 100(5):693-700, 2009
9. Koh DM et al: Pelvic phased-array MR imaging of anal carcinoma before and after chemoradiation. Br J Radiol. 81(962):91-8, 2008
10. Uronis HE et al: Anal cancer: an overview. Oncologist. 12(5):524-34, 2007
11. Cotter SE et al: FDG-PET/CT in the evaluation of anal carcinoma. Int J Radiat Oncol Biol Phys. 65(3):720-5, 2006
12. Trautmann TG et al: Positron Emission Tomography for pretreatment staging and posttreatment evaluation in cancer of the anal canal. Mol Imaging Biol. 7(4):309-13, 2005
13. Ryan DP et al: Carcinoma of the anal canal. N Engl J Med. 342(11):792-800, 2000
14. Klas JV et al: Malignant tumors of the anal canal: the spectrum of disease, treatment, and outcomes. Cancer. 85(8):1686-93, 1999

ANAL CANAL CARCINOMA

Stage II (T2 N0 M0)

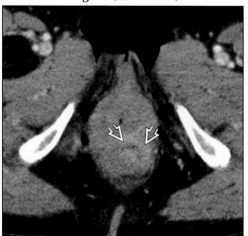

Stage II (T2 N0 M0)

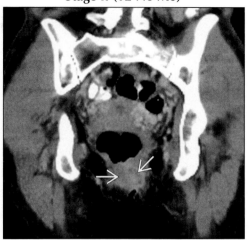

(Left) Axial CECT in a 54-year-old woman who presented because of recurrent rectal bleeding shows a circumferential enhancing anal mass ⮞. (Right) Coronal CECT in the same patient shows an enhancing circumferential anal mass ⮞. The mass measured 3.5 cm, consistent with T2 disease.

Stage II (T2 N0 M0)

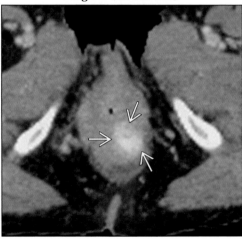

Stage II (T2 N0 M0)

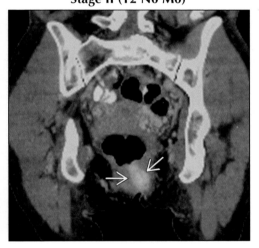

(Left) Axial PET/CT in the same patient shows the anal mass with increased metabolic activity ⮞. The mass is better appreciated on PET/CT, which has a detection rate of 91-100% for primary anal carcinomas. (Right) Coronal PET/CT in the same patient shows the circumferential increased metabolic activity of the anal mass ⮞.

Stage II (T2 N0 M0)

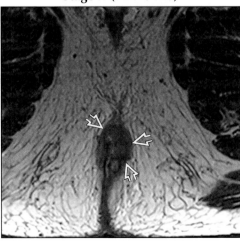

Stage II (T2 N0 M0)

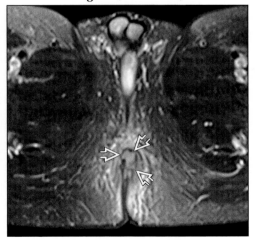

(Left) Axial T1WI MR in a 54-year-old man who presented with rectal bleeding shows an anal mass ⮞ that is slightly hyperintense on T1WI. (Right) Axial T2WI FS MR in the same patient shows an anal mass ⮞ that is hyperintense relative to muscles. Anal carcinomas are usually hyperintense to muscles on T2WI and become isointense or hypointense to muscles when the tumor responds to chemoradiation.

ANAL CANAL CARCINOMA

Stage II (T2 N0 M0)

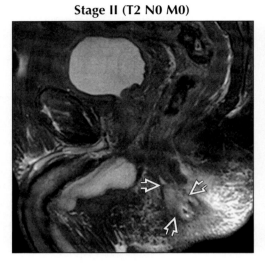

Stage II (T2 N0 M0)

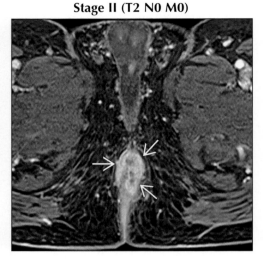

(Left) Sagittal T2WI FS MR in the same patient demonstrates the anal mass ⧁ with higher signal intensity compared to muscles. The mass measured 3 cm, consistent with T2 disease. *(Right)* Axial T1WI C+ FS MR in the same patient shows the anal mass ⧁ with intense enhancement following administration of gadolinium. No inguinal lymph nodes are present.

Stage II (T2 N0 M0)

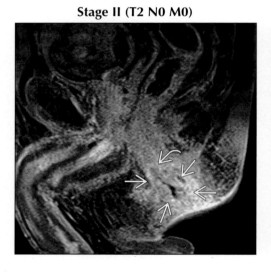

Stage II (T2 N0 M0)

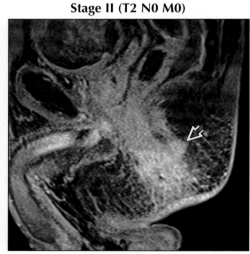

(Left) Sagittal T1WI C+ FS MR in the same patient shows that the enhancing anal mass ⧁ extends to the lower rectum ⧁. Direct extension to the rectum does not constitute T4 disease; the staging from T1-T3 depends on tumor size. *(Right)* Sagittal T1WI C+ FS MR in the same patient shows posterior extension to the perianal fat ⧁, which also does not change the T designation of the tumor.

Stage IIIA (T4 N0 M0)

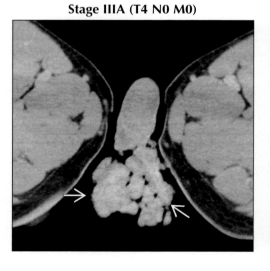

Stage IIIA (T4 N0 M0)

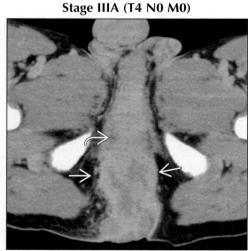

(Left) Axial CECT in a 35-year-old man with history of condyloma acuminatum of the anal canal shows a large polypoid mass ⧁ involving the anal and perineal regions. *(Right)* Axial CECT in the same patient shows the large mass ⧁ infiltrating the perianal fat and completely obliterating the anal canal. The mass extends anteriorly to involve the root of penis ⧁. HPV infection, the cause of vaginal warts, is strongly associated with pathogenesis of anal carcinoma.

ANAL CANAL CARCINOMA

Stage IIIA (T4 N0 M0)

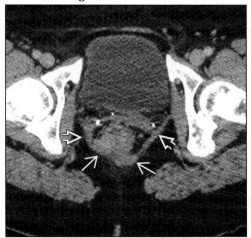

Stage IIIA (T4 N0 M0)

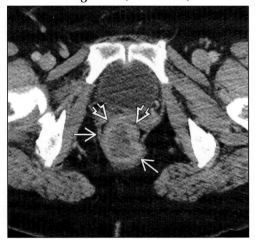

(Left) Axial CECT in a 59-year-old woman who presented with a palpable mass shows the upper extent of anal carcinoma. The tumor ➡ extends laterally to involve the puborectalis muscles ➡ on both sides. Notice, however, that invasion of the sphincter muscle does not constitute T4 disease. *(Right)* Axial CECT in the same patient shows the main bulk of the necrotic mass ➡ separated from the upper part of the vagina ➡.

Stage IIIA (T4 N0 M0)

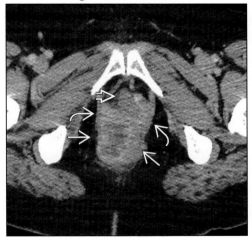

Stage IIIA (T4 N0 M0)

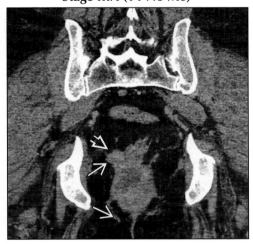

(Left) Axial CECT in the same patient shows the mass ➡ inseparable from the lower vagina ➡ and even encroaching upon the urethra ➡. *(Right)* Coronal CECT in the same patient shows the craniocaudal extent of the mass ➡. The mass extends above the puborectalis muscle into the distal rectum ➡. Rectal invasion does not constitute T4 disease, but vaginal invasion does. The mass measured 7 cm in greatest dimension.

Stage IIIA (T4 N0 M0)

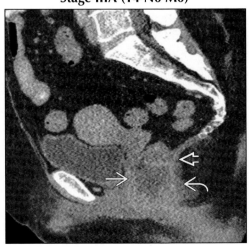

Stage IIIA (T4 N0 M0)

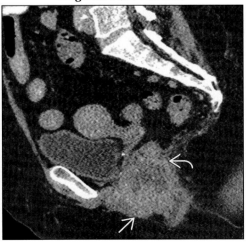

(Left) Sagittal CECT in the same patient shows the rectal mass ➡ invading the distal vagina ➡ and the levator ani muscle ➡. *(Right)* Sagittal CECT in the same patient shows the rectal mass ➡ invading the skin of the perineum ➡.

ANAL CANAL CARCINOMA

Stage IIIA (T4 N0 M0)

Stage IIIA (T4 N0 M0)

(Left) Axial CECT in a 50-year-old woman who presented with rectal bleeding shows the upper end of the anal mass invading the rectum ➡ and extending into the perirectal fat ⮞. (Right) Axial CECT in the same patient shows the main bulk of the mass ➡ contained within the puborectalis muscles ⮞. The mass shows considerable enhancement relative to skeletal muscles.

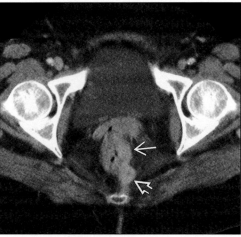

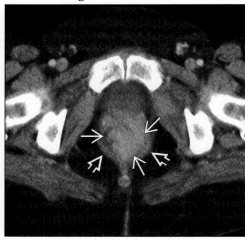

Stage IIIA (T4 N0 M0)

Stage IIIA (T4 N0 M0)

(Left) Axial CECT in the same patient shows the enhancing anal mass ➡ extending anteriorly to involve the vagina ⮞. The extension of the mass in this case is easily identified because of its enhancement. (Right) Axial CECT in the same patient shows the enhancing mass ➡ extending anteriorly to involve the introitus.

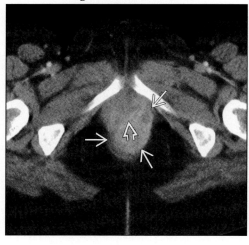

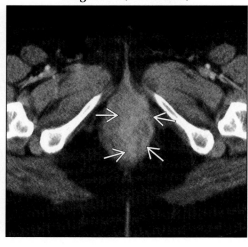

Stage IIIA (T4 N0 M0)

Stage IIIA (T4 N0 M0)

(Left) Axial NECT after administration of rectal contrast in a different 54-year-old woman, who presented due to passage of stool per vagina, shows the contrast within the anal canal ➡ and a filling defect ⮞ representing an anal carcinoma. (Right) Axial NECT in the same patient shows contrast both within the anal canal ➡ and vagina ⮞ due to anovaginal fistula resulting from the anal carcinoma.

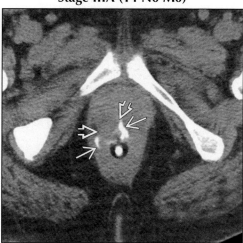

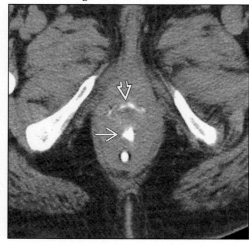

ANAL CANAL CARCINOMA

Stage IIIB (T1 N2 M0)

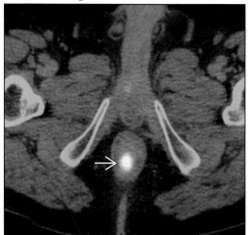

Stage IIIB (T1 N2 M0)

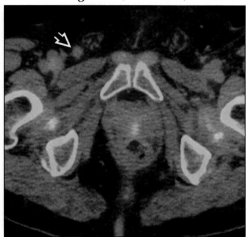

(Left) Axial PET/CT in a 58-year-old man who presented with rectal pain shows increased metabolic activity in an anal mass ➡. The mass measured 18 mm, consistent with T1 disease. *(Right)* Axial PET/CT in the same patient shows increased metabolic activity in a right inguinal lymph node ➡. Metastatic disease to unilateral inguinal nodes constitutes N2 disease.

Stage IIIB (T1 N2 M0)

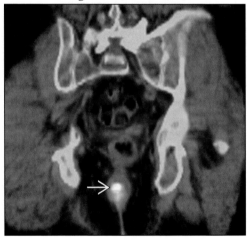

Stage IIIB (T1 N2 M0)

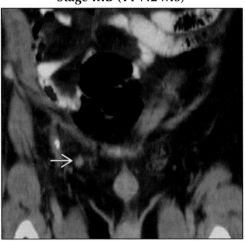

(Left) Coronal PET/CT in the same patient shows marked increase in metabolic activity of the primary anal mass ➡. *(Right)* Coronal PET/CT in the same patient shows increased metabolic activity of the right inguinal lymph node ➡.

Stage IIIB (T4 N3 M0)

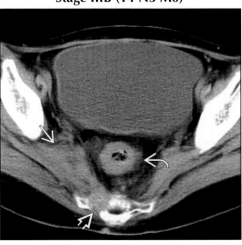

Stage IIIB (T4 N3 M0)

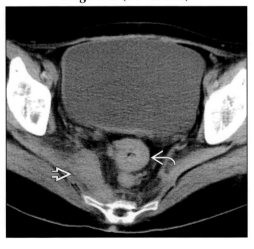

(Left) Axial NECT in a 60-year-old woman with history of hysterectomy, who presented with large bowel obstruction and underwent sigmoid colostomy, shows diffuse concentric thickening of the wall of the distal rectum ➡. There is also tumor invading the right piriformis muscle ➡ and the sacrum ➡. *(Right)* Axial NECT in the same patient shows concentric thickening of the rectum ➡ and tumor invading the piriformis muscle ➡.

ANAL CANAL CARCINOMA

Stage IIIB (T4 N3 M0)

(Left) Axial NECT in the same patient shows a large pelvic mass ⇗ invading the right ischiorectal fossa ➡, vagina ⇉, and coccyx ⤷. Invasion of the vagina, sacrum, and coccyx represents T4 disease. *(Right)* Axial NECT in the same patient shows the large pelvic mass ⇗ reaching to the right pelvic side wall ⇉.

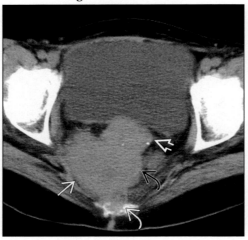

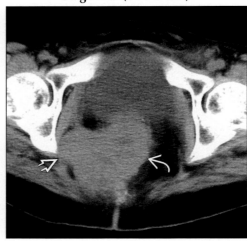

Stage IIIB (T4 N3 M0)

(Left) Axial NECT in the same patient shows the large pelvic mass ⇗ invading the distal vagina ➡. Bilateral enlarged inguinal nodes are also present ⇉. *(Right)* Axial NECT in the same patient shows tumor invading into the introitus ➡. Visible tumor was seen involving both the anal canal and vaginal introitus. There is also an enlarged left inguinal node ⇗. The presence of bilateral inguinal adenopathy represents N3 disease.

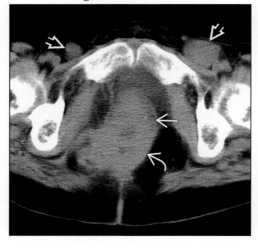

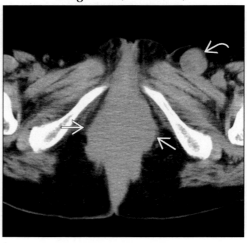

Stage IV (T2 N0 M1)

(Left) Axial CECT in a 52-year-old woman who presented with right upper quadrant abdominal pain shows a hypoattenuating liver lesion ➡. *(Right)* Axial PET/CT in the same patient was performed to work-up the liver lesion, which shows increased metabolic activity of the right lobe liver mass ➡. Later biopsy of the liver lesion revealed metastatic squamous cell carcinoma.

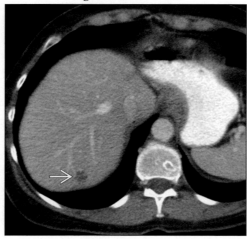

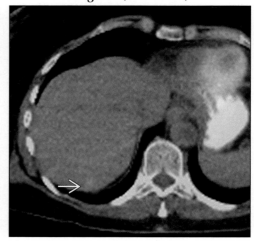

ANAL CANAL CARCINOMA

Stage IV (T2 N0 M1)

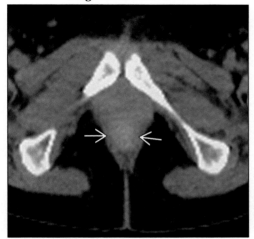

Stage IV (T2 N0 M1)

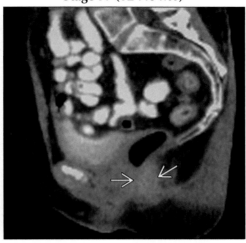

(Left) Axial PET/CT in the same patient shows increased metabolic activity of an anal mass ➡. *(Right)* Sagittal PET/CT in the same patient shows increased metabolic activity of the anal mass ➡. PET/CT is helpful not only for evaluation of local disease but also for detection of distant metastases.

Recurrent Anal Carcinoma

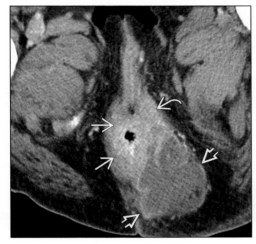

Recurrent Anal Carcinoma

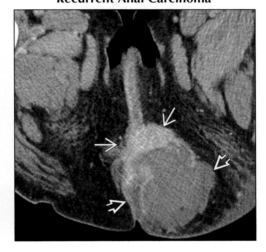

(Left) Axial CECT in a 61-year-old woman, who had a history of anal carcinoma 2 years earlier treated with combined chemoradiation and who presented with fever and septic shock, shows circumferential thickening of the anal canal ➡ with perianal tumor extension ➡ and a large fluid density perianal abscess ➡. *(Right)* Axial CECT in the same patient shows tumor involving the perineum ➡ and a large perianal abscess ➡.

Recurrent Anal Carcinoma

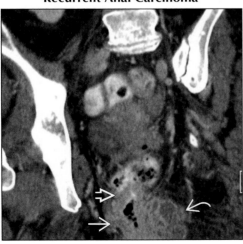

Recurrent Anal Carcinoma

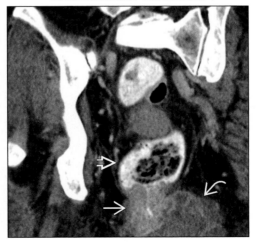

(Left) Coronal CECT in the same patient shows the circumferential thickening of the anal canal ➡ extending to the lower rectum ➡ and a perianal abscess ➡. *(Right)* Coronal CECT in the same patient shows circumferential thickening of the anal canal ➡ with mild dilatation of the proximal rectum ➡ and perianal abscess ➡.

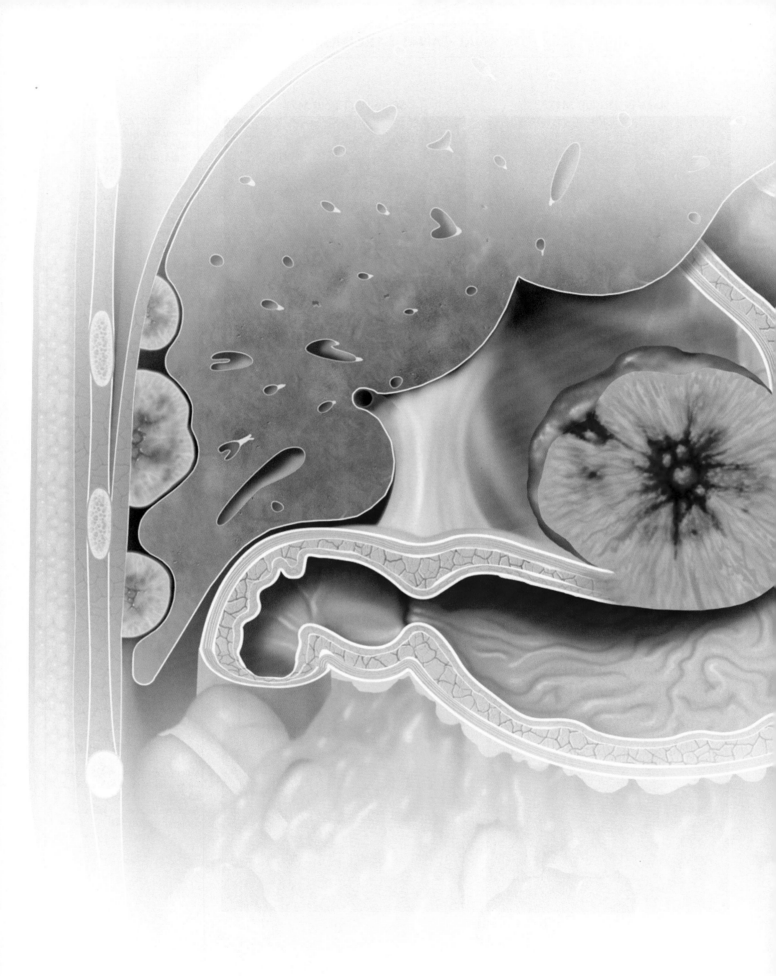

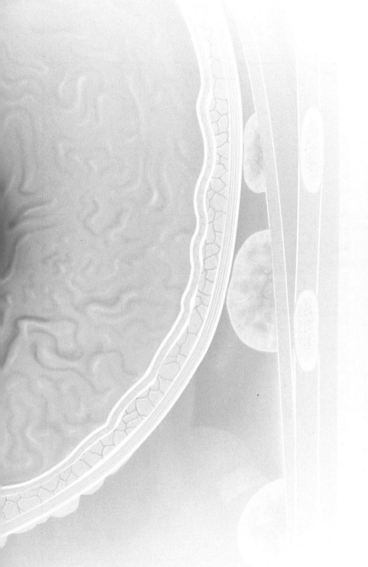

Gastrointestinal Stromal Tumor (GIST)

GASTROINTESTINAL STROMAL TUMOR (GIST)

(T) Primary Tumor	*Adapted from 7th edition AJCC Staging Forms.*

TNM	*Definitions*
TX	Primary tumor cannot be assessed
T0	No evidence of primary tumor
T1	Tumor ≤ 2 cm
T2	Tumor > 2 cm but ≤ 5 cm
T3	Tumor > 5 cm but ≤ 10 cm
T4	Tumor > 10 cm

(N) Regional Lymph Nodes

NX	Regional lymph nodes cannot be assessed
N0	No regional lymph node metastasis
N1	Regional lymph node metastasis

(M) Distant Metastasis

M0	No distant metastasis
M1	Distant metastasis

(G) Histologic Grade

GX	Histologic grade cannot be assessed
G1	Low grade (mitotic rate ≤ 5 per 50 high-power fields)
G2	High grade (mitotic rate > 5 per 50 high-power fields)

Size of tumor is measured in the greatest dimension.

AJCC Stages/Prognostic Groups for Gastric GIST	*Adapted from 7th edition AJCC Staging Forms.*

Stage	*T*	*N*	*M*	*G*
IA	T1	N0	M0	G1
	T2	N0	M0	G1
IB	T3	N0	M0	G1
II	T1	N0	M0	G2
	T2	N0	M0	G2
	T4	N0	M0	G1
IIIA	T3	N0	M0	G2
IIIB	T4	N0	M0	G2
IV	Any T	N1	M0	Any G
	Any T	Any N	M1	Any G

The AJCC stage grouping schema are slightly different for gastric and small bowel GISTs, owing to slightly different biological activities. The staging for gastric GIST should also be used for omentum.

GASTROINTESTINAL STROMAL TUMOR (GIST)

AJCC Stages/Prognostic Groups for Small Intestinal GIST

Adapted from 7th edition AJCC Staging Forms.

Stage	T	N	M	G
I	T1 or T2	N0	M0	G1
II	T3	N0	M0	G1
IIIA	T1	N0	M0	G2
	T4	N0	M0	G1
IIIB	T2	N0	M0	G2
	T3	N0	M0	G2
	T4	N0	M0	G2
IV	Any T	N1	M0	Any G
	Any T	Any N	M1	Any G

The small bowel GIST staging grouping may be applied to esophageal, duodenal, colorectal, and peritoneal GISTs. As there is only minimal data regarding extragastrointestinal GISTs, precise grouping of these rare tumors can be problematic. In cases of extragastrointestinal GISTs and other less common varieties, the staging grouping for small bowel tumors may be used. The T, N, and M criteria reflect imaging findings, whereas tumor grading (G) is based on histologic criteria.

Gastrointestinal Stromal Tumor Prognostic Grouping

Malignancy Risk	Size Criteria	Histologic Criteria
Very low risk	< 2 cm	≤ 5 per 50 HPF
Low risk	2-5 cm	≤ 5 per 50 HPF
Intermediate risk	< 5 cm	6-10 per 50 HPF
	5-10 cm	≤ 5 per 50 HPF
High risk	> 5 cm	> 5 per 50 HPF
	> 10 cm	Any mitotic rate
	Any size	> 10 per 50 HPF

From Levy AD et al: Gastrointestinal stromal tumors: radiologic features with pathologic correlation. Radiographics. 23(2):283-304, 2003.

This system for stratification of aggressive potential in tumors without known metastatic disease was widely used prior to the advent of AJCC TNM staging system and has now been replaced. Size is measured in the greatest dimension. Histologic criteria reflects the number of mitotic figures per 50 high-power fields (HPF).

GASTROINTESTINAL STROMAL TUMOR (GIST)

T2

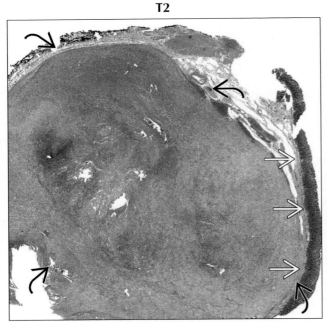

Low magnification of H&E section from the wall of stomach shows gastrointestinal stromal tumor (GIST) ➡. *The tumor measures 2.5 cm in largest dimension. Note the overlying stretched gastric mucosa* ➡. *(Original magnification 10x.)*

T2

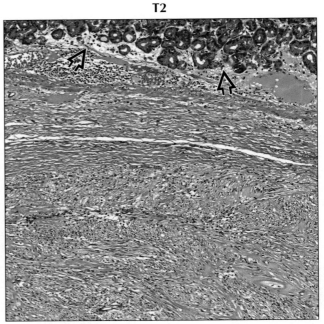

Higher magnification shows a portion of gastric mucosal epithelium in the upper aspect of the photomicrograph ➡. *The lower aspect of the photomicrograph shows a tumor composed of bundles of spindle cells characteristic of GIST. (Original magnification 400x.)*

T2

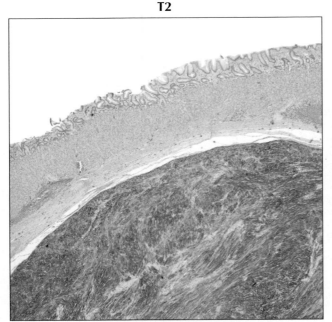

Immunohistochemical stain with antibody against C-kit (CD117) demonstrates positive (brown) staining in the spindle cells. The GIST tumor originates from gastrointestinal pacemaker cells (intercalated cells of Cajal). (Original magnification 100x.)

T2

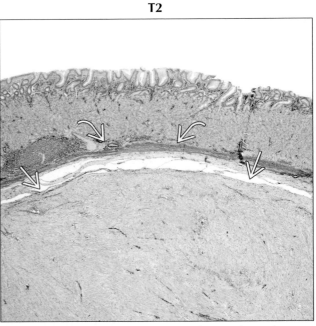

Immunohistochemical stain with antibody for smooth muscle actin (SMA) stains smooth muscle cells brown. The tumor ➡ *is negative for SMA, differentiating GIST from other smooth muscle tumors. Note the positive internal control staining in the smooth muscle cells in the stomach wall* ➡. *(Original magnification 100x.)*

GASTROINTESTINAL STROMAL TUMOR (GIST)

Gastric GIST, Stage I-III

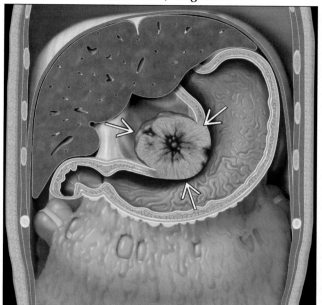

Coronal graphic shows a gastric GIST ➡. Precise staging is based on tumor size and grade in the absence of nodal or metastatic disease.

Metastatic Gastric GIST, Stage IV

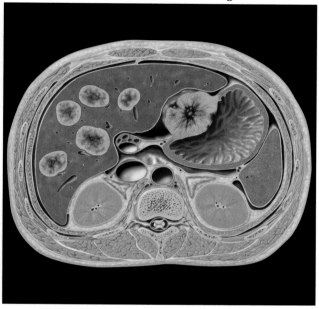

Axial graphic shows a gastric GIST with solid hepatic metastases, representing stage IV.

Metastatic Gastric GIST, Stage IV

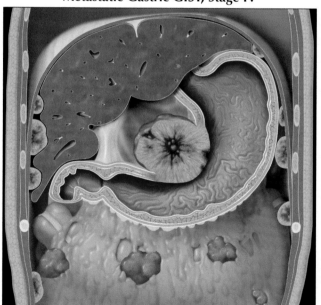

Coronal graphic shows a gastric GIST with peritoneal metastases. This is a stage IV lesion.

Metastatic Small Bowel GIST, Stage IV

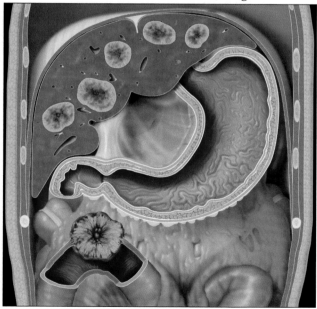

Coronal graphic shows a small bowel GIST with hepatic metastases. This is a stage IV lesion.

GASTROINTESTINAL STROMAL TUMOR (GIST)

Metastatic Small Bowel GIST, Stage IV

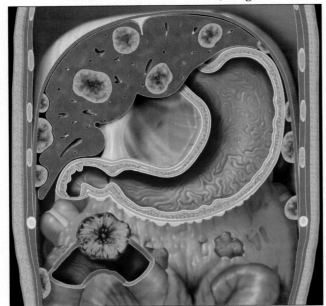

Coronal graphic shows a small bowel GIST with hepatic and peritoneal metastases. This is a stage IV lesion.

Treated Metastatic Small Bowel GIST

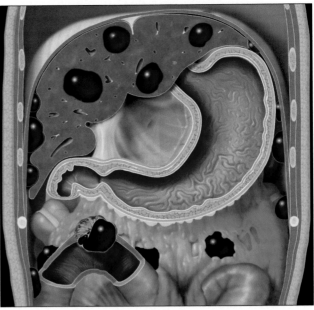

Coronal graphic shows the decrease in size and more cystic nature of primary small bowel GIST after therapy, as well as hepatic and peritoneal metastases.

Esophageal GIST, Stage I-III

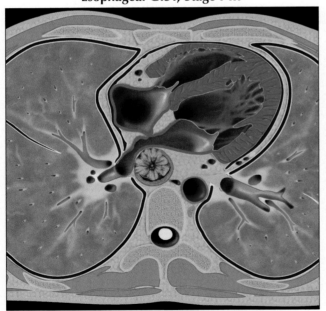

Axial graphic shows mid-esophageal GIST. The small bowel stage grouping should be used in this case. Precise staging is based on lesion size and grade.

Extragastrointestinal GIST, Stage I-III

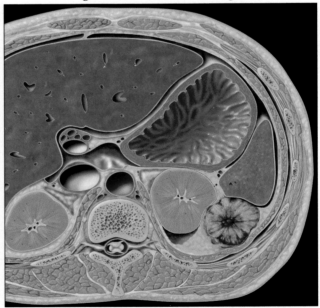

Axial graphic demonstrates a primary retroperitoneal GIST. The small bowel stage grouping should be used in this case. Precise staging is based on lesion size and grade.

GASTROINTESTINAL STROMAL TUMOR (GIST)

Rectal GIST, Stage I-III

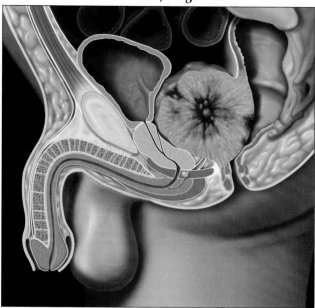

Sagittal graphic shows a rectal GIST. The small bowel stage grouping would be used in this case. Precise staging is based on lesion size and grade.

Treated Rectal GIST

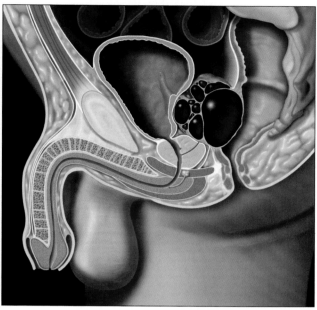

Sagittal graphic shows the decrease in size and more cystic appearance of a rectal GIST after therapy.

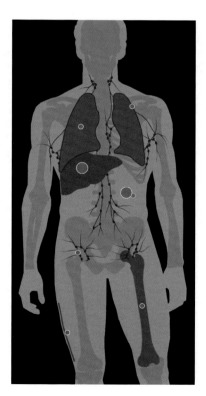

METASTASES, ORGAN FREQUENCY

Liver	46-65%
Peritoneum	21-41%
Retroperitoneum	4%
Lungs	2-6%
Bone	2-6%
Subcutaneous/scar tissue	2%
Pleura	2%
Rare nodal involvement	< 1-6%

GASTROINTESTINAL STROMAL TUMOR (GIST)

OVERVIEW

General Comments
- Most common mesenchymal malignancy of GI tract
  - Represents about 5-6% of all sarcomas
  - 80% of gastrointestinal sarcomas are GISTs
  - Accounts for < 1% of all GI malignancies
- Historically misdiagnosed smooth muscle tumors
  - Diagnosed as leiomyomas, leiomyoblastomas, or leiomyosarcomas
  - Improved immunohistological and electron microscopy techniques allowed for accurate characterization of GISTs after 1983
- AJCC TNM staging criteria
  - Recently established; took effect January 1, 2010
  - Previously, there was no formal TNM staging system, and risk stratification for metastatic potential was based on tumor size and mitotic rate
- Minority (20-30%) of GISTs demonstrate malignant behavior
  - Smaller, more homogeneous tumors tend to be benign and have lower histologic grade
  - Tumors < 2 cm rarely demonstrate high histologic grade

Classification
- Soft tissue sarcoma, distinct from leiomyoma/leiomyosarcoma and nerve sheath tumors

PATHOLOGY

Routes of Spread
- Local spread
  - Transperitoneal spread
    - Common pattern of spread, may occur early
  - Invasion of surrounding structures
    - Less common than peritoneal seeding
- Nodal metastasis
  - Very rare in GIST
  - More likely to occur in women and patients < 40 years old
  - More common in gastric epithelioid/mixed-type ulcerated endoluminal GIST
- Distant metastasis
  - Most commonly metastasizes to liver
  - Uncommon to spread to lung or other soft tissue sites

General Features
- Comments
  - Solid, vascular intramural/submucosal mass
  - Exophytic growth pattern (not usually infiltrative)
    - Can demonstrate intra- or extraluminal growth
  - Tumor may be heterogeneous with variable amount of necrosis/hemorrhage
  - Can occur anywhere along GI tract
    - Stomach (50-70%)
    - Duodenum and small intestine (20-25%)
    - Colon and rectum (5-10%)
    - Esophagus (2-5%)
  - In up to 10% of cases, can occur outside gut (extragastrointestinal GIST)
    - Retroperitoneum

- Mesentery
- Omentum
  - Majority (70-80%) of GISTs are benign
    - Risk of malignancy can be difficult to estimate
    - Potential for metastatic spread can be predicted by tumor size and histologic grading
- Genetics
  - c-KIT
    - Tyrosine kinase oncogene
    - Encodes for transmembrane growth factor receptor, CD117
    - More than 90% of patients with GIST have c-KIT mutations
    - Mutation results in upregulation of tyrosine kinase activity and altered cell growth
  - PDGFRA
    - Tyrosine kinase oncogene
    - Less than 10% of patients with GIST harbor a PDGFRA mutation
    - Involved with intracellular signaling pathways similar to c-KIT
- Etiology
  - Believed to arise from interstitial cells of Cajal
    - "Pacemaker" cells of GI tract
    - Thought to regulate peristalsis
  - Result of tyrosine kinase oncogene mutation (c-KIT, PDGFRA)
    - Results in unregulated cellular growth
  - No described environmental risk factors
- Epidemiology & cancer incidence
  - 4,500-6,000 new cases each year in USA
  - Equal sex predilection
  - Wide age range at presentation (typically 40-70 years but can occur earlier)
    - 75% of cases in patients > 50 years of age
    - Median age at presentation: 58-63 years
- Associated diseases, abnormalities
  - Vast majority of GISTs are sporadic and isolated
  - Carney triad
    - Association between GIST, pulmonary chondroma, and extraadrenal paraganglioma
    - Likely sporadic; no known genetic abnormality
    - Typically epithelioid variant of GIST
    - Strong female predilection (up to 85%)
    - Usually occur in stomach and may be multifocal
    - Minority of patients will have all 3 tumor types at presentation
    - GIST is often 1st tumor to present
  - Increased risk of GIST in patients with neurofibromatosis type 1 (NF1)
    - 5-25% of patients with NF1 will develop a GIST
    - Often multifocal
    - Predominate in small bowel (as opposed to stomach in sporadic GIST)
    - < 20% of lesions in NF1 patients with GIST will have typical c-KIT or PDGFRA mutations
    - Tumor may show S100 positivity (cell marker associated with neural differentiation)
    - Tend to be of low histologic grade and rarely metastatic
  - Familial GIST syndromes
    - Rare; due to inherited germline mutation of c-KIT or PDGFRA
    - Autosomal dominant mode of inheritance

GASTROINTESTINAL STROMAL TUMOR (GIST)

- GISTs tend to occur at younger age compared to nonfamilial GISTs
- Often associated with dermatological abnormalities

Gross Pathology & Surgical Features
- Friable, well-circumscribed mass
- Unencapsulated but may have pseudocapsule
- Larger tumors may demonstrate central necrosis, cystic degeneration, or hemorrhagic components
- Measure between 2-30 cm at presentation

Microscopic Pathology
- H&E
  - Spindle cell variant (70%)
  - Epithelioid variant (20%)
  - Mixed cell type (10%)
- Special stains
  - Immunophenotyping essential to differentiate from other mesenchymal tumors
    - CD117 (c-*KIT*) positive in nearly 100% of tumors
    - CD34 positive in 70-80% of tumors

IMAGING FINDINGS

Detection
- CECT of abdomen and pelvis
  - Primary imaging modality for tumor detection
  - Triple-phase examination may be helpful to evaluate tumor vascularity, but single portal venous phase acquisition with oral contrast is usually adequate for diagnosis
  - Mass arising from gut wall
    - Intramural growth pattern for small lesions, transmural appearance in larger masses
    - May also demonstrate intra- or extraluminal predominant growth pattern
    - Smaller tumors are often well defined
    - Larger tumors and those of higher grade often have more irregular margins
    - Invasion of adjacent structures not common and may suggest higher grade lesion
    - Larger lesion with extraluminal growth may appear as a nonspecific abdominal mass with originating loop of bowel draped along periphery
  - "Embedded organ" sign
    - Helpful in identifying organ of origin when large mass is found
      - Compressed hollow organ adjacent to mass → organ is not site of origin
      - When part of hollow organ appears embedded within mass → organ is likely site of origin
  - Avid contrast enhancement
    - Small tumors show homogeneous enhancement
    - Central necrosis and cystic changes are common in larger tumors (> 3 cm)
    - More heterogeneous enhancement may suggest higher grade tumor
  - Extragastrointestinal GISTs appear as nonspecific soft tissue density enhancing masses
    - Wide DDx necessitates biopsy
    - May be difficult to differentiate from metastatic disease; entire gut must be examined closely to exclude a small primary tumor

- Upper GI fluoroscopic examination
  - Smooth submucosal/mural mass lesion
  - May have irregular contour if necrotic or ulcerated
  - Necrotic components may communicate with gut lumen
  - Larger masses may displace adjacent bowel loops
  - Findings may be suggestive, but cross-sectional imaging necessary for complete characterization and evaluation for metastatic disease
- Endoscopy
  - Often an incidental finding
  - Mural/submucosal mass
  - Cross-sectional imaging necessary to evaluate extraluminal extent and presence of metastatic disease
- Ultrasound typically not helpful for characterization of primary tumor
  - Well-marginated masses closely associated with bowel
    - Often with preservation of typical gut wall signature
  - Smaller masses are typically homogeneously hypoechoic
  - May show internal heterogeneity with central anechoic components, representing hemorrhage/necrosis
  - Association between larger more heterogeneous tumors and higher malignant potential
  - Hepatic or peritoneal metastatic disease may be identified, though nonspecific in appearance
  - Hepatic metastatic disease may demonstrate a simple cystic appearance after therapy
- MR
  - Variable appearance based on degree of necrosis/hemorrhage
  - Solid portions of tumor will typically demonstrate ↓ T1 and ↑ T2 signal
  - Necrotic/hemorrhagic components will have variable signal intensity
  - Viable tumor enhances avidly
  - Hepatic and peritoneal/serosal metastatic disease may be appreciated

Staging
- Local staging (T)
  - T staging depends solely on maximum tumor size
    - T1: Tumor size ≤ 2 cm
    - T2: Tumor size > 2 cm but ≤ 5 cm
    - T3: Tumor size > 5 cm but ≤ 10 cm
    - T4: Tumor size > 10 cm
  - Diameter may be necessarily estimated in case of ruptured tumor
  - Depth of gut wall invasion not useful metric as most GISTs are transmural
  - Invasion of adjacent organs should be described, though does not influence tumor staging
- Nodal staging (N)
  - Lymph node involvement is rare
  - Nodal dissection usually not indicated at time of surgical resection unless suspicious nodes are seen at imaging
- Metastatic staging (M)
  - Intraabdominal spread (liver or peritoneum/serosa) most common

GASTROINTESTINAL STROMAL TUMOR (GIST)

- o Adherence of primary mass to liver does not constitute hepatic metastatic disease
- o Multiple primary GISTs (in setting of familial GIST or NF1) may be difficult to distinguish from metastases
- o Single omental, peritoneal, or retroperitoneal mass may represent primary GIST vs. metastatic spread from unknown primary
  - Extragastrointestinal GIST should be diagnosis of exclusion, and great care should be taken to evaluate for gut primary
- o Liver metastasis
  - Metastases are frequently hypervascular and may be missed if imaging is performed only during portal venous phase
- Histologic grading (G)
  - o Based on number of mitotic figures per 50 high-power fields (HPF)
    - ≤ 5 per 50 HPF = low grade (G1)
    - \> 5 per 50 HPF = high grade (G2)
- Imaging modalities
  - o CECT of abdomen and pelvis for staging
    - Single portal venous phase examination with oral and IV contrast is adequate
    - Baseline density measurements of mass (in Hounsfield units) should be noted, avoiding overtly necrotic components
    - Identification of hepatic metastatic disease critical
    - Careful attention should be paid to mesentery and peritoneum to evaluate for soft tissue nodular implants
    - While nodal involvement is rare, suspicious lymph nodes should be described
  - o CECT of chest often not necessary as GIST rarely demonstrates extraabdominal spread
  - o PET
    - Evaluate baseline SUV(max)
    - Evaluate for additional foci of uptake suggestive of metastatic disease
  - o Contrast-enhanced MR
    - Most helpful in evaluation of known/suspected rectal GIST
    - Pelvic sidewall and adjacent organ involvement should be noted
    - Early peritoneal or hepatic metastatic disease may be detected

Restaging

- No clear consensus on restaging interval, but therapy response can be seen as early as 1 week
- CECT is modality of choice for evaluating response to treatment
  - o Size and density (Hounsfield units) of primary tumor should be described and compared with pre-therapy values
  - o Size and density (Hounsfield units) of hepatic and mesenteric/peritoneal disease should be reported and compared with pre-therapy values
  - o Evaluate primary tumor for new enhancing nodular components (which suggest disease progression)
  - o Evaluate for new metastatic disease
- Pattern of response to imatinib on CECT
  - o ↓ tumor size

- Response typically takes several months before satisfying traditional tumor response criteria, such as the Response Evaluation Criteria in Solid Tumors (RECIST)
  - Restaging/evaluation for treatment response using RECIST criteria (tumor size only) may underestimate response
- o Transition from heterogeneously hyperattenuating pattern → homogeneously hypoattenuating pattern
- o Resolution of enhancing tumor nodules
- o ↓ tumor vascularity
- o ↓ tumor attenuation with development of myxoid degeneration and, occasionally, hemorrhage or necrosis
  - Term cyst or cystic change should be avoided when describing appearance of treated tumors at imaging
- o Paradoxically, tumors may ↑ in size during treatment
  - If associated with ↓ in tumor enhancement, does not indicate progression
  - Can be due to development of intratumoral hemorrhage or to myxoid degeneration
- Modified CT Response Evaluation Criteria were proposed because tumor response to therapy cannot be determined based on size alone
  - o Complete response
    - Resolution of all previously seen lesions
    - No new lesions
  - o Partial response
    - 10% or greater decrease in size of target lesions
    - 15% or greater decrease in density (measured in Hounsfield units) of target lesions
    - No obvious progression of nonmeasurable disease
    - No new lesions
  - o Stable disease
    - Not meeting criteria for either response or progression of disease
    - No symptomatic deterioration attributed to tumor progression
  - o Progressive disease
    - ≥ 10% increase in size of target lesions and absence of ≥ 15% drop in density (measured in Hounsfield units)
    - New lesions
    - New intratumoral nodules or increase in size of existing nodules
- PET
  - o Reevaluate SUV(max)
    - Grading of response based on changes in SUV(max) when compared with pre-therapy values
      - Grade 1: 25% or greater increase in SUV(max)
      - Grade 2: 15% decrease in SUV(max) to 25% increase in SUV(max)
      - Grade 3: 15% decrease in SUV(max) to 60% decrease in SUV(max)
      - Grade 4: 61% or greater decrease in SUV(max)
  - o Evaluate additional target lesions
  - o Evaluate for new foci of FDG uptake

GASTROINTESTINAL STROMAL TUMOR (GIST)

CLINICAL ISSUES

Presentation
- Anemia secondary to gastrointestinal bleeding, melena
- Palpable abdominal mass, often with obstructive symptoms
  - Abdominal pain, bloating
  - Nausea and vomiting
- Often incidentally detected in asymptomatic patients imaged for other reasons

Cancer Natural History & Prognosis
- Every GIST is considered potentially malignant, though most are benign
- Malignant potential may be predicted by tumor size and mitotic rate
- Site of origin may help predict malignant potential
  - Gastric tumors tend to have lower risk for metastasis, even for tumors > 5 cm (T3 and T4)
- Local recurrence occurs in up to 40-50% of patients after surgical resection
- Unresectable or metastatic disease can be treated with chemotherapy, often with significant reduction in tumor bulk
  - Recurrent or refractory tumors are common

Treatment Options
- Major treatment alternatives
  - Percutaneous or endoscopic biopsy often 1st step in diagnosis/management of suspected GIST
  - Most GISTs are surgical lesions
    - Often treated with wedge or segmental resection of affected organ owing to exophytic growth pattern
    - Wide resection is often necessary for esophageal or rectal GISTs
    - En bloc resection required for omental or mesenteric lesions
    - Laparoscopic resection may be considered for small tumors
    - Infiltrative/invasive growth may preclude complete surgical resection
    - Primary treatment goal is complete macro- and microscopic surgical resection
  - Lymph node dissection not routinely performed owing to rarity of lymph node metastasis
  - Traditional chemotherapy for sarcomas are largely ineffective against GIST
  - Imatinib mesylate (Gleevec or Glivec)
    - One of 1st "molecularly targeted" chemotherapeutics
    - ATP analog that binds to and inhibits intracellular portion of c-KIT-encoded cell membrane protein
    - Indicated for treatment of unresectable or metastatic disease
    - Well tolerated with minimal side effects
    - Resistance to therapy can occur
    - Also used in treatment of chronic myeloid leukemia
    - Often very rapid response to therapy with significant decrease in tumor burden over weeks to months
  - Sunitinib malate (Sutent)
    - Treatment alternative to imatinib mesylate
    - Inhibits multiple tyrosine kinases
    - May inhibit growth of imatinib-resistant GISTs
    - Second-line therapy for tumors resistant or unresponsive to imatinib mesylate
  - Adjuvant chemotherapy (with imatinib mesylate) for tumors thought to be high risk for metastasis, but without radiographic/pathologic evidence, remains experimental
- Major treatment roadblocks
  - Positive resection margins increase risk of subsequent peritoneal disease
    - Reexcision may be warranted if no evidence of serosal transgression
- Treatment options by stage
  - Standardized treatment approach based on stage not yet established owing to novelty of formal TNM stage grouping for GIST
  - Resectable disease (stages I-III)
    - Surgical resection is standard of care
    - If negative surgical margins and no evidence of metastatic or recurrent disease, therapy with imatinib mesylate may not be necessary
    - Stage or grade of tumor does not necessarily preclude surgical resection
  - Unresectable or metastatic disease (stage IV)
    - Surgical debulking may be considered (i.e., for palliative purposes)
    - Targeted chemotherapy with imatinib mesylate
    - Sunitinib malate may be considered for tumors refractory to imatinib mesylate

REPORTING CHECKLIST

T Staging
- Size and location of GIST
- Baseline density (prior to chemotherapy)
- Baseline SUV(max) on PET (prior to chemotherapy)
- Invasion of adjacent organs should be noted

N Staging
- While rare, suspicious lymph nodes are important to describe

M Staging
- Evidence of peritoneal or hepatic metastatic disease

Histologic Evaluation
- Initial staging also requires histologic evaluation for tumor grading

Restaging
- Evidence of recurrent or residual disease at primary mass resection site
- Change in size of unresected primary mass (in greatest dimensions) as marker of response
  - Decrease in size of at least 10% correlates with partial response
- Change in density of unresected primary mass (in Hounsfield units) as marker of response
  - Decrease in density of at least 15% correlates with partial response
- Change in SUV(max) on PET of unresected primary mass as marker of response

GASTROINTESTINAL STROMAL TUMOR (GIST)

- Change in size/density/SUV(max) of previously seen peritoneal or hepatic metastatic disease
- New lesions, or new nodules within existing lesions, which are suggestive of disease progression

SELECTED REFERENCES

1. American Joint Committee on Cancer: AJCC Cancer Staging Manual. 7th ed. New York: Springer. 175-80, 2010
2. Agaimy A et al: Lymph node metastasis in gastrointestinal stromal tumours (GIST) occurs preferentially in young patients < or = 40 years: an overview based on our case material and the literature. Langenbecks Arch Surg. 394(2):375-81, 2009
3. Wronski M et al: Gastrointestinal stromal tumors: ultrasonographic spectrum of the disease. J Ultrasound Med. 28(7):941-8, 2009
4. Choi H: Response evaluation of gastrointestinal stromal tumors. Oncologist. 13 Suppl 2:4-7, 2008
5. Badalamenti G et al: Gastrointestinal stromal tumors (GISTs): focus on histopathological diagnosis and biomolecular features. Ann Oncol. 18 Suppl 6:vi136-40, 2007
6. Choi H et al: Correlation of computed tomography and positron emission tomography in patients with metastatic gastrointestinal stromal tumor treated at a single institution with imatinib mesylate: proposal of new computed tomography response criteria. J Clin Oncol. 25(13):1753-9, 2007
7. Gutierrez JC et al: Optimizing diagnosis, staging, and management of gastrointestinal stromal tumors. J Am Coll Surg. 205(3):479-91 (Quiz 524), 2007
8. Hong X et al: Gastrointestinal stromal tumor: role of CT in diagnosis and in response evaluation and surveillance after treatment with imatinib. Radiographics. 26(2):481-95, 2006
9. Rubin BP: Gastrointestinal stromal tumours: an update. Histopathology. 48(1):83-96, 2006
10. Warakaulle DR et al: MDCT appearance of gastrointestinal stromal tumors after therapy with imatinib mesylate. AJR Am J Roentgenol. 186(2):510-5, 2006
11. King DM: The radiology of gastrointestinal stromal tumours (GIST). Cancer Imaging. 5:150-6, 2005
12. Shankar S et al: Gastrointestinal stromal tumor: new nodule-within-a-mass pattern of recurrence after partial response to imatinib mesylate. Radiology. 235(3):892-8, 2005
13. Burkill GJ et al: Malignant gastrointestinal stromal tumor: distribution, imaging features, and pattern of metastatic spread. Radiology. 226(2):527-32, 2003
14. Levy AD et al: Gastrointestinal stromal tumors: radiologic features with pathologic correlation. Radiographics. 23(2):283-304, 456; quiz 532, 2003
15. Sandberg AA et al: Updates on the cytogenetics and molecular genetics of bone and soft tissue tumors. gastrointestinal stromal tumors. Cancer Genet Cytogenet. 135(1):1-22, 2002
16. DeMatteo RP et al: Two hundred gastrointestinal stromal tumors: recurrence patterns and prognostic factors for survival. Ann Surg. 231(1):51-8, 2000

Duodenal GIST, Stage I (T2 N0 M0 G1)

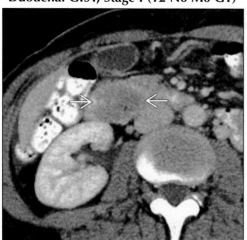

Duodenal GIST, Stage I (T2 N0 M0 G1)

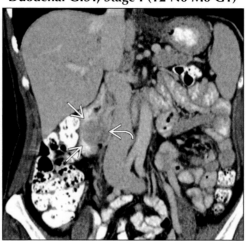

(Left) Axial CECT shows a subtle 3 cm intraluminal mass in the 2nd portion of the duodenum ➡. This was a stage I tumor based on size and low histologic grade. (Right) Coronal CECT in the same patient more clearly demonstrates the intraluminal, mural-based nature of this duodenal GIST ➡. A small extraluminal component is seen as well ➡. It is important to note the presence of hepatic and peritoneal metastatic disease when the presumed diagnosis is GIST.

Duodenal GIST, Stage I (T2 N0 M0 G1)

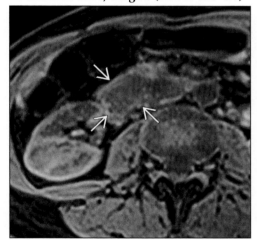

Duodenal GIST, Stage I (T2 N0 M0 G1)

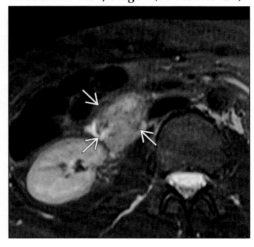

(Left) Axial T1WI FS MR in the same patient demonstrates an intraluminal duodenal GIST ➡ with homogeneously low T1 signal. (Right) Axial T2WI FS MR in the same patient demonstrates slightly increased signal of the GIST ➡ on T2-weighted images. GIST can be heterogeneous on both T1- and T2-weighted sequences secondary to hemorrhage and necrosis, though the solid components are typically T1 hypointense and T2 hyperintense.

Gastric GIST, Stage IA (T2 N0 M0 G1)

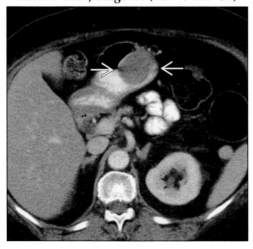

Gastric GIST, Stage IA (T2 N0 M0 G1)

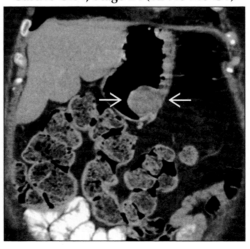

(Left) Axial CECT shows a classic appearance of a gastric GIST ➡. Based on size and low mitotic grade, this was stage IA disease. (Right) Coronal CECT in the same patient again shows the gastric GIST ➡, which tend to have a better prognosis when compared to GISTs arising from other locations.

GASTROINTESTINAL STROMAL TUMOR (GIST)

(Left) *Axial CECT demonstrates a 7 cm gastric GIST* ➡️. *This corresponds with stage IB disease based on lesion size and low histologic grade.* **(Right)** *Axial CECT shows a large intraluminal mass* ➡️ *arising from the gastric antrum. This was a stage II GIST based on size > 10 cm and low histologic grade. In the absence of metastatic disease, this patient may not require therapy with imatinib mesylate.*

Gastric GIST, Stage IB (T3 N0 M0 G1)

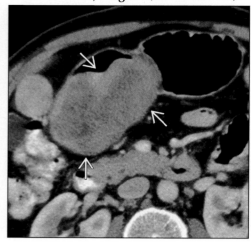

Gastric GIST, Stage II (T4 N0 M0 G1)

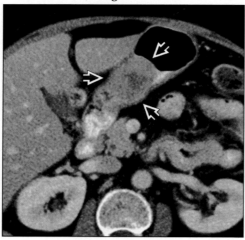

(Left) *Axial CECT shows a highly vascular tumor* ➡️ *supplied by a large mesenteric artery* ➡️ *within the terminal ileum in a 28-year-old woman with a history of neurofibromatosis type 1 who presented with iron deficiency anemia.* **(Right)** *Axial CECT in the same patient shows a large extraluminal component* ➡️ *of the highly vascular tumor within the right lower quadrant.*

**Small Bowel GIST,
Stage II (T3 N0 M0 G1)**

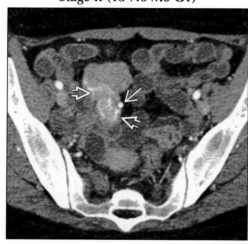

**Small Bowel GIST,
Stage II (T3 N0 M0 G1)**

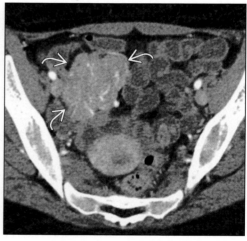

(Left) *Axial CECT in the same patient shows the highly vascular 7.5 cm tumor* ➡️ *with areas of necrosis* ➡️ *adjacent to the uterus* ➡️. **(Right)** *Coronal CECT in the same patient shows the dumbbell-shaped tumor with a small intramural* ➡️ *and larger extramural* ➡️ *components. Mitotic rate of less than 5 per 50 HPF was found on pathological evaluation. GISTs are the most common mesenchymal GI tumors in patients with neurofibromatosis type 1.*

**Small Bowel GIST,
Stage II (T3 N0 M0 G1)**

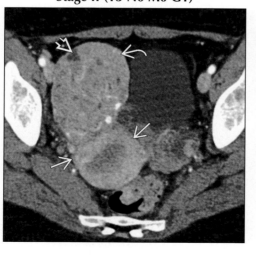

**Small Bowel GIST,
Stage II (T3 N0 M0 G1)**

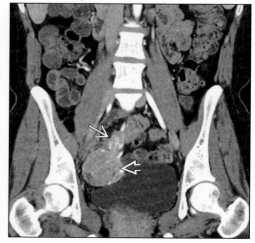

GASTROINTESTINAL STROMAL TUMOR (GIST)

Small Bowel GIST, Stage II (T3 N0 M0 G1)

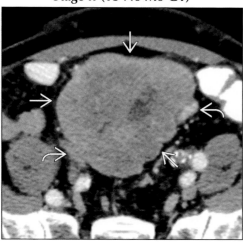

Small Bowel GIST, Stage II (T3 N0 M0 G1)

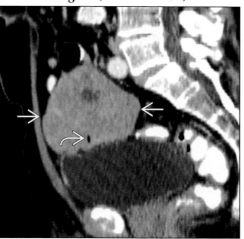

(Left) Axial CECT demonstrates a large, slightly heterogeneous GIST ➡ within the pelvis. The originating loop of small bowel is seen draped about the periphery of the mass ➡. This was stage II based on size and low mitotic grade. *(Right)* Sagittal CECT in the same patient again demonstrates a GIST ➡ arising from the distal small bowel. A punctate focus of air within the mass ➡ suggests fistulization with the bowel lumen.

Gastric GIST, Stage IIIA (T3 N0 M0 G2)

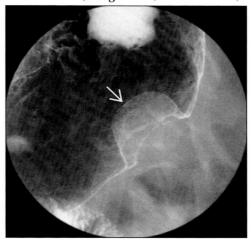

Gastric GIST, Stage IIIA (T3 N0 M0 G2)

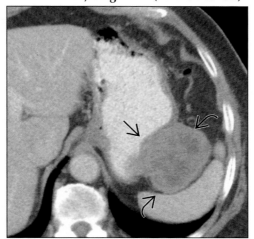

(Left) Frontal image from an upper GI shows a smooth gastric body mass ➡. This has relatively obtuse margins with the gastric contour, suggesting a mural origin. Cross-sectional imaging is required for further characterization and staging. *(Right)* Axial CECT in the same patient shows a heterogeneous GIST with a small intraluminal component ➡ and a larger exophytic component ➡. This was a stage IIIA lesion based on size and high tumor grade.

Sigmoid Colon GIST, Stage IIIA (T4 N0 M0 G1)

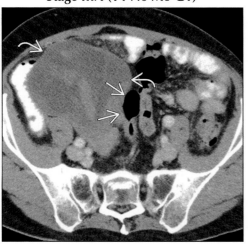

Sigmoid Colon GIST, Stage IIIA (T4 N0 M0 G1)

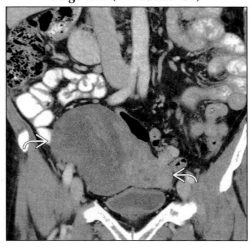

(Left) Axial CECT in a 68-year-old man who presented with anemia shows a 12 cm mass ➡ in the right lower quadrant that has a wide attachment to the sigmoid colon ➡ with a preserved patent lumen. The wall of the colon appears embedded within the mass. *(Right)* Coronal CECT in the same patient shows the large mass ➡ occupying the right lower quadrant. No mitotic figures were identified on pathological examination.

GASTROINTESTINAL STROMAL TUMOR (GIST)

Gastric GIST, Stage IIIB (T4 N0 M0 G2)

(Left) Oblique upper GI image shows mass effect and displacement of the stomach lumen, suggestive of gastric mass ➡️. Cross-sectional imaging is necessary for further evaluation and tumor staging. **(Right)** Axial CECT in the same patient demonstrates a large heterogeneous GIST displacing the stomach anteriorly ➡️. The mass demonstrates central low density ➡️, consistent with necrosis. This was stage IIIB based on tumor size and high histologic grade.

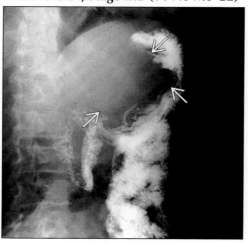

Gastric GIST, Stage IIIB (T4 N0 M0 G2)

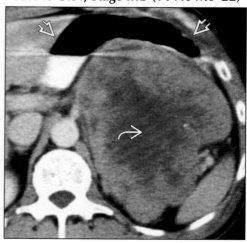

Esophageal GIST, Stage IIIB (T3 N0 M0 G2)

(Left) Axial CECT in a patient with dysphagia demonstrates a heterogeneous esophageal mass ➡️, which was found to be a GIST. Primary esophageal GIST is relatively uncommon. This was stage IIIB based on size and high histologic grade. **(Right)** Coronal fused PET/CT in the same patient shows increased metabolic activity within the esophageal GIST ➡️. It is important to look for hepatic or peritoneal hypermetabolic foci suggestive of metastatic disease.

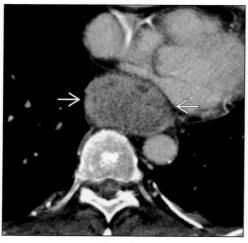

Esophageal GIST, Stage IIIB (T3 N0 M0 G2)

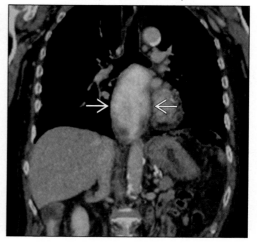

Gastric GIST, Stage IIIB (T4 N0 M0 G2)

(Left) Axial CECT shows a large, predominantly low-density GIST ➡️ within the upper abdomen with anterior displacement of the stomach ➡️. This was a stage IIIB GIST based on size > 10 cm and high mitotic grade. **(Right)** Coronal CECT in the same patient demonstrates the large necrotic GIST ➡️ arising from the stomach. Note the mural thickening and nodularity ➡️, which represents viable tumor.

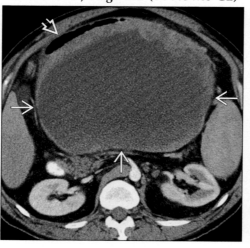

Gastric GIST, Stage IIIB (T4 N0 M0 G2)

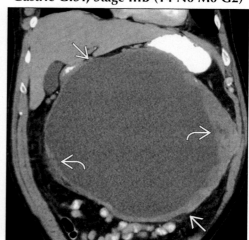

GASTROINTESTINAL STROMAL TUMOR (GIST)

Gastric GIST, Stage IIIB (T4 N0 M0 G2)

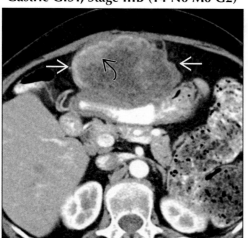

Gastric GIST, Stage IIIB (T4 N0 M0 G2)

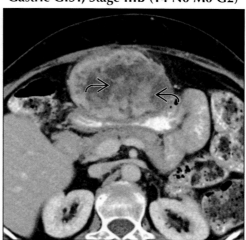

(Left) Axial CECT in the early arterial phase illustrates the hypervascularity of the viable tumor ⮕ in the periphery of this exophytic gastric GIST ⮕. This was stage IIIB based on tumor size and high histologic grade. *(Right)* Axial CECT in the delayed portal venous phase in the same patient shows more gradual enhancement of the partially necrotic tumor ⮕.

Rectal GIST, Stage IIIB (T4 N0 M0 G2)

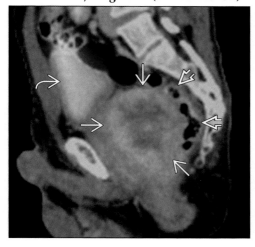

Rectal GIST, Stage IIIB (T4 N0 M0 G2)

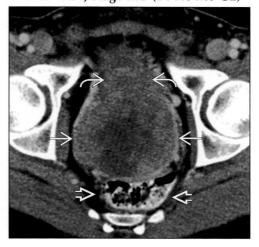

(Left) Sagittal fused PET/CT demonstrates a hypermetabolic mass ⮕ arising from the rectum, with mass effect on the bladder ⮕ and rectal lumen ⮕. This was found to be a GIST on biopsy. Based on size and high tumor grade, this was stage IIIB. *(Right)* Axial CECT in the same patient shows the centrally necrotic rectal GIST ⮕ with mass effect on the adjacent prostate ⮕ and rectum ⮕.

Rectal GIST, Stage IIIB (T4 N0 M0 G2)

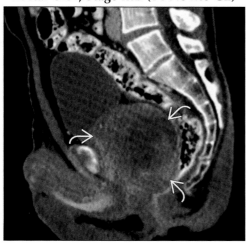

Rectal GIST, Stage IIIB (T4 N0 M0 G2), After Therapy

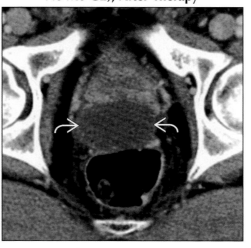

(Left) Sagittal CECT in the same patient demonstrates the relationship of the rectal GIST ⮕ with the adjacent pelvic organs. CE MR of the pelvis can be useful in evaluating for pelvic sidewall and adjacent organ invasion. *(Right)* Axial CECT in the same patient after therapy with imatinib mesylate shows a dramatic decrease in size and attenuation of the rectal GIST ⮕, consistent with a response to therapy.

GASTROINTESTINAL STROMAL TUMOR (GIST)

Recurrent Gastric GIST, Stage IIIB (T4 N0 M0 G2)

(Left) Axial CECT demonstrates a large, heterogeneous recurrent GIST ➡ within the lesser sac. The stomach is displaced anteriorly ➡. The original tumor was stage IIIB based on size and high histologic grade. *(Right)* Coronal CECT in the same patient again demonstrates a recurrent GIST ➡ in the lesser sac. Metallic densities ➡ and associated streak artifact ➡ are related to initial tumor resection.

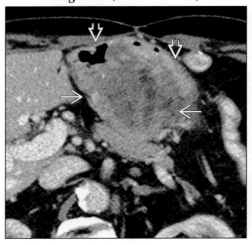

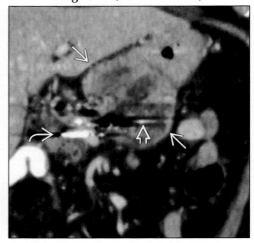

Small Bowel GIST, Stage IV (T3 N0 M1 G2)

(Left) Coronal PET/CT shows a heterogeneous pelvic mass with increased metabolic activity, consistent with a small bowel GIST ➡. A subtle hypoattenuating hypermetabolic right hepatic lobe mass ➡ represents metastatic disease. Note urinary bladder ➡. *(Right)* Axial CECT in the same patient shows a GIST metastasis ➡ to the liver with central necrosis. It is important to note baseline size and density measurements for comparison with post-therapy studies.

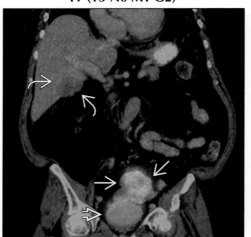

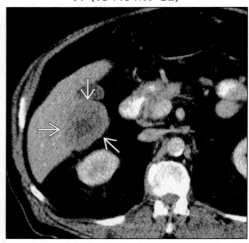

Small Bowel GIST, Stage IV (T3 N0 M1 G2), After Therapy

(Left) Axial CECT in the same patient after therapy with imatinib mesylate shows an interval decrease in size and density of the primary small bowel GIST ➡. *(Right)* Axial CECT in the same patient, after therapy with imatinib mesylate, also shows decreased size and density of the hepatic metastatic lesion ➡. A decrease in size &/or density on follow-up CT, without new lesions, correlates with a partial response to therapy.

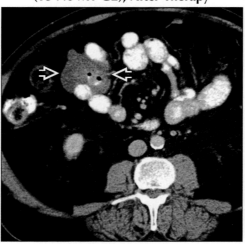

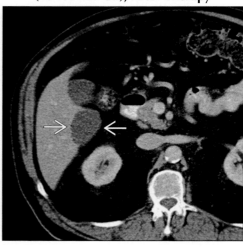

GASTROINTESTINAL STROMAL TUMOR (GIST)

Gastric GIST, Stage IV (T3 N0 M1 G2)

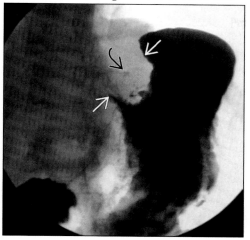

Gastric GIST, Stage IV (T3 N0 M1 G2)

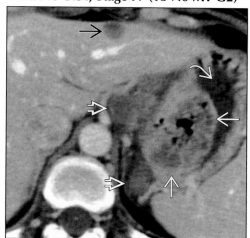

(Left) Frontal image from an upper GI shows an irregular gastric mass ➡ of mural origin. A small focus of contrast centrally within the mass ➡ indicates central necrosis with luminal communication. (Right) Axial CECT in the same patient shows a necrotic gastric GIST ➡ with central air, indicating communication with the gastric lumen ➡. It is important to note the hepatic metastasis ➡ and peritoneal spread ➡. This is a stage IV lesion.

Gastric GIST, Stage IV (T3 N0 M1 G2)

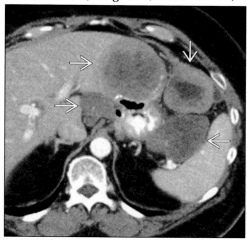

Gastric GIST, Stage IV (T3 N0 M1 G2)

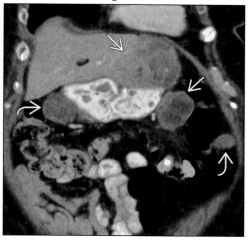

(Left) Axial CECT in a patient status post partial gastrectomy for prior GIST shows several heterogeneous masses ➡ about the resection margin, consistent with recurrent/residual disease. The presence of peritoneal disease makes this a stage IV lesion. (Right) Coronal CECT in the same patient again demonstrates recurrent/residual GIST at the partial gastrectomy surgical margins ➡. Additional peritoneal metastatic disease is also shown ➡.

Gastric GIST, Stage IV (T3 N0 M1 G2), After Therapy

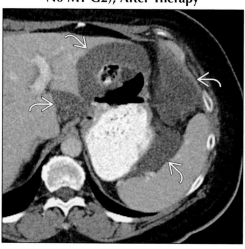

Gastric GIST, Stage IV (T3 N0 M1 G2), After Therapy

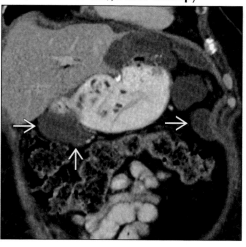

(Left) Axial CECT in the same patient after therapy with imatinib mesylate shows a partial response to therapy with decreased size and density of target lesions ➡. Treated GIST can often appear completely cystic. (Right) Coronal CECT in the same patient after therapy with imatinib mesylate shows a decrease in density of the peritoneal metastases as well ➡, consistent with a partial response to therapy.

GASTROINTESTINAL STROMAL TUMOR (GIST)

Gastric GIST, Stage IV (T2 N0 M1 G2)

Gastric GIST, Stage IV (T2 N0 M1 G2)

(Left) Axial CECT shows a GIST ➡ arising from the lesser curvature of the stomach. This lesion demonstrated an extraluminal growth pattern. *(Right)* Coronal CECT in the same patient again demonstrates a gastric GIST ➡ along the lesser curvature. A solitary liver metastasis ➡ is noted as well, making this stage IV disease.

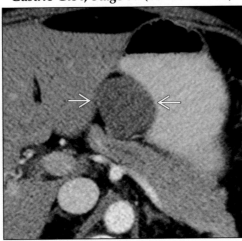

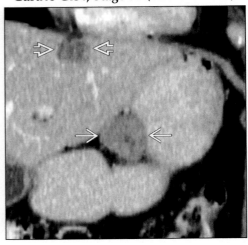

Liver Metastases, Stage IV

Liver Metastases, Stage IV, After Therapy

(Left) Axial CECT demonstrates several necrotic masses ➡ within the liver, representing metastases in this patient with a GIST. *(Right)* Axial CECT in the same patient after therapy with imatinib mesylate demonstrates a decrease in density of the hepatic metastases ➡, consistent with a response to therapy.

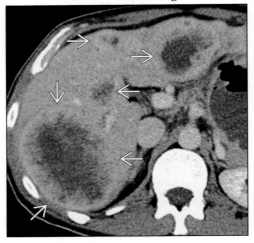

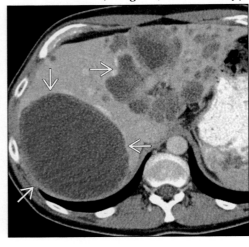

Liver Metastases, Stage IV, After Therapy

Small Bowel GIST, Stage IV

(Left) Longitudinal transabdominal ultrasound in the same patient after treatment with imatinib mesylate illustrates the cystic appearance of treated GIST metastases ➡. A partially treated, more solid-appearing mass is noted as well (calipers). *(Right)* Axial CECT shows a partially necrotic small bowel GIST ➡ with stranding of the superficial soft tissues ➡ from recent biopsy. Peritoneal metastasis ➡ makes this stage IV disease, regardless of GIST origin.

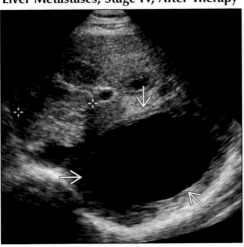

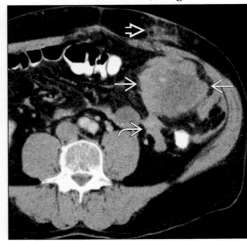

GASTROINTESTINAL STROMAL TUMOR (GIST)

Esophageal GIST, Stage IV (T2 N0 M1 G2)

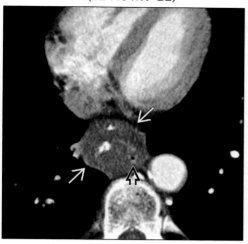

Esophageal GIST, Stage IV (T2 N0 M1 G2)

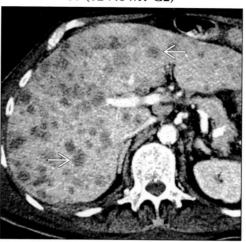

(Left) Axial CECT shows a low-density GIST arising from the mid esophagus ➡. GISTs may occasionally show calcification. The eccentric nature of the mass, with displacement of the esophageal lumen ⤶, suggests a mural origin. *(Right)* Axial CECT in the same patient shows hypoattenuating lesions throughout the liver ➡, representing metastatic GIST and making this a stage IV tumor. Metastatic disease is an indication for imatinib mesylate therapy.

Gastric GIST, Stage IV (T2 N0 M1 G2)

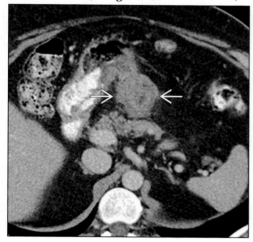

Gastric GIST, Stage IV (T2 N0 M1 G2)

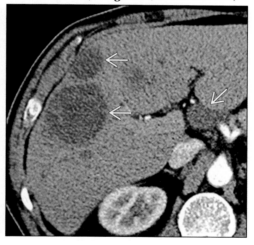

(Left) Axial CECT demonstrates a gastric GIST ➡ arising from the lesser curvature with an extraluminal growth pattern. Concurrent hepatic metastatic disease makes this a stage IV lesion. *(Right)* Axial CECT in the same patient demonstrates several hepatic metastases ➡. The liver is the most common site of metastasis from GIST.

Gastric GIST, Stage IV (T2 N0 M1 G2), After Therapy

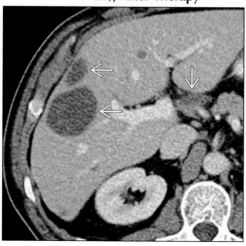

Gastric GIST, Stage IV (T2 N0 M1 G2), Recurrence After Therapy

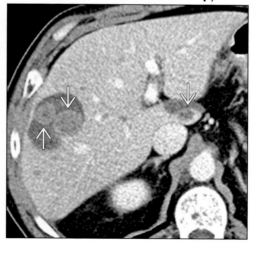

(Left) Axial CECT in the same patient after therapy with imatinib mesylate demonstrates a decrease in size and density of the hepatic metastases ➡, consistent with a response to therapy. *(Right)* Axial CECT in the same patient at follow-up demonstrates the development of enhancing intratumoral nodules ➡, representing recurrent disease. This patient developed resistance to imatinib mesylate and could be a candidate for sunitinib malate.

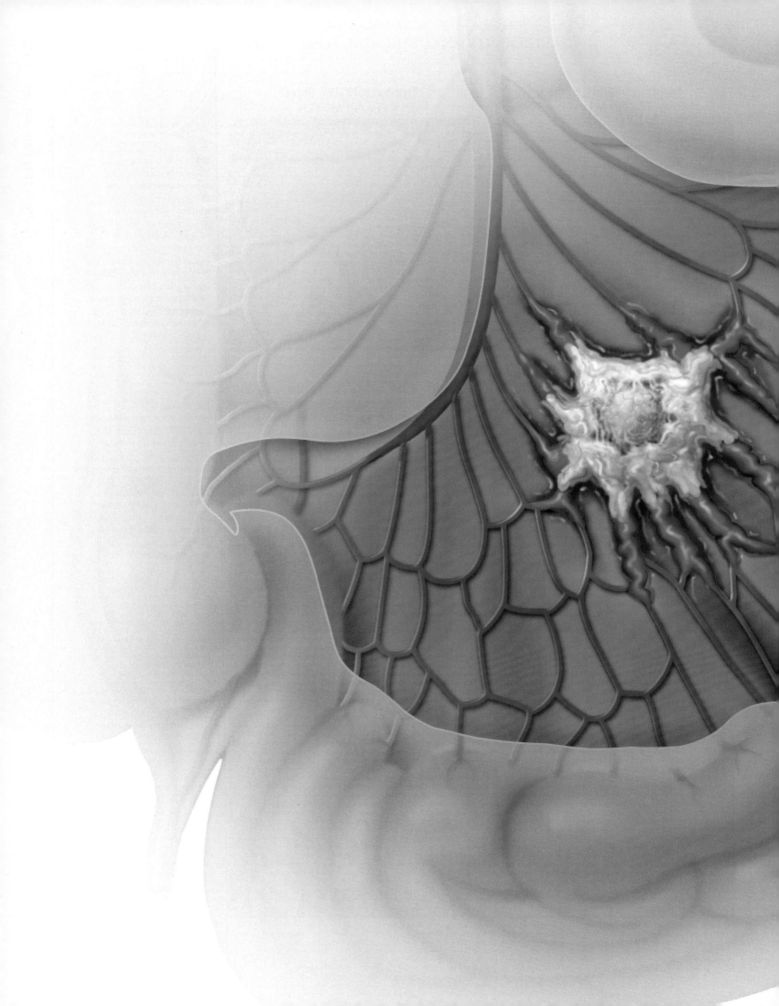

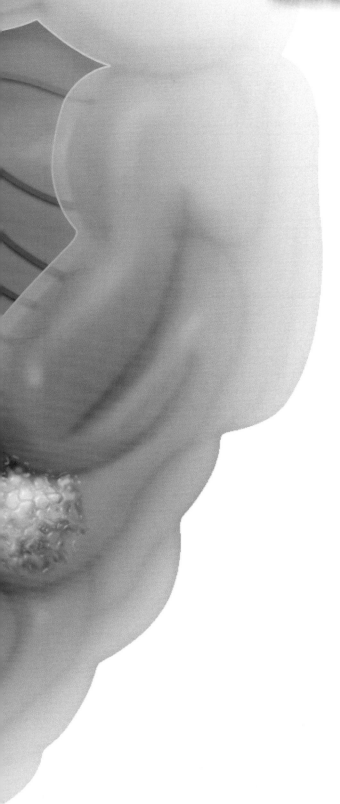

Neuroendocrine Tumors

NEUROENDOCRINE TUMORS

(T) Primary Tumor, Neuroendocrine Tumors of Stomach

Adapted from 7th edition AJCC Staging Forms.

TNM	Definitions
TX	Primary tumor cannot be assessed
T0	No evidence of primary tumor
Tis	Carcinoma in situ/dysplasia (tumor size < 0.5 mm), confined to mucosa
T1	Tumor invades lamina propria or submucosa and ≤ 1 cm in size
T2	Tumor invades muscularis propria or > 1 cm in size
T3	Tumor penetrates subserosa
T4	Tumor invades visceral peritoneum (serosal) or other organs or adjacent structures

For any T, add (m) for multiple tumors.

(T) Primary Tumor, Neuroendocrine Tumors of Duodenum/Ampulla/Jejunum/Ileum

Adapted from 7th edition AJCC Staging Forms.

TNM	Definitions
TX	Primary tumor cannot be assessed
T0	No evidence of primary tumor
T1	Tumor invades lamina propria or submucosa and size ≤ 1 cm* (small intestinal tumors); tumor ≤ 1 cm (ampullary tumors)
T2	Tumor invades muscularis propria or size > 1 cm (small intestinal tumors); tumor > 1 cm (ampullary tumors)
T3	Tumor invades through the muscularis propria into subserosal tissue without penetration of overlying serosa (jejunal or ileal tumors) or invades pancreas or retroperitoneum (ampullary or duodenal tumors) or into nonperitonealized tissues
T4	Tumor invades visceral peritoneum (serosa) or invades other organs

For any T, add (m) for multiple tumors.

*Tumor limited to ampulla of Vater for ampullary gangliocytic paraganglioma.

(T) Primary Tumor, Neuroendocrine Tumors of Colon or Rectum

Adapted from 7th edition AJCC Staging Forms.

TNM	Definitions
TX	Primary tumor cannot be assessed
T0	No evidence of primary tumor
T1	Tumor invades lamina propria or submucosa and size ≤ 2 cm
T1a	Tumor size < 1 cm in greatest dimension
T1b	Tumor size 1-2 cm in greatest dimension
T2	Tumor invades muscularis propria or size > 2 cm with invasion of lamina propria or submucosa
T3	Tumor invades through the muscularis propria into the subserosa or into nonperitonealized pericolic or perirectal tissues
T4	Tumor invades peritoneum or other organs

For any T, add (m) for multiple tumors.

NEUROENDOCRINE TUMORS

(N) Regional Lymph Nodes for All Neuroendocrine Tumors

Adapted from 7th edition AJCC Staging Forms.

TNM	Definitions
NX	Regional lymph nodes cannot be assessed
N0	No regional lymph node metastasis
N1	Regional lymph node metastasis

(M) Distant Metastasis for All Neuroendocrine Tumors

Adapted from 7th edition AJCC Staging Forms.

TNM	Definitions
M0	No distant metastases
M1	Distant metastasis

AJCC Stages/Prognostic Grouping for All Neuroendocrine Tumors

Adapted from 7th edition AJCC Staging Forms.

Stage	T	N	M
0	Tis	N0	M0
I	T1	N0	M0
IIA	T2	N0	M0
IIB	T3	N0	M0
IIIA	T4	N0	M0
IIIB	Any T	N1	M0
IV	Any T	Any N	M1

NEUROENDOCRINE TUMORS

Stomach NET: T1

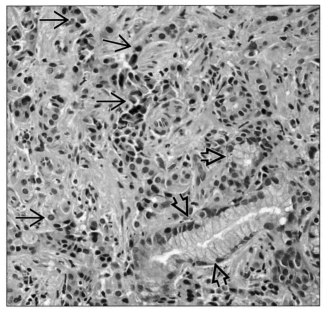

H&E of gastric mucosa shows neoplastic cells ⇨ arranged in small nests, cords, and single cells infiltrating the lamina propria in between benign glands ⧨. The cells show abundant eosinophilic cytoplasm and small round nuclei suggesting neoroendocrine differentation. (Original magnification 400x.)

Stomach NET: T1

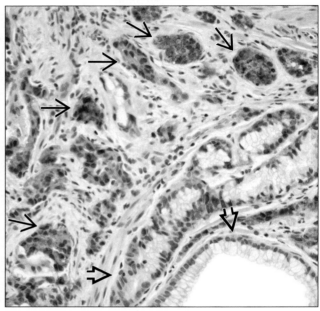

Immunohistochemically stained section for synaptophysin antibody in the same case shows positive (brown) staining of neoplastic cells ⇨. Cells were also positive for chromogranin. Note negative staining of the epithelial cells of benign glands ⧨. (Original magnification 400x.)

Duodenal NET: T1

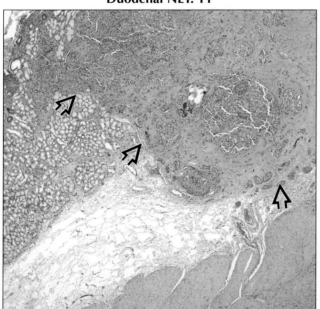

H&E shows a duodenal invasive neuroendocrine tumor. The tumor ⧨ is < 1 cm in the largest dimension and involves both the mucosa as well as the submucosa but does not extend to involve the muscularis propria. (Original magnification 40x.)

Duodenal NET: T1

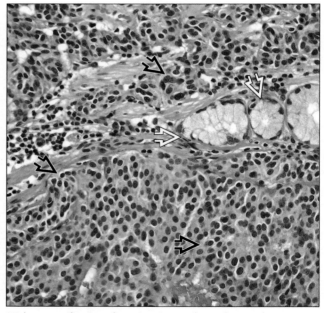

Higher magnification of previous image shows the neoplastic cells ⧨ arranged in nests and sheets in both the mucosa and the submucosa with adjacent Brunner glands ⇨. (Original magnification 400x.)

Ileal NET: T2

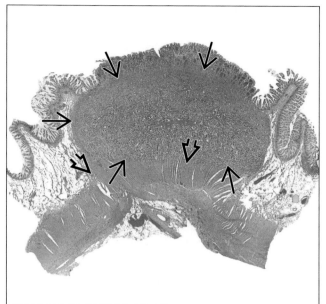

Whole mount of an H&E stained section of full thickness from ileum shows the tumor ⇲ occupies most of the thickness, including the lower aspect of the mucosa and submucosa, and infiltrates the inner circular muscle of the muscularis propria ⇲. The tumor is 13 mm in its largest dimension.

Ileal NET: T2

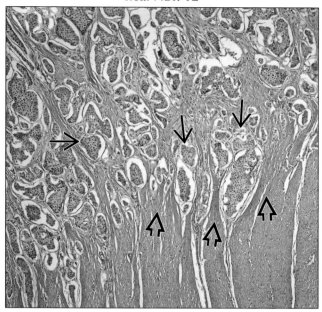

Higher magnification of previous image shows nests of neoplastic cells ⇲ infiltrating the thick bundles of the inner circular layer of the muscularis propria ⇲. (Original magnification 100x.)

Rectal NET: T1a

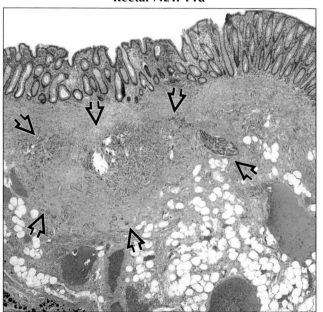

H&E stained section of rectum with invasive neuroendocrine carcinoma shows a 4 mm tumor ⇲ limited to the submucosa. (Original magnification 40x.)

Rectal NET: T1a

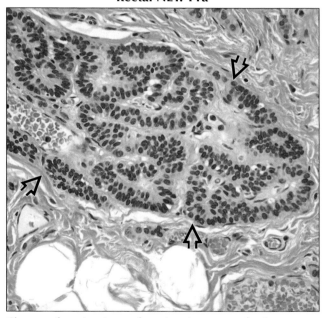

Close-up of previous image shows invasive neuroendocrine carcinoma ⇲ composed of small cells with bland round nuclei arranged in ribbons. (Original magnification 400x.)

NEUROENDOCRINE TUMORS

Stomach NET: Tis and T1

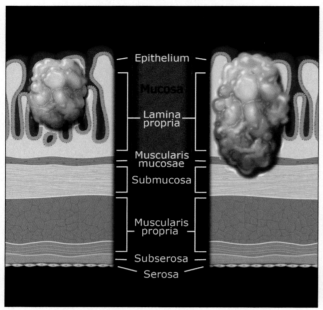

Graphic illustrates Tis (left) and T1 (right) gastric NETs. Tis (carcinoma in situ/dysplasia) is a tumor < 5 mm, limited to the mucosa. T1 is a tumor that invades lamina propria or submucosa and is ≤ 1 cm in size.

Stomach NET: T2 and T3

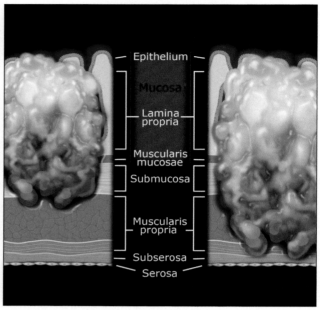

Graphic illustrates T2 (left) and T3 (right) gastric NETs. T2 is a tumor that invades the muscularis propria or is > 1 cm. T3 is a tumor that invades subserosa.

Stomach NET: T4

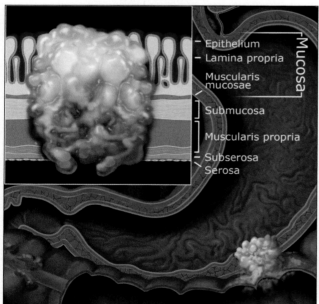

Graphic illustrates a T4 gastric NET invading the transverse colon. T4 is a tumor that invades visceral peritoneum or other adjacent organs and structures.

Stomach NET Nodal Drainage

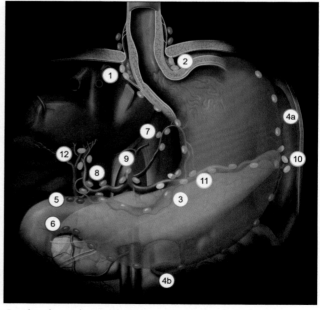

Graphic shows the nodal stations of the stomach: Perigastric nodes of lesser curvature (1, 3, and 5); perigastric nodes of greater curvature (2, 4A, 4B, and 6); left gastric nodes (7); nodes along common hepatic artery (8); nodes along celiac artery (9); nodes along splenic artery (10 and 11); and hepatoduodenal nodes (12).

Small Intestinal NET: T1 and T2

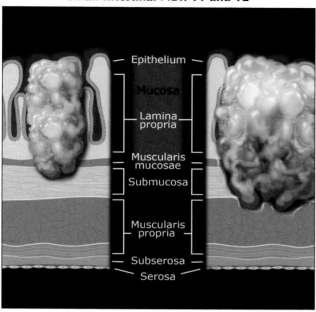

Graphic illustrates T1 (left) and T2 (right) small intestinal (including ampullary) NETs. T1 is a tumor that invades lamina propria or submucosa and is ≤ 1 cm in size. T2 is a tumor that invades muscularis propria or is > 1 cm in size.

Small Intestinal NET: T3

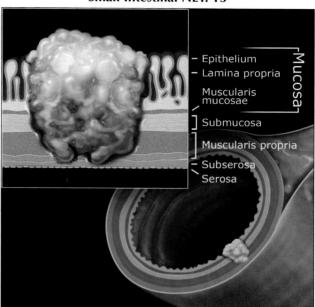

Graphic illustrates a T3 small intestinal (including ampullary) NET. T3 applies to a jejunal or ileal tumor that invades through the muscularis propria into subserosa without penetrating serosa, an ampullary or duodenal tumor that invades pancreas or retroperitoneum, or any NET that invades nonperitonealized tissues.

Small Intestinal NET: T4

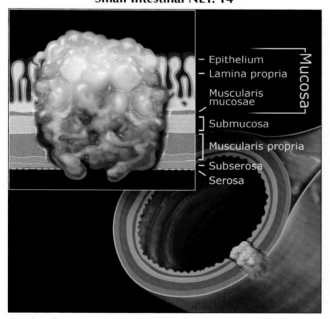

Graphic illustrates a T4 small intestinal (including ampullary) NET. T4 is a tumor that invades visceral peritoneum (serosa) or surrounding structures.

Small Intestinal NET: Mesenteric Metastasis

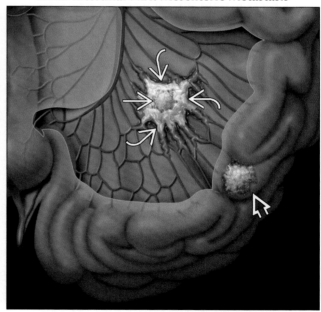

Graphic illustrates a mesnteric nodal mass ➡ surrounded by extensive fibrotic reaction ⇒ resulting from tissue response to substances released by the primary tumor ⇛ or the mesenteric nodal mass.

NEUROENDOCRINE TUMORS

Colorectal NET: T1a and T1b

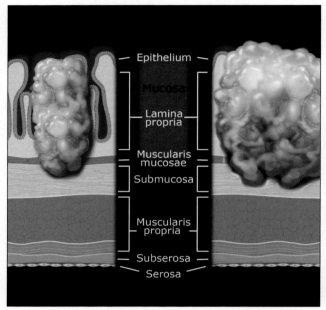

Graphic illustrates T1a (left) and T1b (right) colorectal NETs. T1 is a tumor that invades lamina propria or submucosa and is < 2 cm in size. T1a is < 1 cm and T1b is 1-2 cm in greatest dimensions.

Colorectal NET: T2

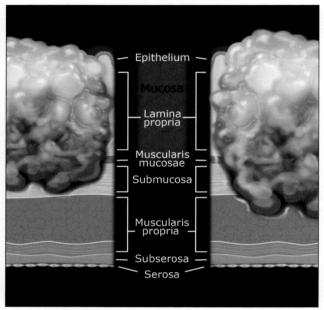

Graphic illustrates T2 colorectal NETs. T2 is a tumor that invades lamina propria or submucosa and is > 2 cm in size (left) or invades muscularis propria (right).

Colorectal NET: T3

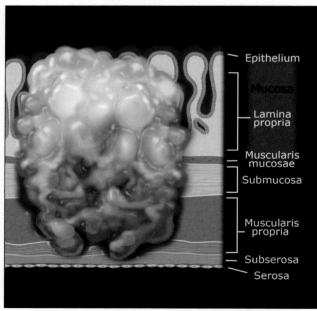

Graphic illustrates a T3 colorectal NET. T3 is a tumor that invades through the muscularis propria into subserosa without penetrating serosa or into nonperitonealized pericolic or perirectal tissues.

Colorectal NET: T4

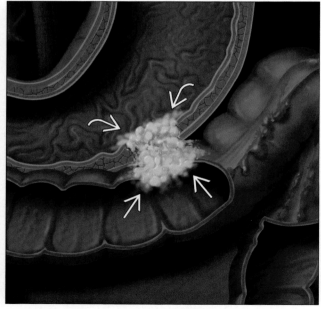

Graphic illustrates a T4 colorectal NET ⇥ invading the gastric body ⇥. T4 is a tumor that invades visceral peritoneum or other adjacent organs and structures.

Colorectal NET Nodal Drainage

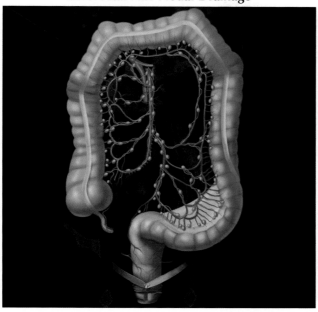

Graphic illustrates colonic nodal drainage. Pericolic nodes drain into the superior mesenteric nodes (along the right and middle colic vessels) for tumors in the ascending and transverse colon and into the inferior mesenteric nodes (along the left colic vessels) for tumors of descending and sigmoid colon.

Lymphatic Drainage of Rectum

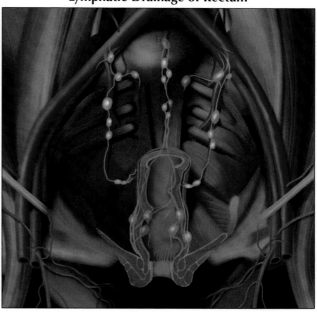

Graphic illustrates nodal drainage of the middle and lower rectum. Perirectal nodes drain into the internal iliac lymph nodes.

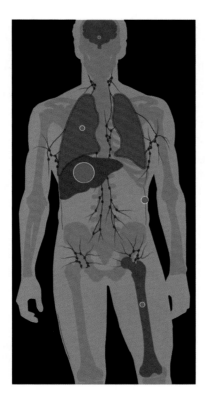

METASTASES, ORGAN FREQUENCY

Liver	85%
Peritoneum	18%
Bone	8-10%
Lung	4%
Brain	1%

NEUROENDOCRINE TUMORS

OVERVIEW

General Comments

- Neuroendocrine tumors (NETs) of the gastrointestinal (GI) tract originate from cells derived from embryonic neural crest, neuroectoderm, and endoderm
  - Usually produce bioactive substances and show immunoreactivity to neuroendocrine markers
- Carcinoids are rare NETs arising from enterochromaffin (Kulchitsky) cells found throughout crypts of Lieberkühn of gut
- This chapter covers gastric, small intestinal, colonic, rectal, and ampulla of Vater carcinoid and malignant carcinoid tumors
  - Pancreatic and appendiceal NETs are staged and discussed separately

Classification

- In clinical practice, terms GI NET and carcinoid are used interchangeably
- World Health Organization classification scheme for neuroendocrine tumors
  - Differentiates NET on basis of biologic behavior (malignant potential)
    - Well-differentiated endocrine tumors (carcinoids)
      - Proliferation index (PI) < 2%
      - Benign behavior or uncertain malignant potential
    - Well-differentiated endocrine carcinomas (malignant carcinoids)
      - PI > 2% but < 15%
      - Low-grade malignancy
    - Poorly differentiated endocrine carcinomas
      - PI > 15%
      - High-grade malignancy
    - Mixed exocrine-endocrine tumors
    - Tumor-like lesions
- Classification schemes contain subdivisions based on location and morphologic criteria
  - Tumor locations include
    - Stomach
      - Type I
      - Type II
      - Type III
      - Type IV
    - Duodenum and proximal jejunum
    - Distal jejunum and ileum
    - Appendix
    - Colorectum
    - Pancreas
  - Morphologic biologic criteria include
    - Tumor size
    - Vascular invasion
    - Mitotic activity
    - Histologic differentiation
    - Presence of metastases
    - Invasion of adjacent organs

PATHOLOGY

Routes of Spread

- Local spread

- Most GI NETs have expansile rather than infiltrative growth pattern
  - Tumor growth by size increase rather than invasion of surrounding structures
- GI NETs differ in their propensity for local spread
  - Gastric carcinoids
    - Types I & II are usually localized to gastric wall
    - Types III & IV are more likely to infiltrate into perigastric tissues
  - Duodenal carcinoids
    - Usually localized to duodenal wall
    - May infiltrate into pancreas and retroperitoneum
  - Jejunoileal carcinoids
    - Infiltrative growth pattern with tumor extension into mesentery
  - Colorectal carcinoids
    - Rarely infiltrate into surrounding structures
- Nodal spread
  - Regional nodal spread can occur with GI NET
    - Rare in types I & II gastric carcinoids
  - Jejunoileal carcinoids
    - Frequently have metastatic foci in mesenteric lymph nodes surrounded by severe fibrotic reaction
    - Possible involvement of serotonin in pathogenesis of fibrosis
    - Probably mediated via 5HT2B receptor
  - Colorectal carcinoids
    - Drain to pericolorectal nodes
      - Eventually to superior and inferior mesenteric nodes with colonic carcinoids
      - Eventually to internal iliac and inguinal nodes with rectal carcinoids
- Distant metastases
  - Liver is most common site of distant metastases
    - Hepatic involvement is usually needed to develop carcinoid syndrome
  - Other sites include lungs, bones, and brain
  - Peritoneal spread
    - Not as common as with adenocarcinoma of GI tract
    - Peritoneal metastases are considered distant metastases

General Features

- Genetics
  - Majority of NETs occur sporadically
  - Can be part of multiple endocrine neoplasia (MEN1) and neurofibromatosis type 1
- Etiology
  - Most GI NETs are sporadic with no obvious underlying etiology
  - Types I & II gastric carcinoids are associated with hypergastrinemia
    - Type I gastric carcinoid
      - Associated with autoimmune chronic atrophic gastritis
      - ↓ hydrochloric acid-producing parietal cells → achlorhydria → ↑ gastrin production → stimulation of enterochromaffin-like (ECL) cell hyperplasia → development of multiple carcinoids
    - Type II gastric carcinoid

NEUROENDOCRINE TUMORS

- Gastrin-producing tumors in Zollinger-Ellison syndrome (ZES) in patients with MEN1
- Gastrin-producing endocrine neoplasm of pancreas or small intestine → hypergastrinemia → stimulation of ECL-cell hyperplasia → development of multiple carcinoids
- Epidemiology & cancer incidence
  ○ Carcinoids most frequently occur in GI tract (66.9%), followed by tracheobronchial system (24.5%)
  ○ 1.2–1.5% of all gastrointestinal neoplasms
  ○ Incidence of 1.6–2.0 new cases per 100,000 persons per year

Gross Pathology & Surgical Features
- General features
  ○ GI carcinoids originate from endocrine cells that populate mucosa and submucosa
  ○ White, yellow, or gray firm nodules in gastric or intestinal wall
  ○ May be intramural masses or intraluminal polypoid nodules
  ○ Overlying mucosa may be intact or have focal ulceration
- Stomach
  ○ Rare
    ▪ < 1% of gastric neoplasms
  ○ 4-9% of all GI NETs
  ○ Main neuroendocrine cells in gastric fundus and body are
    ▪ Enterochromaffin-like (ECL) cells
    ▪ Serotonin-containing enterochromaffin (EC) cells
    ▪ Somatostatin-containing D cells
  ○ 4 types of carcinoids of stomach
    ▪ **Type I gastric carcinoids**
      - Most common type of gastric NET (70–80% of cases)
      - ECL-cell carcinoids
      - Associated with chronic autoimmune atrophic gastritis ± pernicious anemia
      - Grow from fundus and body
      - Small (< 2 cm), often multiple
      - Resembles other more common submucosal tumors at endoscopy and radiology
      - Most are benign, but metastases reported in 3-5% of patients
    ▪ **Type II carcinoids**
      - ECL-cell carcinoids
      - Associated with MEN1 and ZES
      - Least common type of gastric NET (5-10% of cases)
      - ZES–MEN1 patients have 29–34% risk of developing type II gastric carcinoid
      - Small (< 2 cm), often multiple
      - Most are benign, but metastases reported in 10–30% of patients
    ▪ **Type III carcinoids**
      - ECL-cell carcinoids
      - Sporadic tumors, occur in absence of underlying gastric disease or hypergastrinemia
      - 13-20% of gastric carcinoids
      - Usually large (> 2 cm) single
      - Located in body and fundus

- Typically show vascular invasion at time of diagnosis
- Often manifest with metastases, which are found in 50–70% of gastric well-differentiated neuroendocrine carcinomas and in up to 100% of gastric poorly differentiated endocrine carcinomas
    ▪ **Type IV carcinoids**
      - Consist of poorly differentiated endocrine carcinomas and mixed exocrine-endocrine carcinomas
      - Usually > 5 cm, often ulcerating
      - Usually surgically unresectable with poor prognosis
- Duodenum
  ○ Rare: < 3% of GI NETs
  ○ Mostly sporadic, nonfunctioning, and arise in proximal duodenum
  ○ May occasionally be functioning and manifest with Zollinger-Ellison syndrome
  ○ May be seen with neurofibromatosis type 1 or MEN1
    ▪ 30% of patients with periampullary carcinoid tumors also have neurofibromatosis type 1
  ○ Rarely > 2 cm in size
    ▪ Large tumors may metastasize to regional lymph nodes or liver in 40% of patients
- Jejunum and ileum
  ○ Most frequently arise in submucosa of terminal ileum
  ○ Multiple primary tumor sites are found in 29–41% of cases
  ○ Size of small intestine carcinoids is unreliable predictor of metastatic potential
  ○ Metastatic spread is common
    ▪ Regional nodal disease occurs in 70% of patients
    ▪ Liver metastases in > 50%
  ○ Desmoplastic reaction induced around mesenteric nodal metastases → contraction of mesentery and kinking of bowel
    ▪ Mesenteric vessels become occluded from this desmoplastic reaction → chronic bowel
- Colorectum
  ○ Colonic NETs are very rare
  ○ Histologically, these are poorly differentiated neuroendocrine carcinomas
    ▪ Almost all have already metastasized at time of diagnosis
    ▪ Poor prognosis
- Hepatic metastases are generally required for serotonin to access systemic circulation in patients with NETs arising from gut
  ○ Liver deactivates serotonin before reaching systemic circulation
  ○ Carcinoid syndrome can occur without liver metastases in following situations
    ▪ Tumor extending into retroperitoneal tissues
      - Drainage by systemic circulation bypassing liver
    ▪ Large tumor burden
    ▪ Liver dysfunction

Microscopic Pathology
- H&E
  ○ Solid acinar or insular nests of closely packed cells that are uniform in size

NEUROENDOCRINE TUMORS

- ○ Nests may be arranged in glandular rosettes or trabeculae separated by delicate stroma
- ○ Nuclei are round or oval with finely stippled chromatin with no hyperchromasia or significant mitotic activity
- ○ Cytoplasm contains secretory granules seen easily with electron microscopy
  - If numerous, seen easily with light microscopy, on which granules appear as lightly eosinophilic to bright red
- Special stains
  - ○ Positive immunohistochemical staining for 1 or more neuroendocrine markers
    - Chromogranin A: Best general marker of endocrine cells
    - Synaptophysin
    - Neuron-specific enolase
    - Protein gene product
    - Specific peptide hormone markers (e.g., serotonin and gastrin)
  - ○ Historically, argentaffin and argyrophil silver impregnation techniques were employed to diagnose NET
    - Argentaffin marks serotonin-containing granules of EC cells
    - Argyrophil is generally positive in all endocrine cells
    - Enterochromaffin refers to ability to stain with chromium or chrome salts, a common feature of serotonin-containing cells
    - Granules of carcinoid tumors have high affinity for silver stains
      - Argentaffin marks serotonin-containing granules of EC cells
      - Hence the name argentaffinoma, which was used interchangeably with carcinoid tumor years ago
  - ○ Electron microscopy
    - Cells in most tumors contain membrane-bound secretory granules with cytoplasmic dense-core granules

IMAGING FINDINGS

Detection

- **Gastric and duodenal carcinoids**
  - ○ Endoscopic ultrasonography
    - Most sensitive imaging technique for detection of duodenal and gastric carcinoids
    - Tumor appears as small, polypoid, submucosal hypoechoic lesion
  - ○ Double contrast barium studies
    - Mural mass or polypoid mass projecting within lumen
      - Type I and II gastric carcinoids: Usually small (< 1 cm) and multifocal in gastric body and fundus
      - Type III gastric carcinoids: Solitary, large mural masses in body and fundus
    - Overlying mucosa may show ulcerations
      - Occur regardless of malignant potential in large tumors

- Focal irregular collections of barium or air on tumor surface
  - In patients with ZES and MEN1
    - Diffusely thickened gastric folds
    - Nodular gastric mucosa
    - Multiple erosions and ulcers may be present
    - Hypersecretion of gastric fluids may cause flocculation of barium and poor gastric mucosal coating
  - Type III gastric carcinoids
    - Usually appear as large fungating intraluminal mass ± ulceration
- ○ CECT
  - Enhancing mucosal or submucosal masses
    - Small lesions (< 1 cm) may be difficult to detect
  - May also appear as eccentric mural thickening
  - In patients with ZES and MEN1
    - Multiple nodular mucosal and mural masses may be present
    - Marked gastric mural thickening
- **Small intestine NET**
  - ○ Enteroclysis or small bowel series
    - Primary tumor
      - Usually very difficult to detect
      - Single or multiple mural or polypoid nodules projecting within lumen usually in distal ileum
      - Overlying mucosa may ulcerate
    - Mesenteric fibrosis
      - Effects of mesenteric fibrosis are more likely to be visible than primary tumor
      - Appear as thickening, angulation, tethering, and fixation of ileal loops
  - ○ CECT
    - Primary tumor
      - Small solitary carcinoids are difficult to identify
      - Usually appear as small enhancing nodules or focal eccentric wall thickening
      - Larger polypoid lesions may be identified
      - Occasionally produce intussusception
    - Mesenteric fibrosis
      - May occur in absence of mesenteric extension or nodal metastases
  - ○ MR
    - Small solitary carcinoids are difficult to identify
    - Well-defined nodule or focal mural thickening
    - Signal characteristics
      - T1WI: Homogeneous and isointense
      - T2WI: Homogeneously isointense or inhomogeneously hyperintense
      - Gadolinium-enhanced T1-weighted MR images: Moderately intense gadolinium, homogeneous or patchy enhancement
  - ○ Somatostatin-receptor scintigraphy (SRI)
    - Indium-111 pentetreotide
    - Only imaging modality that helps distinguish sclerosing mesenteritis from metastatic carcinoid because
      - Most small bowel carcinoid tumors will be positive with somatostatin-receptor scintigraphy
    - SRI has diagnostic accuracy and positive predictive value of 83% and 100%, respectively
  - ○ 5-HTP PET
    - More sensitive than SRI and CT

NEUROENDOCRINE TUMORS

- Not widely available

Staging

- **Local spread**
  - Stomach
    - Type I & II tumors are usually localized to gastric wall
    - Type III may infiltrate into perigastric tissues and act like gastric adenocarcinoma
  - Duodenum
    - May infiltrate into surrounding structures including pancreas and retroperitoneum
  - Jejunoileal carcinoid
    - Tumor invasion of mesentery is common
    - Difficult to differentiate tumor invasion into mesentery from metastatic nodes on imaging
      - Mesenteric invasion usually contiguous with primary tumor
  - Colorectal NET
    - May infiltrate into pericolic tissues and act like colonic adenocarcinoma
- **Nodal metastases**
  - Nodal metastases from jejunoileal carcinoid is characteristic of disease
    - May be evident even when primary tumor is not seen
    - CT appearance
      - Spiculated infiltrative mesenteric mass
      - Poorly enhancing, radiating fibrotic strands/bands (64-76%)
      - Calcification in 40-70% of mesenteric masses
      - Patterns of calcification varies: Stippled, coarse, or diffuse
      - Mesenteric retraction and fibrosis → bowel angulation, bowel obstruction, and secondary bowel ischemia
    - MR appearance
      - Nodular, spiculated mesenteric mass
      - T1WI: Hypo- to isointense signal intensity
      - T2WI: Heterogeneous or homogeneous, iso- or hyperintense
      - Gadolinium-enhanced MR: Moderate to intense enhancement on early post-contrast images
      - Fibrotic bands or strands are of low signal intensity on T1 and T2WI and do not show enhancement following contrast administration
- **Liver metastases**
  - CT
    - NECT
      - Usually hypoattenuating to liver
      - May be hemorrhagic and show high-attenuation blood or hematocrit level
    - CECT
      - Usually hypervascular; show intense enhancement during arterial phase
  - MR
    - T1WI
      - Usually homogeneous low signal intensity
    - T2WI
      - Homogeneous or heterogeneous high signal intensity
    - Gadolinium-enhanced T1WI
      - Moderately intense enhancement during hepatic arterial phase

- Larger metastases may show heterogeneous enhancement due to central necrosis
  - Somatostatin-receptor scintigraphy (SRI)
    - Radiotracer uptake within liver metastases
      - Unless lesions are predominantly cystic
- **Bone metastases**
  - Bone metastases can be sclerotic or mixed lytic/sclerotic
  - Incidence of skeletal metastases in NETs has been reported to be approximately 10%
  - Axial skeleton is most commonly affected site
  - Bone scintigraphy is most sensitive nuclear imaging technique to detect bone metastases
    - Superior to indium-111 pentetreotide (OctreoScan) and iodine-131 metaiodobenzylguanidine (I-131 MIBG) scintigraphy
  - Ga-68-DOTATOC PET is reliable novel method for early detection of bone metastases
    - Sensitivity of 97%
    - Specificity of 92%

Restaging

- Elevated plasma chromogranin A is 1st indication of recurrence in radically resected jejunoileal tumors

CLINICAL ISSUES

Presentation

- Stomach
  - Type I carcinoid
    - Usually no clinical symptoms directly related to tumor
    - Usually found coincidentally during endoscopy performed for dyspepsia
    - Achlorhydria and, less commonly, pernicious anemia may be present
    - Hypergastrinemia or evidence of antral G-cell hyperplasia is usually observed
  - Type II carcinoid
    - Recurrent peptic ulcers: Abdominal pain or bleeding
    - Diarrhea
    - ↑ serum levels of gastrin
  - Type III carcinoid
    - Presentation resembles that of patients with other gastric neoplasms: Bleeding, abdominal pain, anorexia, and weight loss
- Duodenum
  - Most tumors are discovered coincidentally during endoscopy
- Small intestine
  - Patients usually have symptoms for ~ 5 years before diagnosis is made
    - Nonspecific symptoms and indolent tumor behavior
  - 40% of small intestine GIST patients are discovered during emergency surgery for small bowel obstruction
  - Nonspecific abdominal pain due to chronic intermittent ischemia
  - May be asymptomatic, found incidentally on imaging studies
  - Carcinoid syndrome

NEUROENDOCRINE TUMORS

- Occurs in 20-30% of patients with small bowel carcinoids
- Results from excessive secretion of biogenic amines, peptides, and other factors including serotonin, tachykinins, and bradykinins

- Colorectal NET
  - Majority are asymptomatic, discovered incidentally during colonoscopy
  - May present with rectal bleeding or obstructive symptoms

Cancer Natural History & Prognosis
- Overall 5-year survival for GI NETs
  - Stage I (86%)
  - Stage IIA (75%)
  - Stage IIB (72%)
  - Stage IIIA (59%)
  - Stage IIIB (70%)
    - Better prognosis compared to stage IIIA
    - Represents N1 disease with any T, while stage IIIA is advanced local disease (T4)
  - Stage IV (40%)
- Gastric NET
  - Type I
    - Rarely metastasizes
      - ~ 1-3% metastasizes
    - 5-year survival rate (~ 100%)
  - Type II
    - Infrequently metastasizes
      - ~ 10-30% metastasizes
    - 5-year survival rate (~ 60-90%)
  - Type III
    - Frequently metastasizes
      - ~ 50% metastasizes
    - 5-year survival rate (< 50%)
- Duodenal NET
  - 5-year survival rate (~ 60%)
  - Poor prognosis if
    - Tumor > 2 cm
    - Involvement of muscularis propria
    - Presence of mitotic figures
- Jejunoileal NET
  - 5-year survival rate (~ 61%)
  - Typically presents at advanced stage
  - Tumor size is most predictive factor for prognosis
- Colonic NET
  - 5-year survival rate (~ 33-42%)
- Rectal NET
  - 5-year survival rate (~ 88%)
  - Poor outcome if
    - Tumor > 2 cm
    - Invasion of muscularis propria

Treatment Options
- Stomach
  - Type I and II gastric carcinoids
    - < 1-2 cm: Clinically observed or removed endoscopically
    - > 2 cm: Surgical excision
    - Antrectomy
      - Eliminates trophic effect of gastrin
      - Useful for large, multiple, or recurrent type I carcinoids
  - Type III gastric carcinoids
    - Radical gastrectomy, regardless of tumor size

- Small intestine
  - Tumors < 1 cm in greatest dimension without regional lymph node metastases
    - Segmental resection alone with close postoperative surveillance
  - Tumors > 1 cm, those with mesenteric or lymph node metastases
    - Resection of primary tumor and mesenteric nodes
      - Effective in relieving obstructive and ischemic symptoms
  - Distant metastases
    - Resection of primary tumor and mesenteric nodes whenever possible
      - Improved survival in patients who undergo surgical resection
      - Relieves obstructive and ischemic symptoms
- Colon
  - Formal hemicolectomy with mesenteric resection is preferred treatment for colonic carcinoids
    - Nearly 55% of patients with carcinoid tumors involving colon present with liver or nodal metastases
- Rectum
  - Tumors < 2 cm
    - Endoscopic or surgical local excision
  - Tumors > 2 cm
    - Low anterior resection or abdominal perineal resection with locoregional nodal dissection
- Liver metastases
  - Resection or ablation of hepatic metastases
    - Surgery should be considered 1st treatment option
      - Unfortunately, < 20% of patients present with potentially resectable disease
      - Most patients present with extensive bilobar disease
    - Improvement of symptoms of carcinoid syndrome in 67-96% of patients
    - Survival benefit
      - 83% of patients treated with surgical resection survived for 3 years, compared with 31% of patients treated with medical therapy or embolization
  - Hepatic interventional procedures
    - Hepatic transcatheter arterial embolization (TAE)
      - Hypervascular liver metastases are primarily supplied by hepatic artery
      - TAE → ischemia of tumor cells → ↓ hormone output and tumor necrosis
      - Utilize polyvinyl alcohol and gel foam
      - Overall objective response in 50-80% of patients
    - Transcatheter arterial chemoembolization (TACE)
      - Ischemia of tumor cells → ↑ sensitivity to chemotherapeutic substances
      - Regional delivery of chemotherapy → ↑ intratumoral drug concentration
    - Radiofrequency ablation
      - Most commonly used ablative technique in metastatic NETs
      - Used for treatment of unresectable tumor or palliation of tumor-related symptoms
- Medical treatment
  - Somatostatin analogues

- ▪ Mainstay of symptomatic therapy in patients with carcinoid syndrome
- ▪ Symptomatic response of 50-75% and biochemical response in 40-60% of patients
- ▪ True tumor response (> 50% reduction in tumor volume) is rarely seen
  - – Tumor stability is reported in up 50% of patients
- ▪ Median duration of response is 12 months (thereafter patients develop tachyphylaxis)
- ○ Interferon-α (IFN)
  - ▪ Symptomatic and biochemical response rates ranging from 8-70%
  - ▪ Mechanism of action is still not fully understood
- ○ Chemotherapy
  - ▪ First-line therapy for poorly differentiated midgut carcinoid

REPORTING CHECKLIST

T Staging

- • Tumor appears as well-defined mural lesion or enhancing diffuse wall thickening
- • Only type III gastric carcinoid is likely to invade perigastric tissues
- • Mesenteric invasion is common in ileojejunal carcinoids
- • Depth of tumor invasion is determined on pathological examination and is difficult to determine on imaging
  - ○ Unless tumor invades visceral peritoneum or adjacent organs or structures (T4)

N Staging

- • Mesenteric nodal metastases are hallmark of midgut carcinoids
  - ○ May be visible even when primary tumor is small and not detected on imaging

M Staging

- • Hypervascular liver metastases are common
- • Bone metastases are usually sclerotic

SELECTED REFERENCES

1. American Joint Committee on Cancer: AJCC Cancer Staging Manual. 7th ed. New York: Springer. 181-9, 2010
2. Druce MR et al: Intra-abdominal fibrosis in a recent cohort of patients with neuroendocrine ('carcinoid') tumours of the small bowel. QJM. 103(3):177-85, 2010
3. Pasieka JL: Carcinoid tumors. Surg Clin North Am. 89(5):1123-37, 2009
4. Putzer D et al: Bone metastases in patients with neuroendocrine tumor: 68Ga-DOTA-Tyr3-octreotide PET in comparison to CT and bone scintigraphy. J Nucl Med. 50(8):1214-21, 2009
5. Welin S et al: Elevated plasma chromogranin A is the first indication of recurrence in radically operated midgut carcinoid tumors. Neuroendocrinology. 89(3):302-7, 2009
6. Pape UF et al: Prognostic factors of long-term outcome in gastroenteropancreatic neuroendocrine tumours. Endocr Relat Cancer. 15(4):1083-97, 2008
7. Pinchot SN et al: Carcinoid tumors. Oncologist. 13(12):1255-69, 2008
8. Steward MJ et al: Neuroendocrine tumors: role of interventional radiology in therapy. Radiographics. 28(4):1131-45, 2008
9. Chang S et al: Neuroendocrine neoplasms of the gastrointestinal tract: classification, pathologic basis, and imaging features. Radiographics. 27(6):1667-79, 2007
10. Hou W et al: Treatment of gastric carcinoids. Curr Treat Options Gastroenterol. 10(2):123-33, 2007
11. Levy AD et al: From the archives of the AFIP: Gastrointestinal carcinoids: imaging features with clinicopathologic comparison. Radiographics. 27(1):237-57, 2007
12. Scarsbrook AF et al: Anatomic and functional imaging of metastatic carcinoid tumors. Radiographics. 27(2):455-77, 2007
13. Elsayes KM et al: MRI of the peritoneum: spectrum of abnormalities. AJR Am J Roentgenol. 186(5):1368-79, 2006
14. Zuetenhorst JM et al: Metastatic carcinoid tumors: a clinical review. Oncologist. 10(2):123-31, 2005
15. Horton KM et al: Carcinoid tumors of the small bowel: a multitechnique imaging approach. AJR Am J Roentgenol. 182(3):559-67, 2004
16. Klöppel G et al: The gastroenteropancreatic neuroendocrine cell system and its tumors: the WHO classification. Ann N Y Acad Sci. 1014:13-27, 2004
17. Bader TR et al: MRI of carcinoid tumors: spectrum of appearances in the gastrointestinal tract and liver. J Magn Reson Imaging. 14(3):261-9, 2001

NEUROENDOCRINE TUMORS

(Left) Axial CECT during arterial phase in a 35-year-old woman who presented with right lower quadrant abdominal pain shows an intensely enhancing 1 cm duodenal mural nodule ➡️. *Differential possibilities for such lesions include duodenal GIST, heterotopic pancreas, and other submucosal lesions, but biopsy revealed carcinoid tumor. (Right) Axial CECT during portal venous phase in the same patient shows persistant enhancement of the duodenal mural lesion* ➡️.

Duodenal Carcinoid, Stage I (T1 N0 M0)

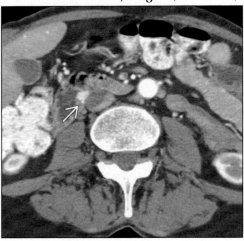

Duodenal Carcinoid, Stage I (T1 N0 M0)

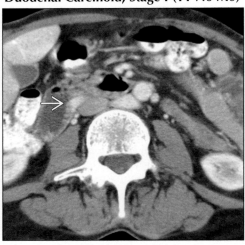

(Left) Axial T1WI C+ FS MR in the same patient shows the intensely enhancing duodenal mural nodule ➡️ *during the arterial phase. (Right) Axial T1WI C+ FS MR in the same patient shows persistent enhancement of the duodenal mural nodule* ➡️ *during the portal venous phase.*

Duodenal Carcinoid, Stage I (T1 N0 M0)

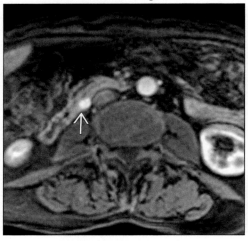

Duodenal Carcinoid, Stage I (T1 N0 M0)

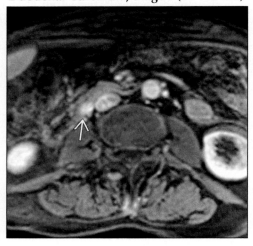

(Left) Axial CECT in a 45-year-old man who presented with right upper quadrant pain shows a distended gallbladder ➡️ *containing a gallstone* ➡️. *Stranding is seen in the fat surrounding the gallbladder* ➡️ *due to acute cholecystitis. (Right) Axial CECT in the same patient shows a round, 2.3 cm polyploid lesion* ➡️ *discovered incidentally in the gastric cardia. On histological examination, the lesion was found to be carcinoid tumor penetrating the muscularis propria. Either size or invasion makes this T2 disease.*

Gastric Carcinoid, Stage IIA (T2 N0 M0)

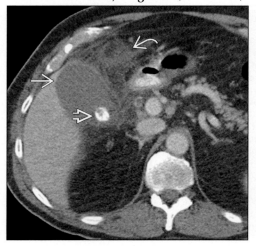

Gastric Carcinoid, Stage IIA (T2 N0 M0)

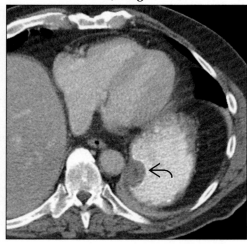

NEUROENDOCRINE TUMORS

**Duodenal Carcinoid,
Stage IIA (T2 N0 M0)**

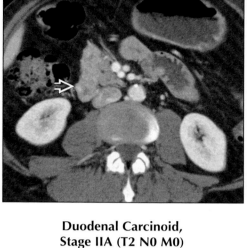

**Duodenal Carcinoid,
Stage IIA (T2 N0 M0)**

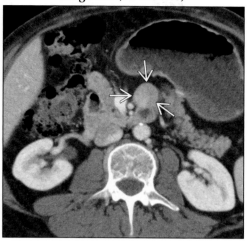

(Left) Axial CECT in a 26-year-old man with a history of neurofibromatosis type 1 shows a small mural enhancing lesion ➡ that on biopsy was found to be a well-differentiated carcinoid. *(Right)* Axial CECT in the same patient shows an exophytic distal duodenal enhancing mass ➡ that was found to be a gatrointestinal stromal tumor (GIST).

**Duodenal Carcinoid,
Stage IIA (T2 N0 M0)**

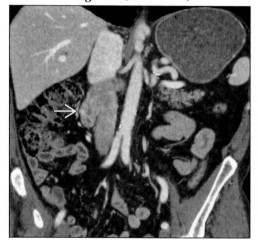

**Duodenal Carcinoid,
Stage IIA (T2 N0 M0)**

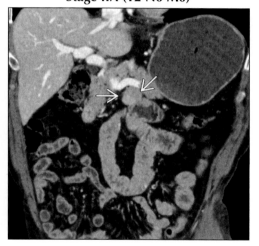

(Left) Coronal CECT in the same patient shows the enhancing mural nodule ➡ in the 2nd part of the duodenum. *(Right)* Coronal CECT in the same patient shows an enhancing exophytic GIST ➡. Both duodenal carcinoids and GISTs are common in patients with neurofibromatosis type 1.

**Colonic Carcinoid,
Stage IIIA (T4 N0 M0)**

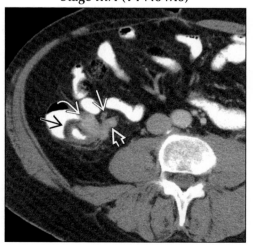

**Colonic Carcinoid,
Stage IIIA (T4 N0 M0)**

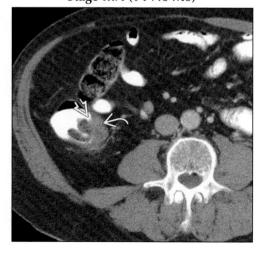

(Left) Axial CECT in a 75-year-old man who presented with vague abdominal pain shows a 3 cm cecal enhancing mass ➡ adjacent to the ileocecal valve ➡. The tumor extends to involve the mesentery ➡. The appendix ➡ is not involved. *(Right)* Axial CECT in the same patient shows a tumor involving the ascending colon ➡ and the outer aspect of the ileocecal valve ➡.

NEUROENDOCRINE TUMORS

(Left) Axial CECT in a 63-year-old man with a long history of epigastric pain shows an infiltrating enhancing gastric fundal mass ⇨ causing gastric wall thickening. *(Right)* Axial CECT in the same patient shows the gastric infiltrative mass ⇨ extending into the perigastric fat ⇨. Type III gastric carcinoid is not associated with hypergastrinemia and is more likely to be infiltrative and to metastasize to the liver.

Type III Gastric Carcinoid, Stage IIIA (T4 N0 M0)

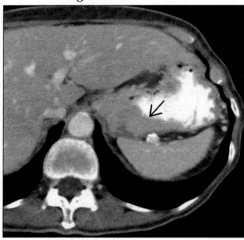

Type III Gastric Carcinoid, Stage IIIA (T4 N0 M0)

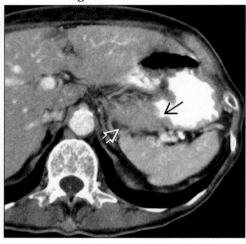

(Left) Axial CECT in a 59-year-old woman who presented with rectal fullness shows a polypoid mass ⇨ of the right posterolateral wall of the rectum. *(Right)* Axial PET/CT in the same patient shows increased metabolic activity of the rectal mass ⇨ and increased metabolic activity of a right inguinal lymph node ⇨.

Rectal Carcinoid, Stage IIIB (T2 N1 M0)

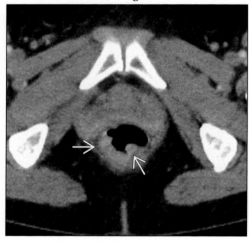

Rectal Carcinoid, Stage IIIB (T2 N1 M0)

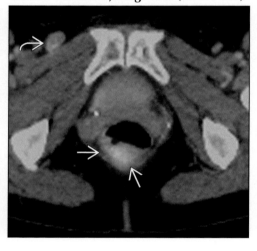

(Left) Axial PET/CT in the same patient shows an additional left perirectal lymph node ⇨ with increased metabolic activity. *(Right)* Sagittal PET/CT in the same patient shows increased metabolic activity within the polypoid rectal mass ⇨. The tumor measured 2.4 cm and invaded the lamina propria, consistent with T2 disease.

Rectal Carcinoid, Stage IIIB (T2 N1 M0)

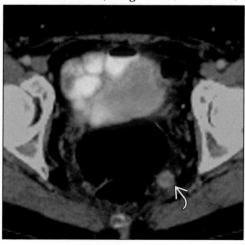

Rectal Carcinoid, Stage IIIB (T2 N1 M0)

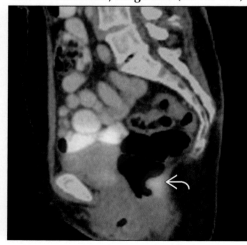

Ileal Carcinoid, Stage IIIB (T3 N1 M0)

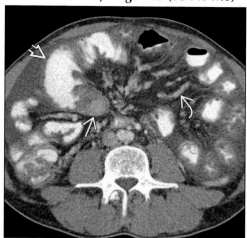

Ileal Carcinoid, Stage IIIB (T3 N1 M0)

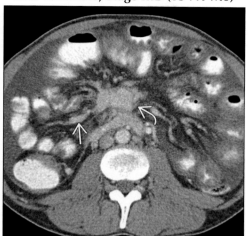

(Left) Axial CECT in a 54-year-old man who presented with abdominal pain and worsening abdominal distension shows an obstructing enhancing intraluminal ileal mass ➡ with dilatation of the proximal ileum ➡ and mesenteric vascular congestion ➡. *(Right)* Axial CECT in the same patient shows large enhancing mesenteric lymph nodal mass ➡ occluding both superior mesenteric artery and vein with radiating fibrous bands ➡ within the mesentery.

Ileal Carcinoid, Stage IIIB (T3 N1 M0)

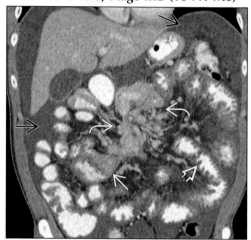

Ileal Carcinoid, Stage IIIB (T3 N1 M0)

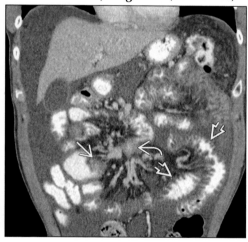

(Left) Coronal CECT in the same patient shows obstructing ileal enhancing mass ➡, desmoblastic mesenteric mass ➡, small bowel fold thickening ➡ due to chronic ischemia, and large amount of ascites ➡. *(Right)* Coronal CECT in the same patient shows the enhancing ileal mass ➡, mesenteric mass ➡, and small bowel wall & fold thickening ➡ due to chronic ischemia resulting from superior mesenteric artery and vein occlusion.

Ileal Carcinoid, Stage IIIB (T3 N1 M0)

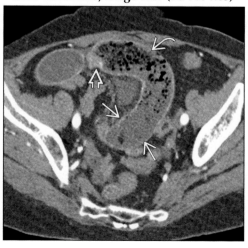

Ileal Carcinoid, Stage IIIB (T3 N1 M0)

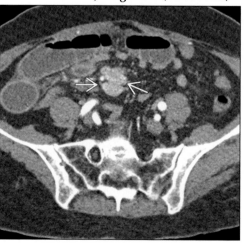

(Left) Axial CECT in a 65-year-old woman who presented with intestinal obstruction shows an enhancing ileal mass ➡ causing small bowel dilatation ➡ and small bowel feces sign ➡. *(Right)* Axial CECT in the same patient shows enhancing central mesenteric lymph nodes ➡. The presence of regional nodal metastases with any GI carcinoid warrants classification as stage IIIB.

(Left) Axial CECT in the same patient shows the tumor extending to the cecum ➡ and an enhancing regional lymph node ➡. **(Right)** Coronal CECT in the same patient shows a tumor of the distal ileum ➡ extending into the cecum ➡. Punctate calcification ⧉ is seen within the tumor, a common finding in carcinoids.

Ileal Carcinoid, Stage IIIB (T4 N1 M0)

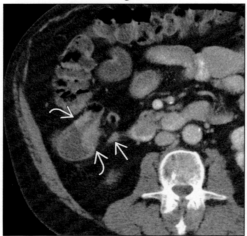

Ileal Carcinoid, Stage IIIB (T4 N1 M0)

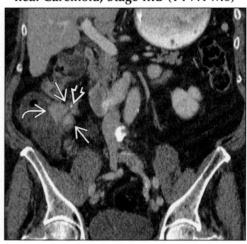

(Left) Axial CECT in a 59-year-old man who presented with abdominal pain shows a distal ileal enhancing mass ➡. **(Right)** Axial CECT in the same patient shows an enhancing nodule ➡ on the serosal aspect of the cecum adjacent to the terminal ileum ➡. Two enhancing ileocolic nodes ⧉ are also present.

Ileal Carcinoid, Stage IIIB (T4 N1 M0)

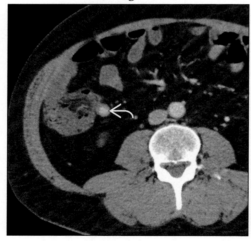

Ileal Carcinoid, Stage IIIB (T4 N1 M0)

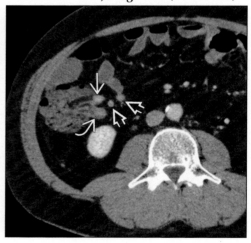

(Left) Coronal CECT in the same patient shows a distal ileal enhancing mass ➡, which is better seen on the coronal reformatted image than on the previous axial image. **(Right)** Coronal CECT in the same patient shows the cecal serosal module ➡ and the regional metastatic lymph node ➡. Pathology showed this tumor invading the serosa with cecal serosal metastasis and metastatic regional nodes.

Ileal Carcinoid, Stage IIIB (T4 N1 M0)

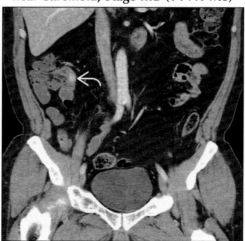

Ileal Carcinoid, Stage IIIB (T4 N1 M0)

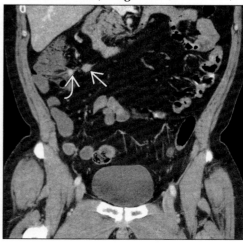

NEUROENDOCRINE TUMORS

Ileal Carcinoid, Stage IIIB (T4 N1 M0)

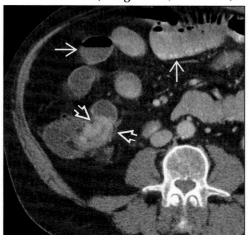

Ileal Carcinoid, Stage IIIB (T4 N1 M0)

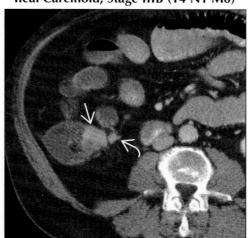

(Left) Axial CECT in a 78-year-old man who presented with abdominal pain and a 3-day history of constipation shows enhancing concentric thickening of the distal ileum ➡ and proximal small bowel dilatation ➡. *(Right)* Axial CECT in the same patient shows the distal ileal mass extending into the cecum ➡ and an enhancing ileocolic lymph node ➡.

Ileal Carcinoid, Stage IIIB (TX N1 M0)

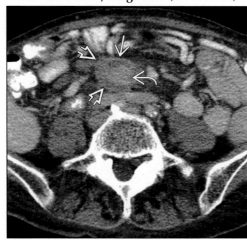

Ileal Carcinoid, Stage IIIB (TX N1 M0)

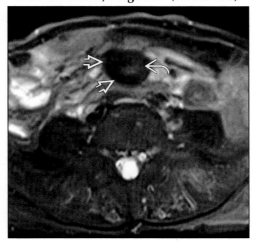

(Left) Axial CECT in a 74-year-old woman shows a central mesenteric mass ➡. The primary tumor was not detected. The mesenteric mass shows an enhancing central component ➡ and a relatively hypoenhancing peripheral component ➡. *(Right)* Axial T2WI FS MR in the same patient shows an isointense component ➡ of the mesenteric mass and a very hypointense component ➡.

Ileal Carcinoid, Stage IIIB (TX N1 M0)

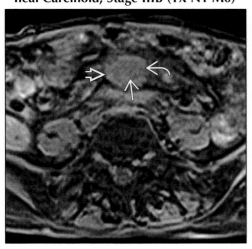

Ileal Carcinoid, Stage IIIB (TX N1 M0)

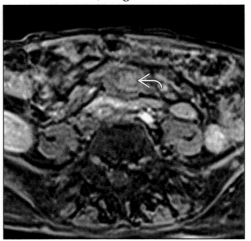

(Left) Axial T1WI MR in the same patient shows an intermediate signal mesenteric mass ➡ with the periphery ➡ slightly hyperintense relative to the central component ➡. *(Right)* Axial T1WI C+ FS MR in the same patient after contrast administration shows relative hyperenhancement of the central component ➡. It is presumed that the enhancing central component represents metastatic nodal disease while the hypoenhancing component represents fibrosis.

NEUROENDOCRINE TUMORS

Ileal Carcinoid, Stage IV (TX N1 M1)

Ileal Carcinoid, Stage IV (TX N1 M1)

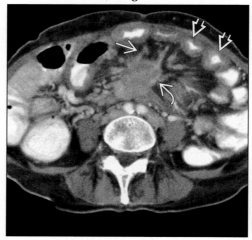

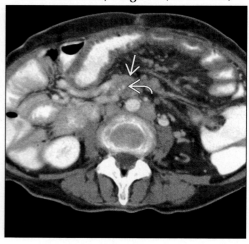

(Left) Axial CECT in a 60-year-old woman who presented with a 5-year history of abdominal pain shows a large central mesenteric mass ➡ with soft tissue bands ➡ radiating from the mesenteric mass toward the small bowel loops. The small bowel walls are thickened ➡. *(Right)* Axial CECT in the same patient shows the mesenteric mass ➡ extending superiorly and causing occlusion of the superior mesenteric artery ➡. The artery was completely occluded below this level.

Ileal Carcinoid, Stage IV (TX N1 M1)

Ileal Carcinoid, Stage IV (TX N1 M1)

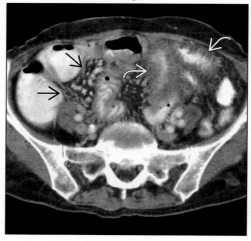

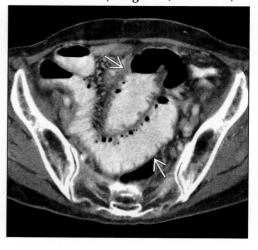

(Left) Axial CECT in the same patient shows wall thickening of multiple loops of small bowel ➡ due to chronic arterial and portal venous occlusion resulting in chronic ischemia. Note the dilated mesenteric vessels ➡ due to venous congestion and arterial collaterals. *(Right)* Axial CECT in the same patient shows mutiple dilated small bowel loops ➡. The primary carcinoid tumor could not be identified.

Ileal Carcinoid, Stage IV (TX N1 M1)

Ileal Carcinoid, Stage IV (TX N1 M1)

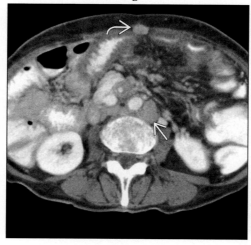

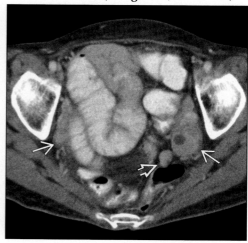

(Left) Axial CECT in the same patient shows an enhancing peritoneal metastasis ➡ as well as retroperitoneal periaortic lymph node ➡. *(Right)* Axial CECT in the same patient shows bilateral ovarian metastases ➡ as well as a peritoneal implant ➡.

Ileal Carcinoid, Stage IV (TX N1 M1)

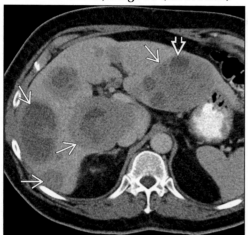

Ileal Carcinoid, Stage IV (TX N1 M1)

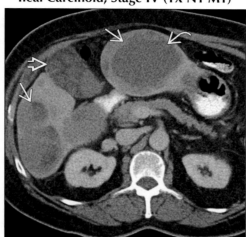

(Left) Axial CECT in a 68-year-old man who presented with carcinoid syndrome shows multiple liver lesions ➡, some of which ⧐ exhibit cystic/necrotic changes. (Right) Axial CECT in the same patient shows multiple metastatic liver lesions ➡ with prominent central necrosis ⧐. Multiple large polypoid masses are also seen within the gallbladder ⧐. The liver lesions were biopsied and revealed a neuroendocrine tumor.

Ileal Carcinoid, Stage IV (TX N1 M1)

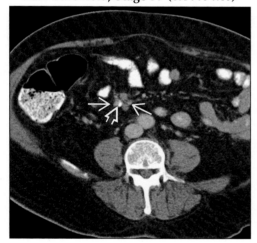

Ileal Carcinoid, Stage IV (TX N1 M1)

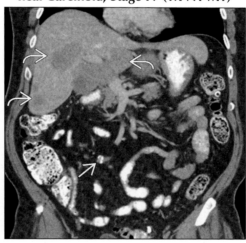

(Left) Axial CECT in the same patient shows an aggregate of multiple mesenteric lymph nodes ➡ with 1 of them showing calcifications ⧐. The primary tumor was not identified on imaging. (Right) Coronal CECT in the same patient shows the mesenteric lymph nodes ➡ and hepatic metastases ➡.

Ileal Carcinoid, Stage IV (TX N1 M1)

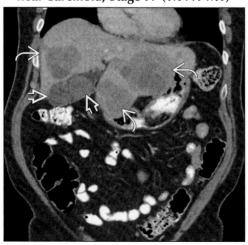

Ileal Carcinoid, Stage IV (TX N1 M1)

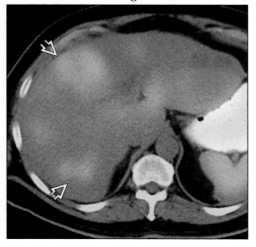

(Left) Coronal CECT in the same patient shows multiple hepatic metastases ➡ and multiple gallbladder polypoid masses ⧐ that have the same appearance of the liver metastases and were presumed to be metastatic lesions to the gallbladder. (Right) Axial fused octreotide SPECT/CT in the same patient shows octreotide uptake by multiple liver lesions ⧐. An octreotide scan is highly sensitive for the detection of carcinoid tumors, with reported sensitivities of 80-100%.

(Left) Axial CECT in a 39-year-old woman who presented with abdominal pain shows multiple hypoattenuating liver lesions ➡ involving the right and left lobe. The gallbladder ➡ is decompressed and appears normal. *(Right)* Axial CECT in the same patient shows a large mass ➡ in the porta hepatis, separate from the liver and closely associated with the duodenum ➡. The mass is mostly cystic with a large solid component ➡.

Malignant Carcinoid in a Duodenal Duplication Cyst, Stage IV (T3 N0 M1)

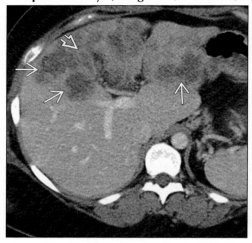

Malignant Carcinoid in a Duodenal Duplication Cyst, Stage IV (T3 N0 M1)

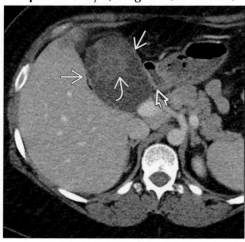

(Left) Coronal CECT in the same patient shows the mixed solid/cystic mass ➡ separate from the liver and closely related to the duodenum ➡. *(Right)* Coronal CECT in the same patient shows the mass ➡ separate from the liver and gallbladder ➡. Pathology revealed a poorly differentiated neuroendocrinal tumor arising in a duodenal duplication cyst.

Malignant Carcinoid in a Duodenal Duplication Cyst, Stage IV (T3 N0 M1)

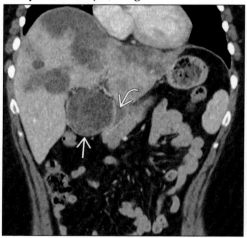

Malignant Carcinoid in a Duodenal Duplication Cyst, Stage IV (T3 N0 M1)

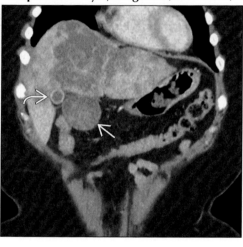

(Left) Axial PET/CT in the same patient shows increased metabolic activity of multiple hepatic lesions ➡. *(Right)* Axial PET/CT in the same patient shows increased metabolic activity of the solid component within the duodenal duplication cyst ➡. Tumors arising in duplication cysts are rare and are more likely to be adenocarcinomas than neuroendocrine tumors.

Malignant Carcinoid in a Duodenal Duplication Cyst, Stage IV (T3 N0 M1)

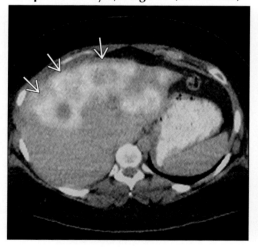

Malignant Carcinoid in a Duodenal Duplication Cyst, Stage IV (T3 N0 M1)

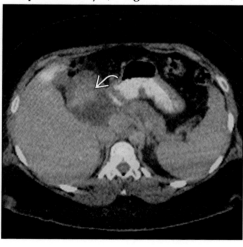

NEUROENDOCRINE TUMORS

Gastric Carcinoid, Stage IV (T3 N1 M1)

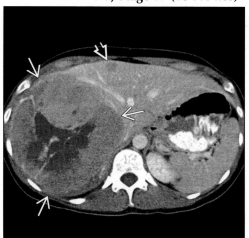

Gastric Carcinoid, Stage IV (T3 N1 M1)

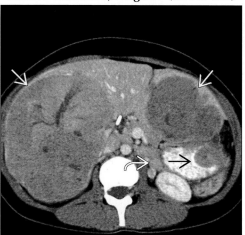

(Left) Axial CECT in a 56-year-old man who presented with right upper quadrant abdominal pain shows a large hepatic mass ➡ almost replacing the entire right lobe and a smaller hypoattenuating nodule ➡ in the left lobe. (Right) Axial CECT in the same patient shows large liver masses ➡, a polypoid gastric mass ➡, and a perigastric lymph node ➡. Biopsy of 1 of the liver masses and the gastric mass revealed carcinoid tumors.

Colonic Carcinoid, Stage IV (T4 N1 M1)

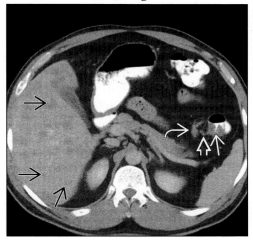

Colonic Carcinoid, Stage IV (T4 N1 M1)

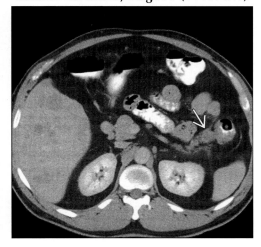

(Left) Axial CECT in a 47-year-old woman shows a polypoid lesion ➡ within the descending colon with tumor strands extending into the pericolonic fat ➡ as well as pericolonic adenopathy ➡. Multiple hypoattenuating liver metastatic lesions ➡ are also present. (Right) Axial CECT in the same patient shows extensive peritoneal tumor extension ➡. The appearance is indistinguishable from invasive colonic carcinoma; however, biopsy revealed high-grade NET.

Colonic Carcinoid, Stage IV (T4 N1 M1)

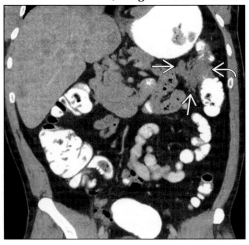

Colonic Carcinoid, Stage IV (T4 N1 M1)

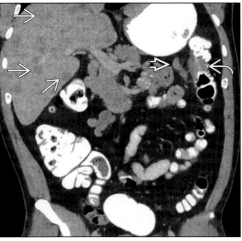

(Left) Coronal CECT in the same patient shows an annular lesion of the descending colon ➡ with extensive pericolonic peritoneal extension ➡. (Right) Coronal CECT in the same patient shows an annular lesion ➡ of the descending colon with peritoneal nodules ➡ and multiple liver metastases ➡.

NEUROENDOCRINE TUMORS

Ileal Carcinoid, Stage IV (T4 N1 M1)

Ileal Carcinoid, Stage IV (T4 N1 M1)

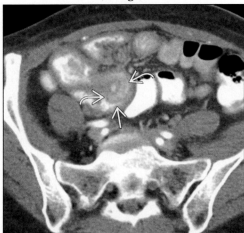

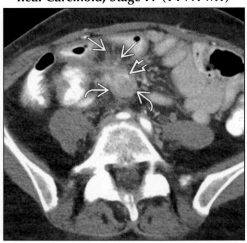

(Left) Axial CECT in a 55-year-old woman who presented with abdominal pain, diarrhea, and flushing characteristic of cacinoid syndrome shows eccentric thickening and enhancement ⇒ of the wall of the ileum with luminal narrowing ➡. *(Right)* Axial CECT in the same patient shows a large mesenteric mass ➡ with radiating strands ➡ and stippled calcifications ⇒.

Ileal Carcinoid, Stage IV (T4 N1 M1)

Ileal Carcinoid, Stage IV (T4 N1 M1)

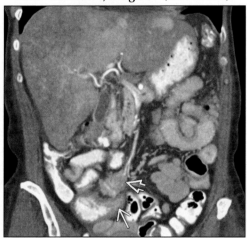

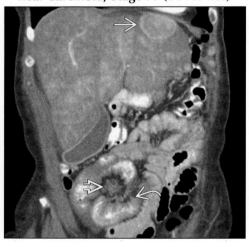

(Left) Coronal CECT in the same patient shows enhancement and thickening of the wall of the ileum ➡ and a central mesenteric mass ⇒. *(Right)* Coronal CECT in the same patient shows the desmoplastic reaction within the mesentery ⇒ with tethering ➡ of the surrounding ileal loops. The liver shows heterogeneous enhancement and a large, peripherally enhancing left lobe metastatic lesion ➡.

Ileal Carcinoid, Stage IV (T4 N1 M1)

Ileal Carcinoid, Stage IV (T4 N1 M1)

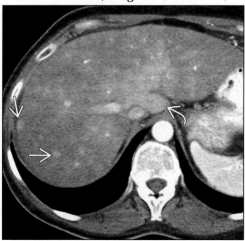

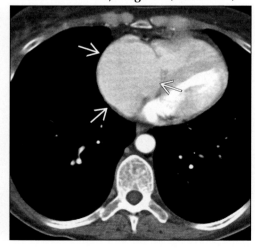

(Left) Axial CECT in the same patient shows heterogeneous liver enhancement with increased enhancement of the caudate lobe ➡ due to hepatic congestion. Multiple enhancing lesions ➡ are seen within the liver. *(Right)* Axial CECT in the same patient shows an enlarged heart with marked dilatation of the right atrium ➡ due to carcinoid tricuspid valve disease. Carcinoid syndrome and heart disease usually develop only in patients with liver metastases.

Rectal Carcinoid, Stage IV (T4 N1 M1)

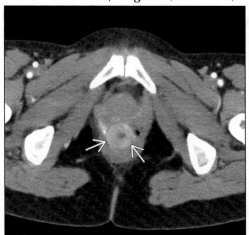

Rectal Carcinoid, Stage IV (T4 N1 M1)

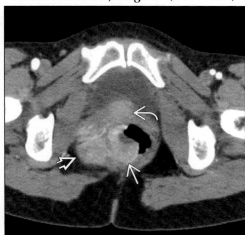

(Left) Axial CECT in a 47-year-old woman who presented with bowel obstructive symptoms shows circumferential thickening and enhancement of the distal rectum ➡. *(Right)* Axial CECT in the same patient shows a large rectal mass ➡ invading into the vagina ➡ and into the fat of the ischiorectal fossa ➡. This is an unusual appearance of rectal carcinoid, which are generally localized and not infiltrative.

Rectal Carcinoid, Stage IV (T4 N1 M1)

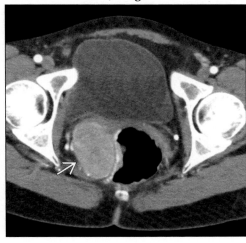

Rectal Carcinoid, Stage IV (T4 N1 M1)

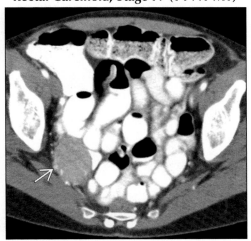

(Left) Axial CECT in the same patient shows a large perirectal enhancing lymph node ➡. *(Right)* Axial CECT in the same patient shows a large enhancing internal iliac lymph node ➡. Risk factors for lymph node metastasis for rectal carcinoid include tumor size ≥ 1.0 cm and lymphovascular invasion. Tumors ≥ 2.0 cm have a 60-89% incidence of metastasis.

Rectal Carcinoid, Stage IV (T4 N1 M1)

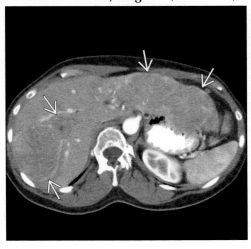

Rectal Carcinoid, Stage IV (T4 N1 M1)

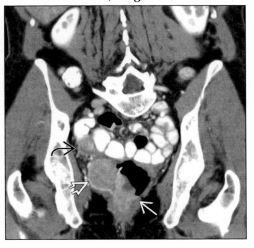

(Left) Axial CECT in the same patient shows multiple large metastatic lesions ➡ in the liver. Interestingly, patients with rectal carcinoids and liver metastases do not usually present with carcinoid syndrome, as is the case with this patient. *(Right)* Coronal CECT in the same patient shows the rectal mass ➡, perirectal lymph node ➡, and internal iliac node ➡.

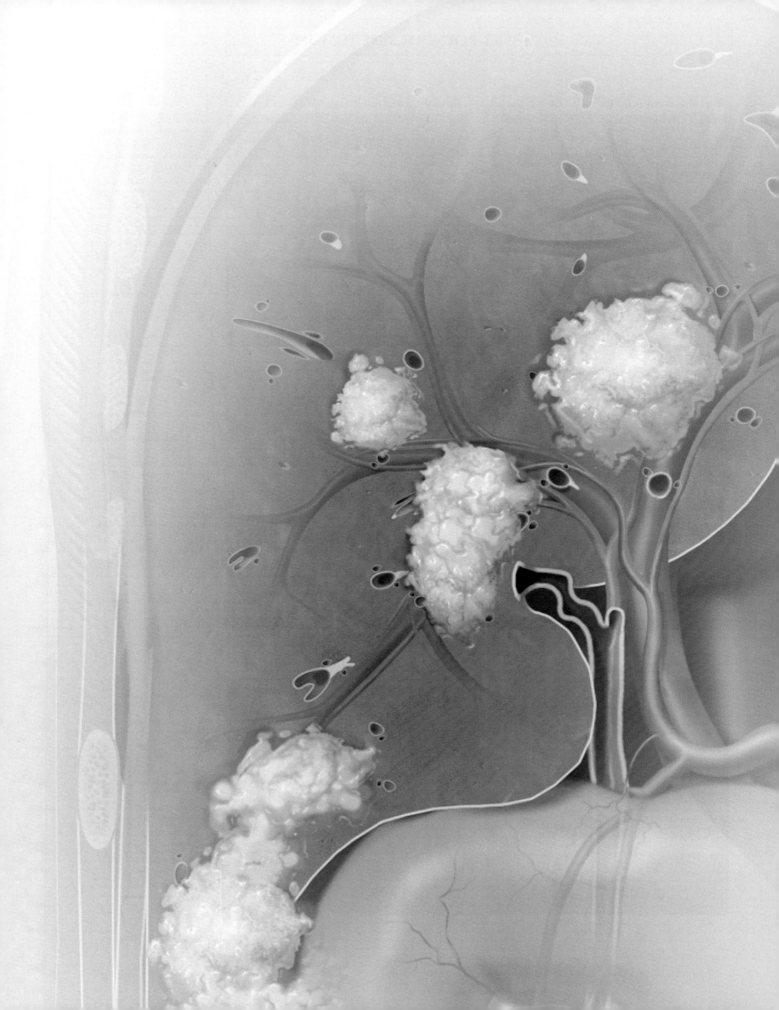

Hepatocellular Carcinoma

HEPATOCELLULAR CARCINOMA

(T) Primary Tumor

Adapted from 7th edition AJCC Staging Forms.

TNM	Definitions
TX	Primary tumor cannot be assessed
T0	No evidence of primary tumor
T1	Solitary tumor without vascular invasion
T2	Solitary tumor with vascular invasion or multiple tumors, none > 5 cm
T3a	Multiple tumors > 5 cm
T3b	Single tumor or multiple tumors of any size involving a major branch of the portal vein or hepatic vein
T4	Tumor(s) with direct invasion of adjacent organs other than the gallbladder or with perforation of visceral peritoneum

(N) Regional Lymph Nodes

NX	Regional lymph nodes cannot be assessed
N0	No regional lymph node metastasis
N1	Regional lymph node metastasis

(M) Distant Metastasis

M0	No distant metastasis
M1	Distant metastasis

(G) Histologic Grade

G1	Well differentiated
G2	Moderately differentiated
G3	Poorly differentiated
G4	Undifferentiated

AJCC Stages/Prognostic Groups

Adapted from 7th edition AJCC Staging Forms.

Stage	T	N	M
I	T1	N0	M0
II	T2	N0	M0
IIIA	T3a	N0	M0
IIIB	T3b	N0	M0
IIIC	T4	N0	M0
IVA	Any T	N1	M0
IVB	Any T	Any N	M1

T1

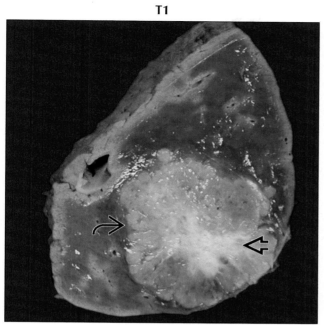

Gross specimen shows a solitary fibrolamellar hepatocellular carcinoma without vascular invasion. Note well-circumscribed tumor ⊅ with radiating fibrous septa that merge to form a central scar ⊅.

T1

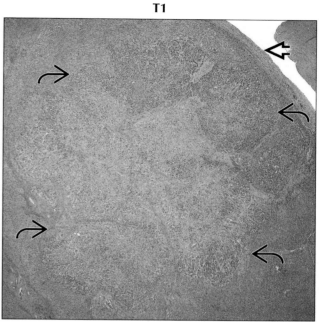

Micrograph of H&E stained section of a solitary HCC shows fairly well-defined tumor margins ⊅. The tumor is immediately deep to the liver capsule ⊅. (Original magnification 10x.)

T1

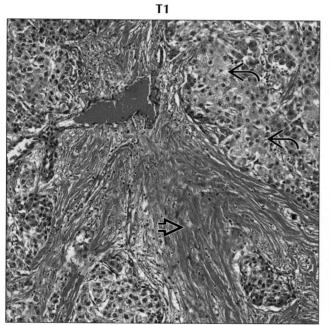

Higher magnification of the preceding figure shows sheets and nests of small neoplastic cells with abdundant eosinophilic cystoplasm ⊅. Lamellar pink fibrous strands ⊅ are seen separating nests and sheets of malignant cells. (Original magnification 400x.)

T2

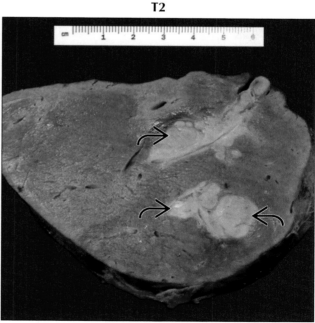

Gross specimen shows multiple small tumor nodules ⊅, none measuring more than 5 cm.

HEPATOCELLULAR CARCINOMA

T2

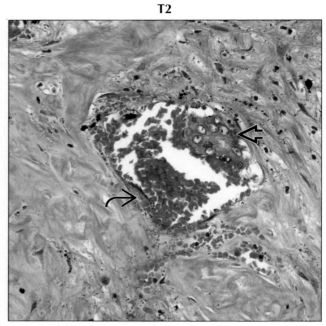

Micrograph of H&E stained section of a solitary hepatocellular carcinoma shows tumor cells ⇨ infiltrating a fibrotic background ⇨. Tumor cells ⇨ are likewise seen infiltrating dilated vascular spaces. The presence of vascular invasion makes this tumor T2. (Original magnification 100x.)

T2

Higher power micrograph of preceding image shows a small blood vessel lined by endothelial cells ⇨. There is direct vascular infiltration of neoplastic hepatocellular carcinoma cells ⇨.

T3a

Gross specimen shows multiple discrete tumor nodules ⇨, some of which measure more than 5 cm.

T3b

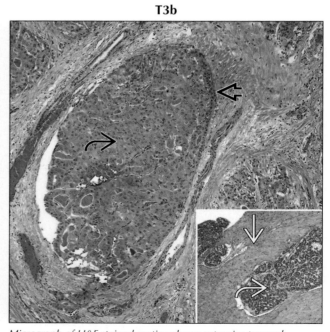

Micrograph of H&E stained section shows extensive tumoral invasion ⇨ into the distended portal vein ⇨. Inset shows a major hepatic vessel wall ⇨ with extensive tumoral infiltration of the vessel lumen ⇨. Invasion of large vessels constitutes T3b disease. (Original magnification 100x.)

T1

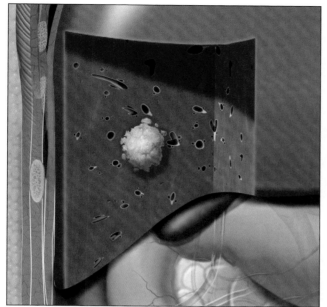

Graphic shows a solitary tumor without vascular invasion, consistent with T1 disease.

T2

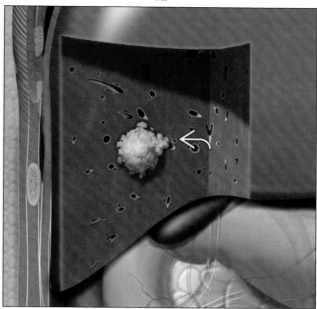

Graphic shows a solitary tumor with small vessel invasion ➔, consistent with T2 disease.

T2

Graphic shows multiple tumors throughout the liver, all of which are smaller than 5 cm. No vascular invasion is seen, consistent with T2 disease.

T3a

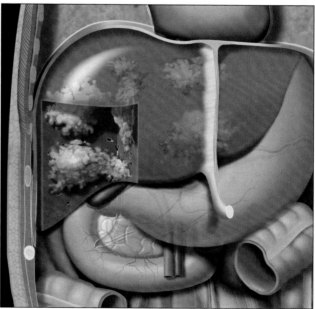

Graphic shows multiple tumors throughout the liver measuring more than 5 cm, consistent with T3a disease.

T3b

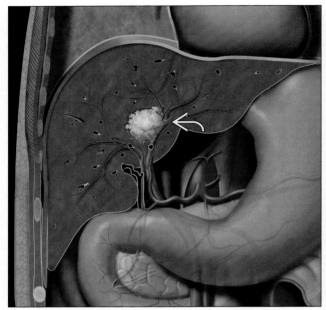

Graphic shows a solitary tumor with adjacent invasion of the portal vein ➔, consistent with T3b disease.

T3b

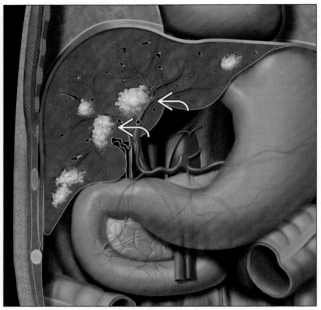

Graphic shows multiple tumors throughout the liver with portal venous invasion ➔. The presence of major vascular invasion, whether associated with a single or multiple tumors, is considered T3b disease.

T4

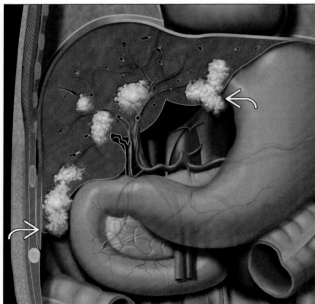

Graphic shows multiple tumors throughout the liver, some of which demonstrate extracapsular extension ➔. Extracapsular tumoral extension with perforation of the visceral peritoneum is consistent with T4 disease.

T4

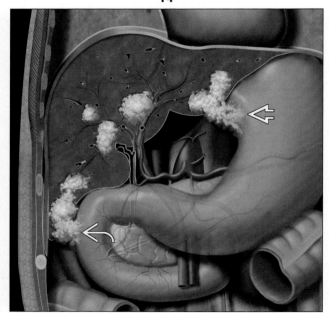

Graphic shows multiple tumors throughout the liver. There is extracapsular tumor extension with invasion of the adjacent duodenum ➔ and stomach ➔, consistent with T4 disease. Invasion of the gallbladder wall would not be classified as T4.

Regional Lymphadenopathy

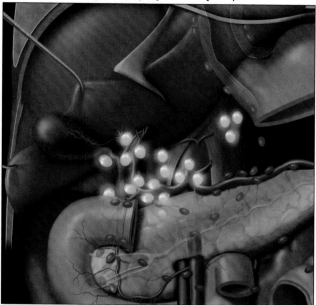

Graphic shows regional lymphadenopathy for metastatic hepatocellular carcinoma. These include paraceliac, hilar (common bile duct, hepatic artery, portal vein, and cystic duct), paraaortic, and portocaval lymph nodes.

Thoracic Lymphadenopathy

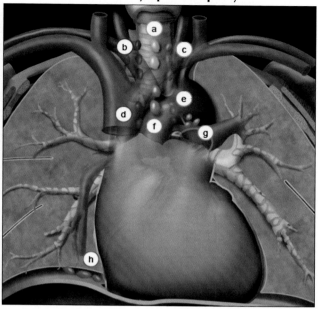

Graphic shows thoracic lymph nodes in metastatic hepatocellular carcinoma. These include a) pretracheal, b) right paratracheal, c) left paratracheal, d) right hilar, e) aortopulmonary, f) anterior mediastinal, g) left hilar, and h) cardiophrenic lymph nodes.

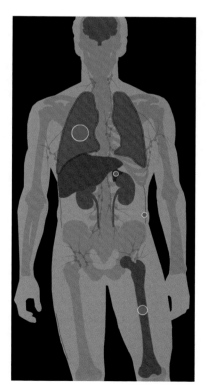

METASTASES, ORGAN FREQUENCY

Lung	55%
Bone	28%
Adrenal gland	11%
Peritoneum/omentum	11%

HEPATOCELLULAR CARCINOMA

OVERVIEW

General Comments
- Most common primary hepatic malignant tumor
- Synonymous with hepatoma

Classification
- Hepatocellular carcinoma (HCC)
  ○ Usually occurs in setting of cirrhosis
  ○ Poor prognosis
- Fibrolamellar carcinoma
  ○ Relatively rare variant of HCC
  ○ Does not occur in setting of cirrhosis
  ○ Better prognosis than conventional HCC

PATHOLOGY

Routes of Spread
- Local spread
  ○ 3 distinct intrahepatic forms have been commonly described
    ▪ Solitary massive tumor
    ▪ Multiple nodules scattered throughout liver
    ▪ Diffuse infiltration of liver
  ○ Vascular invasion commonly seen
    ▪ Hepatic vein invasion leads to Budd-Chiari syndrome
    ▪ Portal venous invasion
- Lymphatic spread
  ○ Regional lymphadenopathy implies N1 disease by TNM criteria
  ○ Regional nodal involvement (in order of prevalence)
    ▪ Periceliac
    ▪ Portohepatic
    ▪ Paraaortic
    ▪ Portocaval
    ▪ Peripancreatic
    ▪ Aortocaval
    ▪ Retrocaval
  ○ Distant lymphadenopathy (in order of prevalence)
    ▪ Mediastinal
    ▪ Cardiophrenic
    ▪ Mesenteric
    ▪ Internal mammary
    ▪ Perirectal
    ▪ Retrocrural
    ▪ Iliac
    ▪ Paraspinal
- Distant metastases (in order of prevalence)
  ○ Lungs
  ○ Musculoskeletal sites
  ○ Adrenal gland
  ○ Peritoneum &/or omentum

General Features
- Comments
  ○ Carcinogenesis of HCC in cirrhosis
    ▪ Commonly described as multistep evolution of cirrhotic nodules
  ○ International Working Party nomenclature describes 2 types of cirrhotic nodules
    ▪ Regenerative nodules
      - Localized proliferation of hepatocytes and supporting stroma
      - Occur as response to local hepatocellular damage
      - Undergo hyperplasia due to deficient portal venous perfusion → early arterial neovascularity
    ▪ Dysplastic nodules
      - Composed of hepatocytes that undergo abnormal growth due to genetic alteration
      - Histologic precursor to HCC
      - Small HCCs (< 2 cm) are often histologically indistinguishable from dysplastic nodules
      - Increased arterial neovascularity compared to regenerative nodules
- Genetics
  ○ Hepatitis B virus (HBV) DNA integrated into host's genomic DNA in tumor cells
- Etiology
  ○ HCC usually occurs in setting of underlying cirrhosis (90%)
  ○ Common causes of cirrhosis include
    ▪ Viral hepatitis (individuals with chronic hepatitis are at 20x greater risk of developing HCC)
      - Hepatitis C virus (accounts for 55% of cirrhosis)
      - Hepatitis B virus (accounts for 16% of cirrhosis)
    ▪ Alcoholism
    ▪ Carcinogens
      - Aflatoxins
      - Thorotrast
      - Androgens
      - Hemosiderosis (from repeated blood transfusions)
    ▪ Metabolic disorders
      - α-1 antitrypsin deficiency
      - Hemochromatosis
      - Wilson disease
      - Tyrosinosis
- Epidemiology & cancer incidence
  ○ 3rd leading cause of death from cancer worldwide
  ○ Accounts for 250,000 deaths worldwide each year
  ○ Incidence of HCC in developing nations is over 2x that of developed countries
    ▪ Incidence of HCC is highest in Asia and Africa due to high prevalence of hepatitis B and C
  ○ Frequency in United States
    ▪ Incidence in USA has doubled in last 20 years from 2.6 to 5.2 per 100,000 population
    ▪ Average age at diagnosis is 65 years
    ▪ 75% of cases occur in men
    ▪ Racial distribution
      - Caucasian (48%)
      - Hispanic (15%)
      - African-American (14%)
      - Other, predominantly Asian (24%)
- Associated diseases, abnormalities
  ○ Fibrolamellar carcinoma
    ▪ Variant of hepatocellular carcinoma
    ▪ Relatively rare neoplasm with better prognosis than conventional HCC
    ▪ Occurs most commonly in absence of cirrhosis
    ▪ Affects younger age group with peak incidence at 24.8 ± 8 years
    ▪ Higher incidence among Caucasians
    ▪ No gender predilection

HEPATOCELLULAR CARCINOMA

Gross Pathology & Surgical Features

- Classic macroscopic classification proposed by Eggle in 1901 still used today
  - Nodular
    - Smaller and more distinct than massive lesions
    - Sharper margins
  - Massive: 2 dominant forms
    - Composed of confluent small tumors
    - 1 large lesion occupying almost entire liver
  - Diffuse
    - Multiple infiltrating lesions occupying large part of liver

Microscopic Pathology

- H&E
  - Edmondson grading system widely used to grade histologic tumor differentiation of HCC
    - Grade I
      - Tumor cells similar in size to normal hepatocytes
      - Arranged in relatively thin trabeculae
      - Acini containing bile are rare
    - Grade II
      - Cells larger than normal hepatocytes
      - Hyperchromatic nuclei occupy greater proportion of cells
      - Thicker trabeculae
      - Acini containing bile are common
    - Grade III
      - Hepatocytes with large nuclei that occupy > 50% of cytoplasm
      - Trabeculae still dominant, although isolated cells may be present
      - Giant and bizarre cells common
      - Bile is rarely present
    - Grade IV
      - Cells contain nuclei that occupy most of cytoplasm
      - Predominantly solid areas with little or no bile
      - Intravascular and intrasinusoidal growth common
- Special stains
  - Reticulin stain commonly used to visualize reticular fibers
  - HepPar 1
    - Commonly used immunostain for suspected HCC
    - Highly sensitive and specific for hepatocytic differentiation

IMAGING FINDINGS

Detection

- HCC commonly occurs in setting of chronic liver disease &/or cirrhosis
  - Frequently results as final manifestation in continuum of nodular liver disease
- Cirrhosis alters normal liver morphology with variable degree of
  - Fibrosis
  - Scarring
  - Nodular regeneration
  - Altered hepatic perfusion
    - Portal hypertension
    - Portal venous occlusion ± reversal of flow
- Regenerative nodules
  - Ultrasound
    - Plays little role in detection of discrete liver nodules
    - Liver margins may demonstrate nodular contour in setting of macronodular cirrhosis
  - CT
    - Nodules poorly visualized on NECT
    - Enhancement similar to background parenchyma on CECT
    - Siderotic nodules may be occasionally seen as hyperdense on NECT
  - MR
    - T1WI
      - Nonsiderotic nodules can occasionally be detected as slightly hyperintense
      - Siderotic nodules well visualized on gradient-echo images, but rarely seen on spin-echo images
    - T2WI
      - Nonsiderotic nodules rarely seen
      - Siderotic nodules well visualized as discrete hypointense foci
    - T1 C+
      - Nonsiderotic nodules poorly visualized (may very rarely demonstrate arterial phase enhancement)
      - Siderotic nodules commonly seen as hypointense foci
- Dysplastic nodules
  - Ultrasound
    - Plays little role in detection of liver nodules
  - CT
    - Nodules may occasionally be seen as hyperdense on NECT
    - Generally isodense to liver on CECT
  - MR
    - T1WI
      - Large nodules may be homogeneously hyperintense
    - T2WI
      - Large nodules may be homogeneously hypointense
    - T1 C+
      - Enhancement rare
      - Mimics HCC when seen
- Hepatocellular carcinoma
  - Ultrasound
    - Usual modality of choice for screening of HCC in cirrhotic patient
      - Most affordable imaging modality
      - No ionizing radiation
    - Echogenicity of HCC highly variable
    - Small lesions (< 5 cm) are usually hypoechoic
      - Thin hypoechoic halo corresponding to fibrous capsule commonly seen
    - Larger lesions (> 5 cm) are generally mixed echogenicity
      - Hyperechoic areas can be seen in setting of intratumoral fat
      - Hypoechoic regions commonly seen in setting of necrosis
    - Color Doppler

HEPATOCELLULAR CARCINOMA

- Neovascularity and arteriovenous shunting may be seen
- High velocity waveforms characteristic, albeit nonspecific
- Power Doppler signal variable; cannot be used to reliably distinguish HCC from metastatic disease
- CT
  - NECT
    - Visualization generally limited without IV contrast
    - Lesions are usually hypodense if detected
      - Patchy fat attenuation may be seen in lesions with intratumoral fat
      - Fluid attenuation may be seen with tumoral necrosis
  - CECT
    - Arterial phase
      - Avid homogeneous enhancement in small lesions
      - Heterogeneous enhancement in larger lesions
      - Transient hepatic attenuation difference (THAD) may be seen as wedge-shaped region of increased perfusion from local portal vein occlusion
      - Some investigators advocate both early and late arterial phases in order to overcome differences in blood flow kinetics and tumor characteristics
    - Portal venous phase
      - Small lesions usually not detectable due to washout
      - Larger lesions may retain variable degree of enhancement
    - Delayed phase
      - Both small and large lesions generally not well visualized
    - Hepatic artery catheter CT
      - Invasive procedure requiring selective catheterization of hepatic artery
      - May reveal small lesions not seen during routine intravenous arterial phase studies
      - May potentially alter treatment options
- MR findings
  - Most sensitive and specific imaging modality for detection of HCC
  - Considered gold standard for characterization of liver nodules in setting of cirrhosis
  - T1WI
    - Variable signal, depending on degree of fatty metaplasia, fibrosis, and necrosis
    - Generally iso- to hypointense
    - Rarely hyperintense in presence of fat, copper, or glycoproteins
  - T2WI
    - Variable signal, although generally hyperintense
    - "Nodule within nodule" occasionally seen (small T2 hyperintense focus within uniformly T2 hypointense dysplastic nodule)
  - T1 C+
    - Small lesions (< 2 cm) generally show rapid arterial enhancement with rapid washout in portal venous and delayed phases

- Large lesions (> 2 cm) demonstrate heterogeneous nodular enhancement during both arterial and later phases
  - Diffusion-weighted imaging (DWI)
    - Evolving technology used in conjunction with other imaging sequences
    - Useful tool for lesion detection
    - DWI presently limited for lesion characterization
- Angiography
  - Enlarged arterial feeders
  - Coarse neovascularity
  - Arterioportal shunts
  - "Threads and streaks"
    - Linear parallel vascular channels coursing along portal venous radicles
    - Seen in setting of portal venous involvement
- Nuclear medicine
  - Technetium sulfur colloid
    - Focal defect in cirrhotics
    - Heterogeneous uptake in noncirrhotics
  - Hepatobiliary scan
    - Variable uptake (roughly 50% of lesions)
  - Gallium scan
    - Avid uptake in 90% of cases

Staging

- Multiple staging systems for HCC are currently employed
- Surgical staging
  - American Joint Committee on Cancer/Union Internationale Contre le Cancer (AJCC/UICC) system
    - Most widely used surgical system
    - Incorporates anatomic and histologic findings at tumor resection
    - Based on standard system of tumor, node, and metastasis classification
    - System can be applied after liver resection or transplantation
- Medical and clinical staging
  - Okuda system
    - Earliest medical classification system
    - 1st system to incorporate both
      - Tumor size
      - Liver function parameters
    - Has been largely replaced with newer Cancer of the Liver Italian Program (CLIP) and Barcelona Clinic Liver Cancer (BCLC) systems
    - System parameters include
      - Tumor size
      - Ascites
      - Jaundice
      - Serum albumin
    - Individuals are assigned to stage 1-3 based on above parameters
      - 1 implies best prognosis
      - 3 implies poorest prognosis
    - Limitations of Okuda system
      - Does not categorize tumor as unifocal, multifocal, or diffuse
      - Does not specify presence or absence of vascular invasion
  - Cancer of the Liver Italian Program (CLIP) system
    - Scoring system designed to classify
      - Extent and severity of HCC

- Clinical parameters of underlying liver disease
  - Generally regarded as easier to implement and more accurate than Okuda classification
  - Parameters of CLIP system include
    - Child-Pugh score
    - Tumor morphology
    - α-fetoprotein
    - Portal vein patency
  - Individuals are assigned score between 0-6 according to CLIP system
    - 0 implies best prognosis
    - 6 implies worst prognosis
  - Barcelona Clinic Liver Cancer (BCLC) staging
    - Regarded as highly reliable staging system that includes the following parameters
      - Tumor stage
      - Underlying liver function
      - Physical status
- Assessment of underlying liver disease
  - Child-Pugh score (Child-Turcotte-Pugh score)
    - Not a scoring system for HCC
      - Used to assess severity of cirrhosis
    - Originally used to predict mortality during surgery
    - Often employed in setting of HCC for establishing
      - Disease prognosis
      - Treatment options
      - Necessity of liver transplantation
    - Scoring is based on 5 clinical measures of liver disease
      - Total bilirubin
      - Serum albumin
      - INR (some older references substitute prolongation time [PT])
      - Ascites
      - Hepatic encephalopathy
    - Liver disease is stratified into Child-Pugh class A through C based on summation of above parameters
      - Class A entails 100% 1-year survival and 85% 2-year survival
      - Class B entails 81% 1-year survival and 57% 2-year survival
      - Class C entails 45% 1-year survival and 35% 2-year survival
  - Model of end-stage liver disease (MELD) score
    - Additional scoring system for assessing severity of chronic liver disease
    - Used to predict mortality for patients with chronic endstage disease
    - Utilized by United Network for Organ Sharing (UNOS) and Eurotransplant for prioritizing allocation of liver transplants
    - Scoring is based on 3 clinical parameters
      - Serum bilirubin
      - INR
      - Serum creatinine
  - Fibrosis score
    - Often employed as additional prognostic indicator in setting of HCC
    - Scoring system uses 0-6 scale
    - F0
      - Fibrosis score 0-4 (none to moderate fibrosis)
    - F1

- Fibrosis score 5-6 (severe fibrosis or cirrhosis)
- Imaging techniques for local staging
  - Ultrasound
    - Useful tool for HCC screening
      - Wide availability
      - Low cost
      - Lack of ionizing radiation
    - Plays little role in staging of HCC
  - CT
    - Preferred imaging modality for staging of widespread metastatic disease
    - Useful tool for local staging if MR not feasible
      - Implanted medical devices that are MR incompatible
      - Lack of MR availability
      - Patient claustrophobia
    - Multiplanar capability significantly improved with ongoing evolution of robust post-processing software
  - MR
    - Imaging modality of choice for local staging of HCC
    - Continual evolution of faster pulse sequences provide high quality imaging
    - Excellent intrinsic soft tissue contrast
    - Superb multiplanar capability
    - Multiple contrast agents available allow for greater flexibility of liver imaging
      - Extracellular fluid agents (conventional gadolinium)
      - Hepatobiliary-specific agents
      - Reticuloendothelial agents
      - Blood pool agents
    - Permits serial evaluation of liver lesions following IV contrast administration
- Local staging
  - T1
    - Solitary tumor without vascular invasion
  - T2
    - Solitary tumor with vascular invasion
    - Multiple tumors, none > 5 cm
  - T3a
    - Multiple tumors > 5 cm
  - T3b
    - Single or multiple tumors of any size
    - Vascular invasion involving major branch of portal or hepatic vein
  - T4
    - Direct invasion of adjacent organs
      - Other than gallbladder
    - Perforation of visceral peritoneum

CLINICAL ISSUES

Presentation

- Clinical signs and symptoms vary depending on degree of underlying cirrhosis
  - Right upper quadrant fullness
  - Abdominal pain
  - Weight loss
  - Jaundice
  - Ascites
  - Tumoral rupture with hemoperitoneum

HEPATOCELLULAR CARCINOMA

- More common in Africa and Southeast Asia
- Systemic metabolic complications can include
  - Hypoglycemia
  - Erythrocytosis
  - Hypercalcemia
  - Hyperlipidemia
- Abnormal lab values
  - Elevated α-fetoprotein (AFP)
    - Signifies dedifferentiation of hepatocytes
    - Elevated AFP levels (> 400 µg/mL) seen in 40-65% of patients with HCC
  - Abnormal liver function tests (LFTs)

Cancer Natural History & Prognosis
- 5-year survival < 5% without treatment

Treatment Options
- Surgical therapy
  - Surgical resection
    - Preferred alternative with highest chance of cure
    - Criteria for successful surgical resection include
      - Small, unifocal tumors
      - Absence of vascular invasion
      - Adequate hepatic functional reserve (Child-Pugh class A or well-compensated class B disease)
      - No clinically significant comorbidities
  - Hepatic transplantation
    - Offers good chance for long-term survival
    - Typically reserved for individuals with Child-Pugh class C disease who would not tolerate limited resection
    - Milan criteria for successful transplantation
      - 3 or fewer tumor nodules < 3 cm
      - Solitary tumor < 5 cm
      - No vascular invasion
      - No lymphadenopathy
- Medical therapy
  - Percutaneous ethanol injection
    - Direct injection of ethanol into tumors using CT or US guidance
    - Procedure has been employed for many years with variable success
    - Has largely been replaced with more sophisticated techniques
  - Transcatheter arterial chemoembolization (TACE)
    - Technique is well suited for individuals with large, infiltrative, &/or multifocal disease
    - Involves transarterial administration of various cocktails including
      - Alcohol
      - Acetic acid
      - Doxorubicin
      - Cisplatin
      - Mitomycin C
    - Chemotherapeutic agents are effectively delivered via hepatic arteries
      - Hepatomas derive 80-85% of blood supply via hepatic arterial system
      - Normal hepatic parenchyma primarily supplied via portal venous system
    - Feeding arteries are occluded with gel foam or coils prior to chemotherapeutic delivery in order to prevent systemic toxicity

- Tumor burden reduction seen in 16-61% of patients
- Patients with significant liver impairment (Child-Pugh class C) are generally considered ineligible for TACE
- Other contraindications include
  - Severe thrombocytopenia or leukopenia
  - Cardiac or renal insufficiency
  - Uncorrectable coagulopathy
  - Ascites
  - Portal vein occlusion
  - Atypical or diseased hepatic arterial anatomy that would potentially increase risk of injury to adjacent nontarget organs
- TACE therapy has been shown to prolong survival in patients with HCC who are ineligible for surgical excision
- Reported survival rates following TACE
  - 34-88% at year 1
  - 33-64% at year 2
  - 18-51% at year 3
  - Transarterial internal radiation therapy
    - Delivery of radioactive material into arterial blood supply of tumor after directed catheterization with fluoroscopic guidance
    - Several isotopes have been successfully utilized
      - Yttrium-90 (most commonly used agent to date)
      - Iodine-131
      - Rhenium-188
    - Yttrium-90 has 64.2-hour half-life and decays to stable zirconium-90
    - Radioisotope composition and preparation
      - Particles are embedded in insoluble and nonbiodegradable glass or resin microsphere
      - Particles have mean diameter of 20-40 µg
      - Microspheres help facilitate predictable delivery of agent
    - Radiotherapy is generally delivered over course of 10-12 days for total dose of around 150 Gy
    - Careful pre-procedure planning is essential in order to limit systemic toxicity
      - Regional embolization of feeding vessels is crucial in order to avoid collateral radiation damage to nearby organs
    - Technique shows promise for prolonging survival
      - Agent is still relatively novel
      - Few large scale investigations have been performed to date
  - Radiofrequency ablation (RFA)
    - Generally reserved for treatment of focal or multifocal lesions that are surgically unresectable
    - HCC in cirrhotic liver is particularly well suited for radiofrequency ablation
      - Especially given hard pseudocapsule that often surrounds hepatomas
    - Generally accepted criteria for successful radiofrequency ablation
      - Tumors should not exceed 5 cm in diameter
      - Number of tumors should not exceed 3
    - Technique involves
      - CT- or US-assisted percutaneous placement of probe into tumor

- Administration of electrical current until tumor temperature reaches 50° C
  - ▪ Procedure often employed in operating room in conjunction with partial hepatic resection
  - ▪ Technique has traditionally been effective for small tumors
    - Success rate of tumoral necrosis decreases significantly as tumor volume increases
  - ▪ Recent innovations in probe technology will hopefully permit successful ablation of tumors up to 6-7 cm
  - ▪ RFA advantages include
    - High local efficacy for small lesions
    - Easily repeatable procedure
    - Sparing of adjacent unaffected liver tissue
    - Low complication rate
    - Relatively low cost
- ○ Systemic chemotherapy
  - ▪ Effectiveness is generally minimal
    - High rate of tumoral drug resistance
    - Inherently impaired liver function in setting of advanced HCC prohibits safe administration of systemic agents
  - ▪ Chemotherapeutic agents commonly employed
    - 5-fluorouracil
    - Doxorubicin
    - Cisplatin
    - Etoposide
    - Gemcitabine
    - Vincristine
  - ▪ Biologic agents
    - Composed mainly of interferon
    - Has preventative role in tumorigenesis
    - Particularly useful for patients with active hepatitis with high viral load
  - ▪ Monoclonal antibodies
    - Recently developed for treatment of colon, lung, and breast cancer
    - Promising future agent for treatment of HCC

- ▪ Lung
- ▪ Bone
- ▪ Adrenal gland
- ▪ Peritoneum/omentum

SELECTED REFERENCES

1. American Joint Committee on Cancer: AJCC Cancer Staging Manual. 7th ed. New York: Springer. 191-9, 2010
2. Seale MK et al: Hepatobiliary-specific MR contrast agents: role in imaging the liver and biliary tree. Radiographics. 29(6):1725-48, 2009
3. Hanna RF et al: Cirrhosis-associated hepatocellular nodules: correlation of histopathologic and MR imaging features. Radiographics. 28(3):747-69, 2008
4. Lencioni R et al: Guidelines for imaging focal lesions in liver cirrhosis. Expert Rev Gastroenterol Hepatol. 2(5):697-703, 2008
5. Willatt JM et al: MR imaging of hepatocellular carcinoma in the cirrhotic liver: challenges and controversies. Radiology. 247(2):311-30, 2008
6. Clark HP et al: Staging and current treatment of hepatocellular carcinoma. Radiographics. 25 Suppl 1:S3-23, 2005
7. Iannaccone R et al: Hepatocellular carcinoma: role of unenhanced and delayed phase multi-detector row helical CT in patients with cirrhosis. Radiology. 234(2):460-7, 2005
8. Pawlik TM et al: Staging of hepatocellular carcinoma. Hepatology. 42(3):738-9; author reply 739-40, 2005
9. Laghi A et al: Hepatocellular carcinoma: detection with triple-phase multi-detector row helical CT in patients with chronic hepatitis. Radiology. 226(2):543-9, 2003
10. Martín J et al: Magnetic resonance of focal liver lesions in hepatic cirrhosis and chronic hepatitis. Semin Ultrasound CT MR. 23(1):62-78, 2002
11. Baron RL et al: From the RSNA refresher courses: screening the cirrhotic liver for hepatocellular carcinoma with CT and MR imaging: opportunities and pitfalls. Radiographics. 21 Spec No:S117-32, 2001
12. Katyal S et al: Extrahepatic metastases of hepatocellular carcinoma. Radiology. 216(3):698-703, 2000

REPORTING CHECKLIST

T Staging
- Detection of HCC in setting of regenerative and dysplastic nodules
- Tumor size
- Tumor number
- Tumor morphology
  - ○ Sharply marginated
  - ○ Diffusely infiltrating
- Presence or absence of vascular invasion
- Extracapsular tumor extension

N Staging
- N0
  - ○ No regional lymph node metastases
- N1
  - ○ Regional lymph node metastases

M Staging
- M0
  - ○ No distant metastases
- M1
  - ○ Distant metastases

HEPATOCELLULAR CARCINOMA

Stage I (T1 N0 M0)

Stage I (T1 N0 M0)

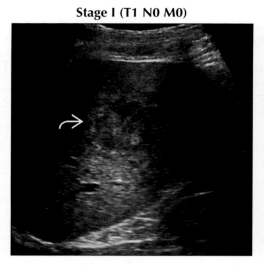

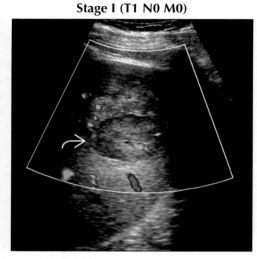

(Left) Transverse transabdominal ultrasound in a patient who presented with jaundice and weight loss shows a mildly heterogeneous, predominantly hypoechoic mass ➔ within the right lobe of the liver. (Right) Transverse color Doppler ultrasound in the same patient shows scattered areas of arterial blood flow within the mass ➔. The tumor proved to be a solitary hepatocellular carcinoma following partial hepatectomy.

Stage I (T1 N0 M0)

Stage I (T1 N0 M0)

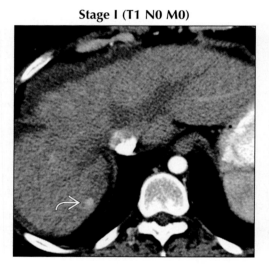

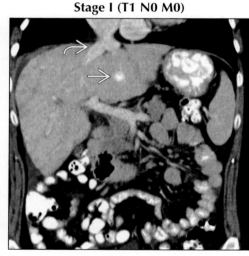

(Left) Axial CECT shows a solitary subcentimeter enhancing lesion ➔ within the posterior segment of the right lobe, representing a small HCC. The liver is diffusely nodular in contour, consistent with cirrhosis. (Right) Coronal CECT shows a solitary 1.2 cm enhancing lesion ➔ within the left liver lobe, consistent with small HCC. Mild hepatic venous congestion and hepatic vein distention ➔ from impaired right heart function is likewise noted.

Stage I (T1 N0 M0)

Stage I (T1 N0 M0)

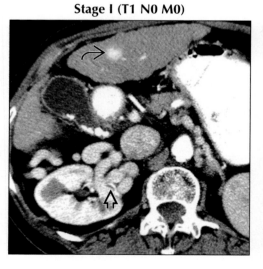

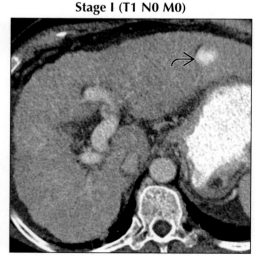

(Left) Axial CECT shows an early enhancing lesion in the lateral segment of the left hepatic lobe ➔, consistent with a small HCC. Morphologic features of cirrhosis and portal hypertension are present, as evidenced by a spontaneous portorenal shunt ➔. (Right) Axial CECT shows an arterially enhancing lesion ➔ within the lateral segment of the left hepatic lobe, consistent with small HCC. Diffusely nodular liver contour is visible, consistent with cirrhosis.

HEPATOCELLULAR CARCINOMA

Stage I (T1 N0 M0)

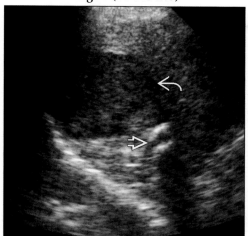

Stage I (T1 N0 M0)

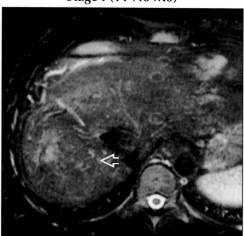

(Left) Transverse transabdominal ultrasound shows a sharply marginated hypoechoic lesion ⮎ within the posterior segment of the right lobe, consistent with HCC. Linear echogenic artifact from a TIPS ⮕ is likewise noted. *(Right)* Axial T2WI FSE MR in the same patient shows a predominantly isointense mass ⮕ within the posterior segment of the right lobe, consistent with HCC.

Stage I (T1 N0 M0)

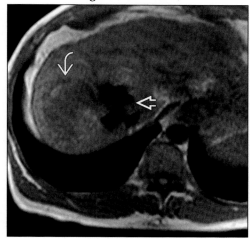

Stage I (T1 N0 M0)

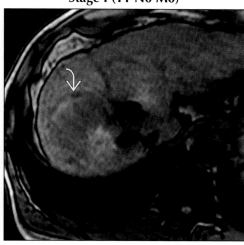

(Left) Axial T1WI in-phase MR in the same patient shows a predominantly hypointense mass ⮕ in the posterior segment of the right lobe of the liver, consistent with HCC. Blooming artifact from a TIPS ⮕ is noted. *(Right)* Axial T1WI out-of-phase MR in the same patient again shows a predominantly hypointense mass ⮕ within the posterior segment of the right lobe of the liver. Nodular liver contour is noted, consistent with cirrhosis.

Stage I (T1 N0 M0)

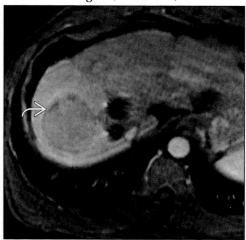

Stage I (T1 N0 M0)

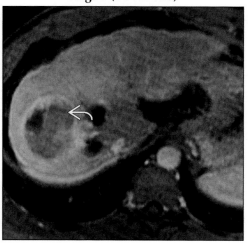

(Left) Axial T1WI C+ MR in the arterial phase in the same patient shows homogeneous enhancement of the right hepatic lobe mass ⮕. The mass is essentially isointense to the liver following IV gadolinium administration. *(Right)* Axial T1WI C+ MR in the portal venous phase in the same patient shows de-enhancement of the mass ⮕ in the posterior segment of the right lobe, consistent with HCC.

HEPATOCELLULAR CARCINOMA

Stage I (T1 N0 M0)

Stage I (T1 N0 M0)

(Left) Axial CECT in the late arterial phase in a cirrhotic patient shows an enhancing mass ➔ within the anterior segment of the right hepatic lobe, consistent with HCC. *(Right)* Axial CECT in the portal venous phase in the same patient shows washout of contrast from the mass ➔ within the anterior segment of the right lobe.

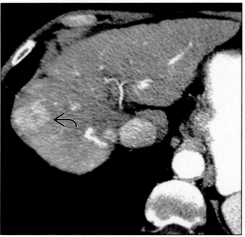
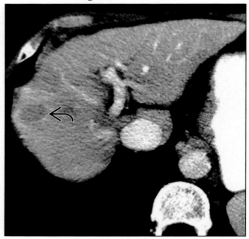

Stage I (T1 N0 M0)

Stage I (T1 N0 M0)

(Left) Axial T1WI MR in the same patient shows a mildly hyperintense mass ➔ within the anterior segment of the right lobe. *(Right)* Axial T2WI FSE MR in the same patient shows a mildly hyperintense mass ➔ within the anterior segment of the right heptic lobe. A small amount of perihepatic ascites ➔ is likewise noted in this cirrhotic patient.

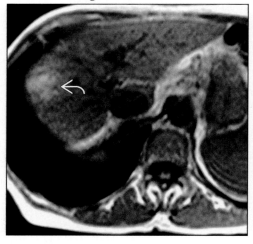
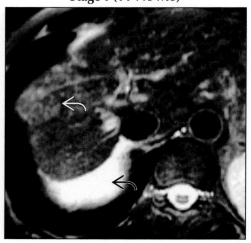

Stage I (T1 N0 M0)

Stage I (T1 N0 M0)

(Left) Axial T1WI C+ MR in the late arterial phase in the same patient shows avid homogeneous enhancement of the mass ➔ in the anterior segment of the right hepatic lobe, consistent with a solitary HCC. *(Right)* Axial T1WI C+ MR in the portal venous phase in the same patient shows de-enhancement of the mass ➔ within the anterior segment of the right hepatic lobe. Note the persistent peripheral enhancement of the lesion.

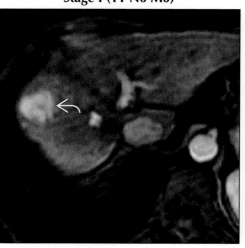
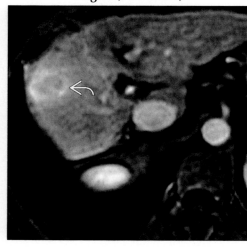

HEPATOCELLULAR CARCINOMA

Stage II (T2 N0 M0)

Stage II (T2 N0 M0)

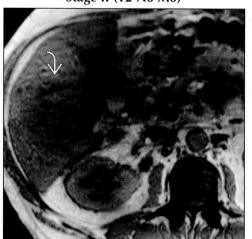 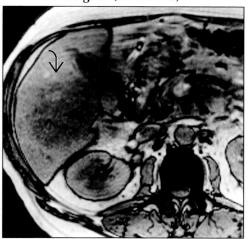

(Left) Axial T1WI in-phase MR shows a large, heterogeneous, poorly marginated mass ➔ within the posterior segment of the right lobe in this patient with hemochromatosis. (Right) Axial T1WI out-of-phase MR in the same patient shows the poorly marginated, heterogeneous mass ➔ in the posterior segment of the right lobe of the liver.

Stage II (T2 N0 M0)

Stage II (T2 N0 M0)

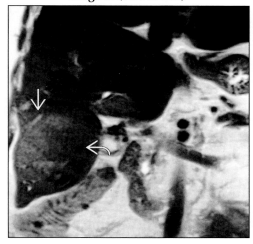 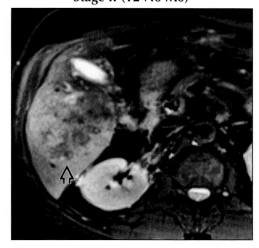

(Left) Coronal T2WI FSE MR in the same patient shows the poorly marginated, mildly hyperintense mass ➔ within the posterior segment of the right lobe of the liver. Vascular invasion is noted involving a small branch of the right portal vein ➔. (Right) Axial T2WI FS MR in the same patient shows the poorly marginated, heterogeneous mass ➔ within the posterior segment of the right lobe of the liver.

Stage II (T2 N0 M0)

Stage II (T2 N0 M0)

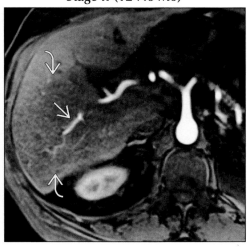 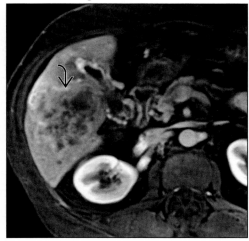

(Left) Axial T1WI C+ MR in the arterial phase in the same patient shows the poorly marginated hypointense mass ➔ within the posterior segment of the right lobe. There is tumoral neovascularity with prominent hepatic arterial branches ➔ within the periphery of the mass. (Right) Axial T1WI C+ MR in the portal venous phase in the same patient shows the heterogeneously enhancing mass within the posterior segment of the right hepatic lobe ➔.

HEPATOCELLULAR CARCINOMA

Stage II (T2 N0 M0)

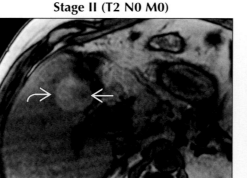

Stage II (T2 N0 M0)

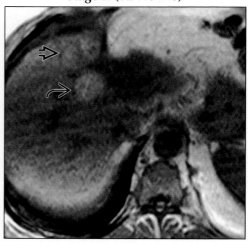

(Left) Axial T1WI out-of-phase MR shows a hyperintense mass ➡, consistent with a dysplastic nodule. A hypointense nodule is noted in the periphery of the mass ➡, consistent with a small HCC within a dysplastic nodule or a "nodule within a nodule" sign. *(Right)* Axial T1WI in-phase MR shows a uniformly hyperintense mass ➡ at a different level in the same patient, consistent with a dysplastic nodule. An additional "nodule within a nodule" lesion ➡ is faintly visualized.

Stage II (T2 N0 M0)

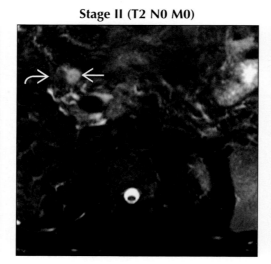

Stage II (T2 N0 M0)

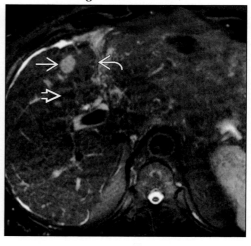

(Left) Axial T2WI FS MR in the same patient shows that the mass is isointense to the background parenchyma ➡, consistent with a dysplastic nodule. A hyperintense nodule is noted within the mass ➡, consistent with a "nodule in a nodule" focus of HCC within a dysplastic nodule. *(Right)* Axial T2WI FS MR shows the same mass with a hyperintense nodule of HCC ➡ within an isointense dysplastic nodule ➡. A 2nd dysplastic nodule is faintly visualized ➡.

Stage II (T2 N0 M0)

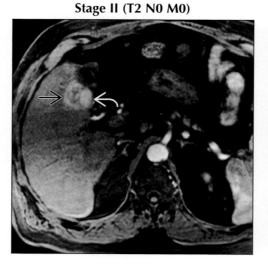

Stage II (T2 N0 M0)

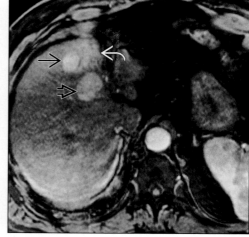

(Left) Axial T1WI C+ MR demonstrates the same mass. Note the "nodule within a nodule" enhancing focus of HCC ➡ within a dysplastic nodule ➡. *(Right)* Axial T1WI C+ MR in the same patient again shows a "nodule within a nodule" enhancing focus of HCC ➡ in a mildly enhancing dysplastic nodule ➡. A 2nd mildly enhancing dysplastic nodule ➡ is again seen.

HEPATOCELLULAR CARCINOMA

Stage II (T2 N0 M0)

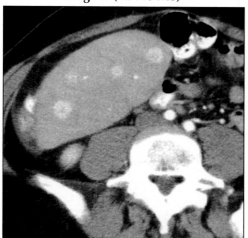

Stage II (T2 N0 M0)

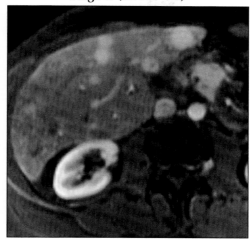

(Left) Axial CECT in the arterial phase shows multiple enhancing masses within the right lobe of the liver; all of the masses measure less than 5 cm. These findings are consistent with stage II multifocal HCC. *(Right)* Axial T1WI C+ MR shows multiple enhancing masses, all of which measure less than 5 cm, consistent with multifocal T2 HCC.

Stage II (T2 N0 M0)

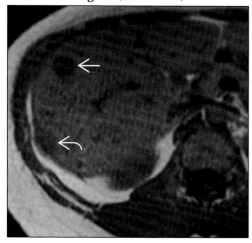

Stage II (T2 N0 M0)

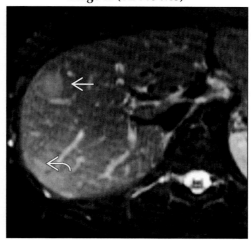

(Left) Axial T1WI MR shows a hypointense intraparenchymal ➡ and subcapsular ➡ mass, consistent with multifocal HCC. *(Right)* Axial T2WI FS MR in the same patient shows a mildly hyperintense intraparenchymal mass ➡ and a faintly visualized subcapsular mass ➡, consistent with multifocal HCC.

Stage II (T2 N0 M0)

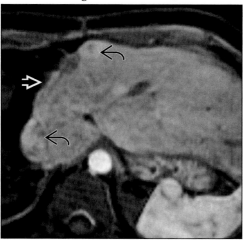

Stage II (T2 N0 M0)

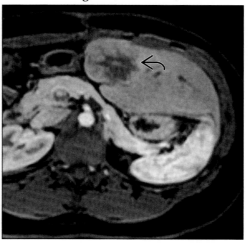

(Left) Axial T1WI C+ MR shows evidence of prior right hepatectomy for a solitary HCC within the right lobe ➡. Heterogeneously enhancing masses are noted at the resection margin ➡, consistent with disease recurrence. *(Right)* Axial T1WI C+ MR in the same patient shows a large HCC adjacent to the resection margin ➡, consistent with disease recurrence.

HEPATOCELLULAR CARCINOMA

**Fibrolamellar HCC,
Stage IIIA (T3a N0 M0)**

**Fibrolamellar HCC,
Stage IIIA (T3a N0 M0)**

(Left) Axial T1WI MR shows a large, sharply marginated, uniformly hypointense mass arising from the right lobe of the liver, consistent with fibrolamellar HCC. *(Right)* Axial T2WI FS MR in the same patient shows a sharply marginated mass that is hyperintense relative to the background liver parenchyma, consistent with fibrolamellar HCC. A characteristic hypointense central scar ➔ is noted.

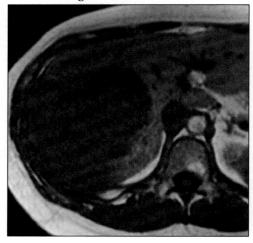

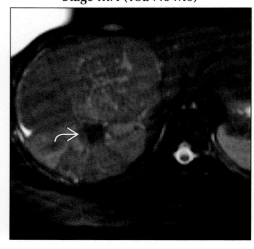

**Fibrolamellar HCC,
Stage IIIA (T3a N0 M0)**

**Fibrolamellar HCC,
Stage IIIA (T3a N0 M0)**

(Left) Axial T1WI C+ MR in the arterial phase in the same patient shows avid heterogeneous enhancement of the mass, consistent with fibrolamellar HCC. There is no enhancement of the central scar ➔. *(Right)* Axial T1WI C+ MR in the portal venous in the same patient shows intravenous contrast washout of the right hepatic lobe fibrolamellar HCC.

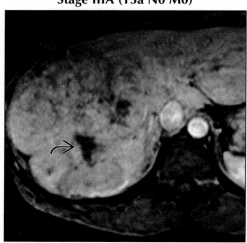

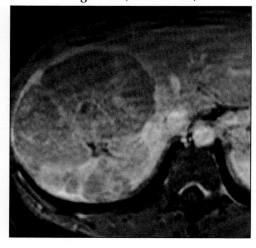

Stage IIIA (T3a N0 M0)

Stage IIIA (T3a N0 M0)

(Left) Axial CECT in the early arterial phase shows multiple large, partially confluent masses that demonstrate heterogeneous enhancement. Extensive abdominal ascites is likewise noted in this patient with advanced cirrhosis and portal hypertension. *(Right)* Axial T1WI MR shows poorly marginated, hypointense masses within the posterior segment of the right lobe ➔ and the caudate lobe ➱, consistent with multifocal HCC.

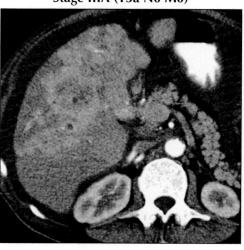

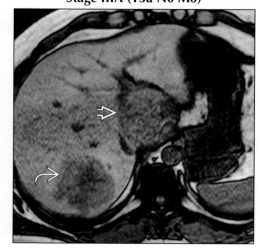

HEPATOCELLULAR CARCINOMA

Stage IIIA (T3a N0 M0)

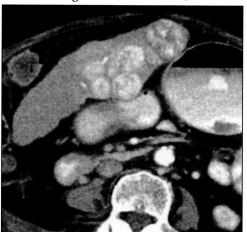

Stage IIIA (T3a N0 M0)

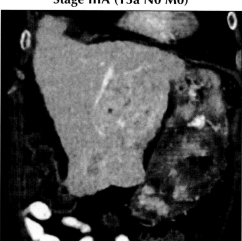

(Left) Axial CECT shows several partially contiguous, heterogeneously enhancing masses within the inferior aspect of the lateral segment of the left hepatic lobe, consistent with multifocal HCC. Diffuse contour nodularity is noted, consistent with advanced cirrhosis. *(Right)* Coronal CECT in the same patient shows partially contiguous, heterogeneously enhancing masses throughout the lateral segment of the left lobe of the liver, consistent with mutifocal HCC.

Stage IIIB (T3b N0 M0)

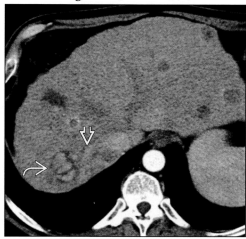

Stage IIIB (T3b N0 M0)

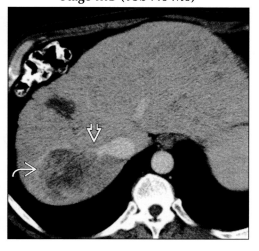

(Left) Axial CECT arterial phase image shows a heterogeneously enhancing mass within the posterior segment of the right hepatic lobe ➔, which partially obscures and expands the right hepatic vein ➔. *(Right)* Axial CECT portal venous image in the same patient shows washout of tumor within the posterior segment of the right lobe ➔. Tumor is clearly seen invading and expanding the left hepatic vein ➔.

Stage IIIB (T3b N0 M0)

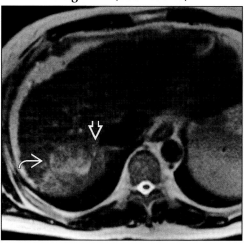

Stage IIIB (T3b N0 M0)

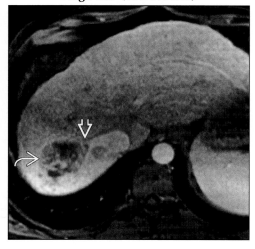

(Left) Axial T2WI FSE MR in the same patient shows the heterogeneous, predominantly hyperintense mass within the posterior segment of the left lobe ➔, consistent with HCC. Tumor extends into the adjacent left hepatic vein ➔. *(Right)* Axial T1WI C+ MR in the same patient again shows the heterogeneous mass within the posterior segment of the right liver lobe ➔. The mass expands and invades the left hepatic vein ➔.

HEPATOCELLULAR CARCINOMA

Stage IIIB (T3b N0 M0)

Stage IIIB (T3b N0 M0)

(Left) Axial T1WI C+ MR shows a heterogeneously enhancing mass within the posterior segment of the right hepatic lobe, consistent with HCC. *(Right)* Axial T1 C+ MR in the portal venous phase in the same patient shows extensive tumoral thrombus expanding the right portal vein ➡ and main portal vein.

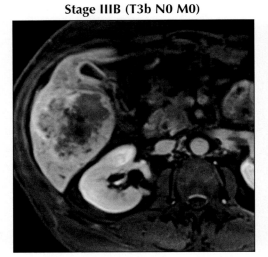

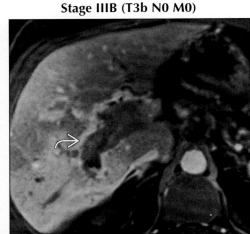

Stage IIIC (T4 N0 M0)

Stage IIIC (T4 N0 M0)

(Left) Axial T1WI C+ MR shows a large exophytic HCC arising from the lateral segment of the left lobe ➡ and invading the splenic hilum ➡. *(Right)* Coronal T2WI MR in the same patient shows the large HCC ➡ invading the upper pole of the spleen ➡.

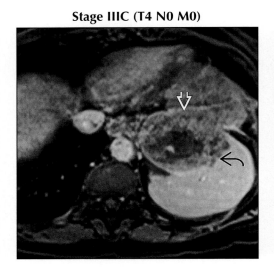

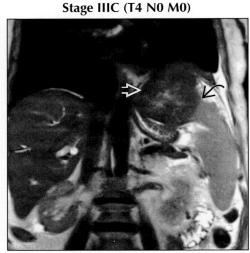

Stage IIIC (T4 N0 M0)

Stage IIIC (T4 N0 M0)

(Left) Axial T2WI FS MR shows a mass arising from the posterior aspect of the medial segment of the left lobe ➡ and extending beyond the visceral peritoneum. There is direct tumoral extension into the left main bile duct ➡. *(Right)* Axial T2WI MR in the same patient shows extensive tumoral invasion of the common hepatic duct ➡.

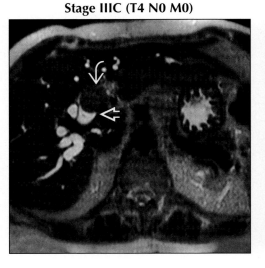

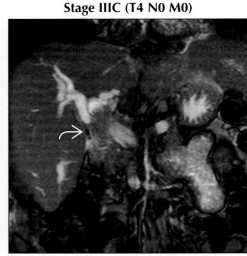

Stage IVA (T1 N1 M0)

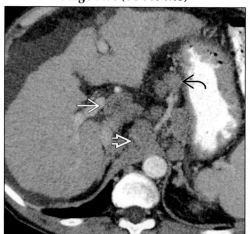

Stage IVA (T2 N1 M0)

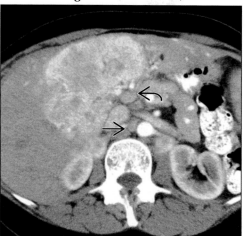

(Left) Axial CECT in the same patient shows extensive gastrohepatic ligament ⇗, porta hepatis ➡, and hepatic artery nodes ⇉. *(Right)* Axial CECT shows a large, avidly enhancing mass predominantly involving the medial segment of the left lobe. There are periportal ⇗ and paraaortic ➡ lymph nodes.

Stage IVB (T2 N1 M1)

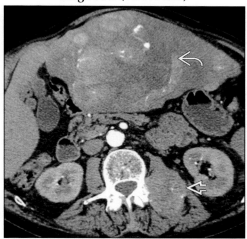

Stage IVB (T2 N1 M1)

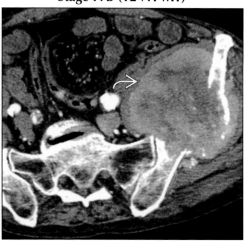

(Left) Axial CECT shows a large, heterogeneously enhancing mass expanding the left lobe of the liver ➡, consistent with a large HCC. Note the left paraspinal mass ⇉ with associated destructive changes of the L2 transverse process. Percutaneous CT-guided biopsy of the paraspinal mass confirmed osseous metastatic HCC. *(Right)* Axial CECT in the same patient shows a very large, lytic soft tissue mass arising from the left iliac bone ⇗.

Stage IVB (T3a N1 M1)

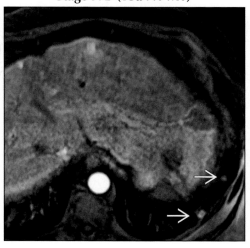

Stage IVB (T3a N1 M1)

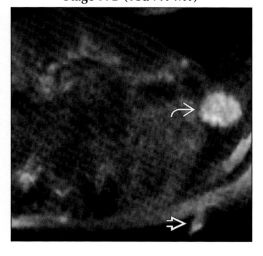

(Left) Axial T1WI C+ MR shows multiple masses throughout the liver that demonstrate variable enhancement, consistent with multifocal HCC. Two lung nodules are noted within the left lower lobe ⇉, consistent with metastatic disease. *(Right)* Axial diffusion-weighted image in the same patient shows an exophytic mass with increased signal intensity ⇗, consistent with HCC. A pulmonary nodule is faintly visualized within the left lower lobe ⇉.

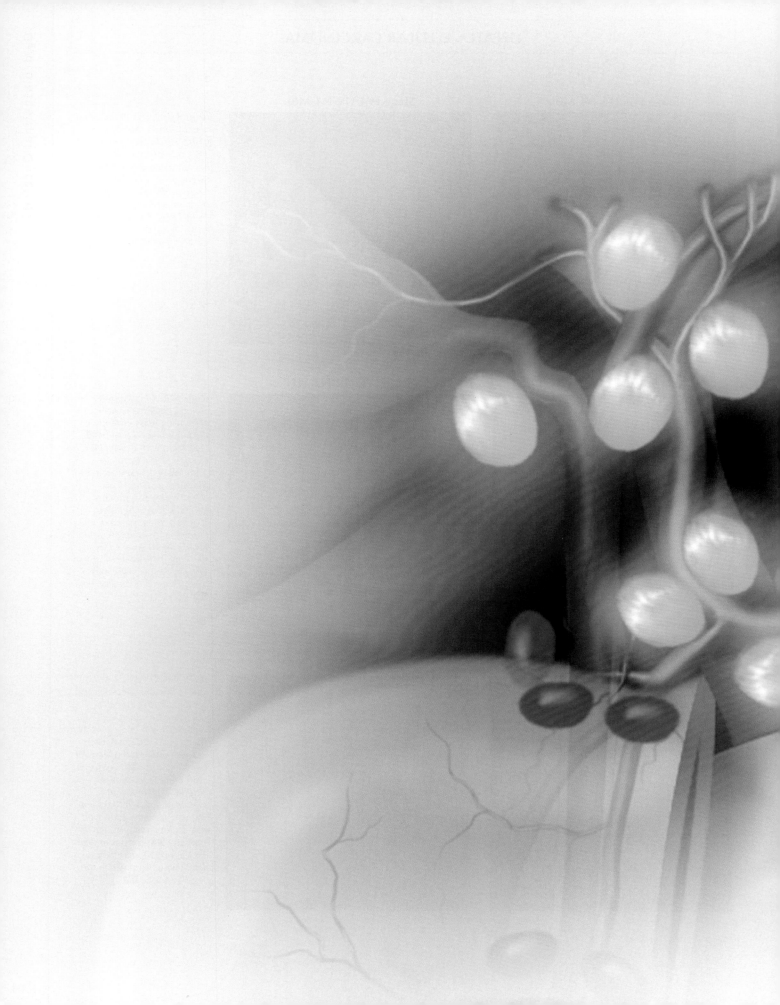

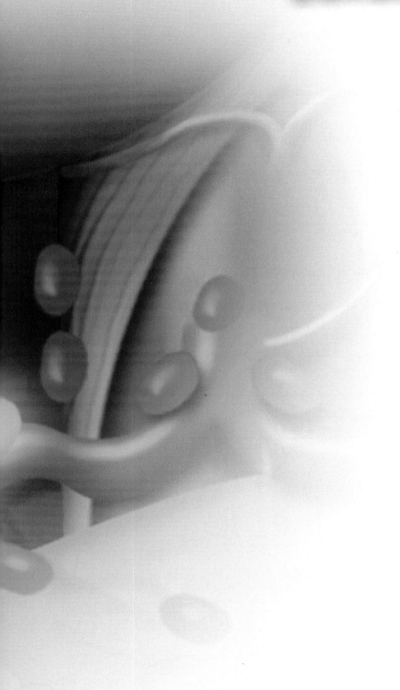

Gallbladder Carcinoma

GALLBLADDER CARCINOMA

(T) Primary Tumor

Adapted from 7th edition AJCC Staging Forms.

TNM	Definitions
TX	Primary tumor cannot be assessed
T0	No evidence of primary tumor
Tis	Carcinoma in situ
T1	Tumor invades lamina propria or muscular layer
T1a	Tumor invades lamina propria
T1b	Tumor invades muscular layer
T2	Tumor invades the perimuscular connective tissue; no extension beyond the serosa or into liver
T3	Tumor perforates the serosa (visceral peritoneum) &/or directly invades the liver &/or 1 other adjacent organ or structure, such as the stomach, duodenum, colon, pancreas, omentum, or extrahepatic bile ducts
T4	Tumor invades main portal vein or hepatic artery or invades ≥ 2 extrahepatic organs or structures

(N) Regional Lymph Nodes

NX	Regional lymph nodes cannot be assessed
N0	No regional lymph node metastasis
N1	Metastases in nodes along the cystic duct, common bile duct, hepatic artery, &/or portal vein
N2	Metastases to periaortic, pericaval, superior mesenteric artery, &/or celiac artery lymph nodes

(M) Distant Metastasis

M0	No distant metastasis
M1	Distant metastasis

AJCC Stages/Prognostic Groups

Adapted from 7th edition AJCC Staging Forms.

Stage	T	N	M
0	Tis	N0	M0
I	T1	N0	M0
II	T2	N0	M0
IIIA	T3	N0	M0
IIIB	T1, T2, T3	N1	M0
IVA	T4	N0, N1	M0
IVB	Any T	N2	M0
	Any T	Any N	M1

Tis

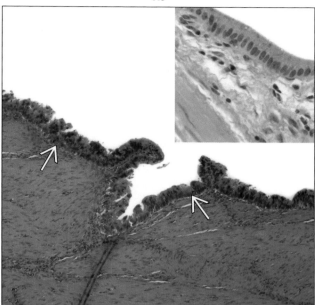

H&E stain shows high-grade dysplasia of the gallbladder epithelium. Neoplastic cells are limited to the mucosa and do not invade through the basement membrane ➡. These cells show crowded and hyperchromatic nuclei. Compare with normal uninvolved gall bladder epithelium (inset). (Original magnification 40x.)

Tis

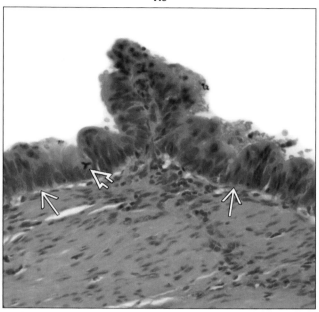

Higher magnification discloses neoplastic cells that have hyperchromatic, crowded, and stratified nuclei and are limited to the basement membrane ➡. Note the triple mitotic figure ➡ within the neoplastic cells. (Original magnification 500x.)

T1a

H&E stained section shows gallbladder carcinoma ➡ that is limited to the lamina propria, which extends from the overlying surface epithelium ➡ to the muscular layer ➡. (Original magnification 50x.)

T1a

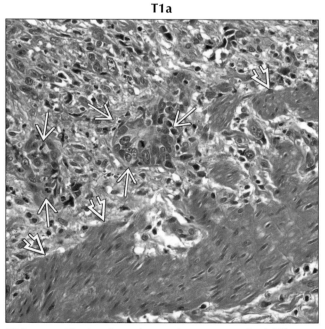

Higher magnification shows the neoplastic invasive glands ➡ in proximity to the muscle bundles ➡. (Original magnification 500x.)

GALLBLADDER CARCINOMA

T1b

T2

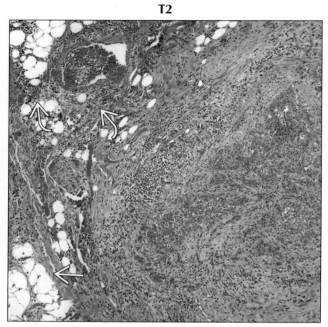

H&E stained section of gallbladder adenocarcinoma shows the neoplastic glands ➔ *infiltrating into the muscular layer. Note uninvolved separated muscle bundles* ➔. *(Original magnification 40x.)*

H&E stained section shows invasive gallbladder carcinoma ➔ *invading into perimuscular connective tissue* ➔, *but the tumor does not extend to the serosal surface. (Original magnification 40x.)*

T3

T3

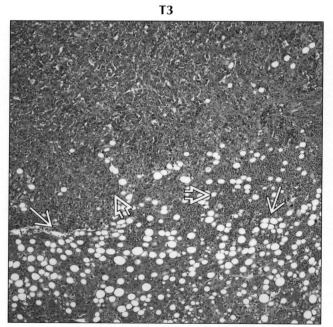

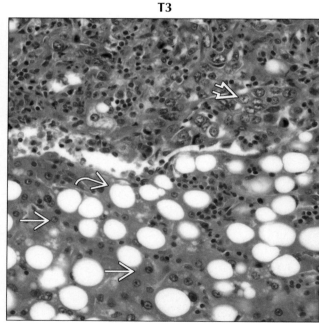

H&E stained section from the liver ➔ *shows invasive gallbladder adenocarcinoma* ➔. *(Original magnification 40x.)*

Higher magnification shows neoplastic glands ➔ *infiltrating into liver tissue. Hepatocytes are polyhedral cells with eosinophilic cytoplasm and round nuclei with occasional prominent nucleoli* ➔. *Note the prominent steatosis showing as a large number of fat clear cells* ➔ *admixed with liver cells. (Original magnification 400x.)*

T1a

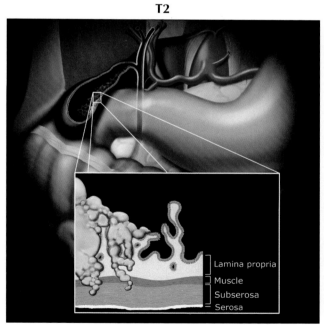

Graphic shows tumor invading the lamina propria, consistent with T1a disease.

T1b

Graphic shows tumor invading the muscle layer, consistent with T1b disease.

T2

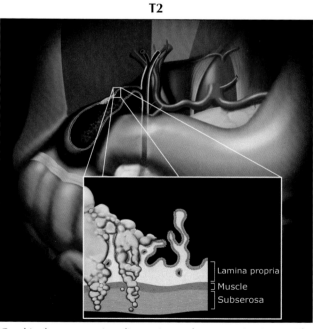

Graphic shows tumor arising from part of the gallbladder with serosal covering (away from the liver bed) and invading the subserosa without extension into the serosa, consistent with T2 disease.

T2

Graphic shows tumor invading perimuscular connective tissue with no extension into the liver, also consistent with T2 disease.

GALLBLADDER CARCINOMA

T3

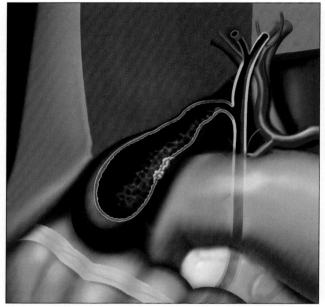

Graphic shows tumor arising from part of the gallbladder with serosal covering (away from the liver bed) and perforating the serosa, consistent with T3 disease.

T3

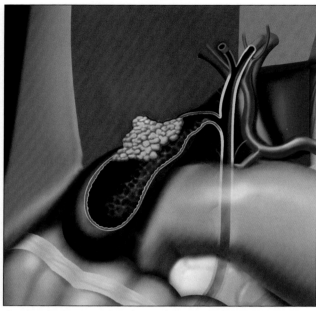

Graphic shows tumor directly invading into the liver in parts of the gallbladder with no serosal covering, also consistent with T3 disease.

T3

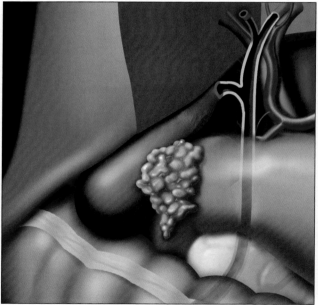

Graphic shows tumor invading the duodenum, consistent with T3 disease. Invasion of 1 adjacent structure, including the stomach, colon, pancreas, omentum, and extrahepatic bile duct, constitutes T3 disease. Invasion of 2 or more would be T4.

T4

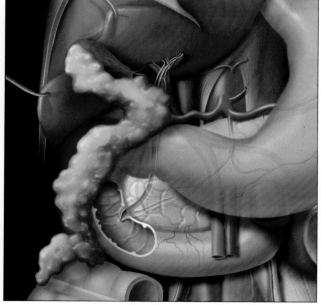

Graphic shows tumor invading the duodenum and the colon. As this represents invasion of 2 or more extrahepatic organs or structures, it is classified as T4 disease. If the tumor invades the main portal vein or hepatic artery, it is also considered T4 disease.

N1

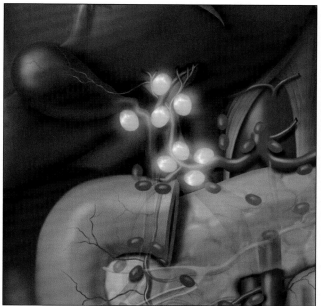

Graphic illustrates regional nodal involvement in gallbladder carcinoma. Regional lymph nodes include nodes along the common bile duct, hepatic artery, portal vein, and cystic duct.

N2

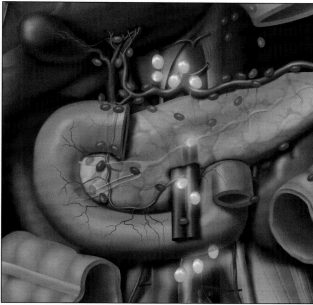

Graphic illustrates N2 nodal metastases in gallbladder carcinoma. N2 nodes include the celiac, periduodenal, peripancreatic, and superior mesenteric nodes.

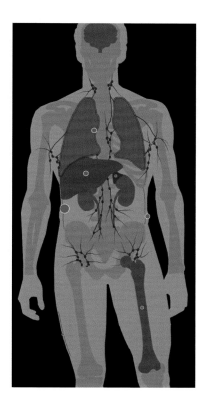

METASTASES, ORGAN FREQUENCY

Peritoneum	31%
Liver (intrahepatic)	10%
Lung or mediastinum	9%
Abdominal wall/incision	9%
Bone	4%
Skin	2.5%
Adrenal gland	2.5%
Distant lymph nodes	1%

GALLBLADDER CARCINOMA

OVERVIEW

General Comments
- Relatively rare neoplasm
- Highly lethal disease

Classification
- Histologic types of gallbladder cancer include
  - Carcinoma in situ
  - Adenocarcinoma, not otherwise specified (NOS) (75.8%)
  - Carcinoma, NOS (7.6%)
  - Papillary carcinoma (5.8%)
  - Mucinous carcinoma (4.8%)
  - Adenosquamous carcinoma (3.6%)
  - Squamous carcinoma (1.7%)
  - Small cell (oat cell) carcinoma (0.5%)
  - Adenocarcinoma, intestinal type
  - Clear cell adenocarcinoma
  - Signet ring cell carcinoma
  - Undifferentiated carcinoma
    - Spindle and giant cell types
    - Small cell types
  - Carcinosarcoma

PATHOLOGY

Routes of Spread
- Direct spread
  - Direct spread is common and occurs early
    - Due to lack of muscularis mucosa and submucosa in gallbladder wall
  - Tumor can spread to following organs
    - Liver
      - In autopsy series, direct extension to liver was present in up to 65% of cases
      - Facilitated by direct venous drainage through liver parenchyma to hepatic veins
      - Gallbladder straddles Couinaud segments 4b and 5, which are segments initially invaded by carcinoma
    - Colon (15%)
    - Duodenum (15%)
    - Pancreas (6%)
- Lymphatic spread
  - Present in > 50% of patients at initial diagnosis
  - Frequency of involvement of lymph nodes is strongly influenced by depth of invasion of primary tumor
  - Regional nodes are those along cystic duct, common bile duct, hepatic artery, and portal vein (N1)
  - Periaortic, pericaval, superior mesenteric, and celiac artery nodes are considered N2
  - More distal nodal metastases are considered M1
- Intraductal spread
  - Tumor extending to cystic duct is indication of poor prognosis
  - Carcinoma of gallbladder neck region frequently involves common bile duct
    - By intraductal extension through cystic duct or by external invasion of hepatoduodenal ligament
  - Results in obstructive jaundice
- Hematogenous spread

- Mainly to liver
  - Hepatic metastatic nodules, away from primary tumor, indicate dismal outcome even after resection
- Other organs affected include lungs and bones
  - Rare at presentation
  - Usually occur in patients with advanced local disease
- Neural pathways
  - Perineural invasion more common in patients with extrahepatic bile duct invasion
    - 96% of patients with extrahepatic bile duct invasion have perineural invasion
    - Worse prognosis than in patients without perineural invasion
- Intraperitoneal "drop" metastases
  - Occur after tumor breaks serosal coverage
  - Peritoneal seeding occurs → peritoneal metastases

General Features
- Etiology
  - Predisposing risk factors include
    - Cholelithiasis
      - Primary risk factor for development of gallbladder carcinoma
      - Gallstones are present in 74–92% of patients with gallbladder cancer
      - Gallstones → chronic irritation and inflammation → mucosal dysplasia → carcinoma
    - Chronic biliary infections (*Opisthorchis viverrini*, *Salmonella typhi*)
      - Risk factor in high-incidence populations of La Paz, Bolivia and Mexico City, Mexico
      - Postulated that chronic *S. typhi* infection is associated with bile carcinogens → ↑ risk of hepatobiliary and gallbladder carcinoma
    - Primary sclerosing cholangitis
    - Porcelain gallbladder
      - Diffuse calcification of gallbladder wall
      - 10–25% of patients have gallbladder carcinoma
    - Postmenopausal status
    - Old age
    - Cigarette smoking
    - Congenital anatomic anomalies of biliary system including
      - Congenital cystic dilatation of biliary tree
      - Choledochal cyst
      - Anomalous junction of pancreaticobiliary ducts (± coexistent choledochal cyst)
      - Low insertion of cystic duct
  - Gallbladder carcinoma represents progression from dysplasia → carcinoma in situ → invasive carcinoma
    - Severe dysplasia and carcinoma in situ have been found in 90% of gallbladders containing carcinomas
- Epidemiology & cancer incidence
  - Most common primary hepatobiliary carcinoma
    - Incidence of 0.8-1.2%
  - 5th most common malignancy of GI tract
  - Estimated 9,760 new cases of gallbladder carcinoma in USA in 2009
    - 2.5 new cases per 100,000 population per year

GALLBLADDER CARCINOMA

- ○ Estimated 3,370 deaths from gallbladder carcinoma in USA in 2009
- ○ Women are affected 2-6x more frequently than men
- ○ More frequently diagnosed in 6th and 7th decades
- ○ Incidence varies among different ethnic groups
  - ▪ Hispanic women have highest incidence rates in USA
- • Associated diseases, abnormalities
  - ○ Cholelithiasis
  - ○ Primary sclerosing cholangitis
  - ○ Porcelain gallbladder

Gross Pathology & Surgical Features

- • 2 main macroscopic patterns
  - ○ Diffusely infiltrating lesions
    - ▪ 68% of gallbladder carcinomas
  - ○ Intraluminal polypoid growth
    - ▪ 32% of gallbladder carcinomas
- • Site of origin
  - ○ Gallbladder fundus (~ 60%)
  - ○ Gallbladder body (~ 30%)
  - ○ Gallbladder neck (~ 10%)

Microscopic Pathology

- • Adenocarcinomas account for 90% of gallbladder carcinomas
  - ○ Characterized by glands lined by cuboidal or columnar cells, which may contain mucin
  - ○ Grading depends on degree of gland formation
    - ▪ Well differentiated
    - ▪ Moderately differentiated
    - ▪ Poorly differentiated
    - ▪ Undifferentiated
- • Several histologic variants of adenocarcinoma
  - ○ Papillary
    - ▪ Branching fibrovascular stalks lined by atypical cuboidal or columnar cells
    - ▪ Tend to fill gallbladder lumen before mural invasion
    - ▪ Better prognosis than other variants
  - ○ Intestinal
    - ▪ Resembles intestinal epithelium and is believed to be variant of well-differentiated adenocarcinoma
    - ▪ 2 subtypes
      - – Lined chiefly by goblet cells
      - – Resembling colonic adenocarcinoma glands
    - ▪ Subtypes are often mixed within same tumor and may contain nests of ordinary well-differentiated adenocarcinoma
  - ○ Mucinous
    - ▪ Tumors consist of > 50% extracellular mucin
    - ▪ 2 histologic variants
      - – Contains large pools of extracellular mucin with small clusters of malignant epithelial cells
      - – Characterized by mucin-filled glands with cystic dilatation
    - ▪ Foci of both variants may be found admixed with conventional well-differentiated adenocarcinoma
  - ○ Signet ring cell
    - ▪ Contains cells with abundant intracytoplasmic mucin, with peripheral displacement of nuclei
    - ▪ Cells grow in cords, nests, and sheets and may form incomplete glandular structures within mucoid stroma

- ▪ Infiltrative submucosal growth can be prominent feature and resemble linitis plastica of stomach
- ○ Clear cell
  - ▪ Composed of cords, sheets, nests, and trabeculae of clear cells with well-defined cytoplasmic borders
  - ▪ May be confused histologically with metastatic renal cell carcinoma
  - ▪ May also contain areas mixed with conventional adenocarcinoma and mucin production, findings that help distinguish these tumors from renal cell carcinoma

IMAGING FINDINGS

Detection

- • Up to 50% of patients with "incidental gallbladder carcinoma" after simple cholecystectomy had radiological findings suspicious for carcinoma on retrospective review of imaging
- • General imaging features
  - ○ Imaging patterns parallel gross pathological patterns of gallbladder carcinoma
    - ▪ Mass replacing gallbladder
      - – 40–65% of cases
    - ▪ Focal or diffuse asymmetric wall thickening
      - – Most difficult to diagnose
      - – Asymmetric, irregular, or extensive thickening
      - – Gallbladder carcinoma may arise as nidus in preexisting background chronic cholecystitis, which can obscure or delay diagnosis
      - – 20–30% of cases
    - ▪ Intraluminal polyp
      - – Malignant lesions are usually > 1 cm in diameter and may have thickened implantation base
      - – 15–25% of cases
  - ○ Biliary dilatation is common imaging finding
- • **Ultrasound**
  - ○ Often 1st imaging technique in cases of suspected gallbladder disease
    - ▪ Relatively low cost
    - ▪ Widespread availability
  - ○ Sensitivity of 85% and accuracy of 80% for diagnosis of gallbladder carcinoma
    - ▪ Limited sensitivity in diagnosis of early lesions
    - ▪ Relatively high sensitivity for detection of tumor at advanced stages
  - ○ Sonographic appearance
    - ▪ Heterogeneous, predominantly hypoechoic tumor fills much or all of gallbladder lumen
      - – Anechoic foci of trapped bile or necrotic tumor may be present
      - – Echogenic shadowing foci from gallstones, porcelain gallbladder, or tumor calcifications
    - ▪ Gallbladder polyp
      - – Immobile polypoid mass, does not move with change of patient's position
  - ○ Color Doppler sonography can help to differentiate between gallbladder carcinoma and polyps
    - ▪ High flow rates have been described in gallbladder carcinoma

- Sensitivity of 96% for diagnosing gallbladder carcinoma using cutoff value of 30 cm/s
- CT
  - Hypoattenuating or isoattenuating mass on unenhanced CT
    - Hyperdense foci from gallstones, porcelain gallbladder, or tumor calcifications
  - Pattern of contrast enhancement
    - Up to 40% of lesions show hypervascular foci with enhancement ≥ that of liver
    - Wall enhancement during arterial phase that persists or becomes isodense to liver during portal venous phase
      - Contrast enhancement may be retained in fibrous stromal components of tumors during portal venous phase
    - Intense irregular enhancement may occur at periphery of large tumors during early arterial phase
- MR
  - T1WI: Hypo- to isointense mass within gallbladder lumen
  - T2WI: Moderately hyperintense mass
  - Gadolinium-enhanced T1WI
    - Intense irregular enhancement at periphery of large tumors during early arterial phase with contrast retention on delayed phases
- FDG PET
  - FDG PET may be helpful in differentiating gallbladder carcinoma from other causes of gallbladder wall thickening
    - Sensitivity of 75% and specificity of 87.5%
  - Delayed FDG PET is more helpful than early FDG PET for evaluating malignant lesions
    - Due to ↑ lesion uptake and ↑ lesion-to-background contrast

Staging

- Ultrasound
  - Unreliable for tumor staging
- MDCT
  - Commonly performed as unenhanced and contrast-enhanced studies during hepatic arterial and portal venous phases
  - Reported accuracy of up to 84% in determining local tumor extension
    - Addition of MPR images to axial CT data improves accuracy
  - Reported accuracy of up to 85% in predicting resectability
    - Due to its ability to delineate hepatic and vascular invasion, lymphadenopathy, and distant metastases
      - Multiplanar and 3D volume-rendered reconstructed images provide vascular road map for surgical planning
  - Local disease (T)
    - T1 disease
      - Polypoid lesions without focal thickening of gallbladder wall
      - Nodular or flat lesions with mucosal enhancement or focal thickening of inner enhancing layer of gallbladder wall with clear, low-attenuation outer wall
    - T2 disease

- Nodular or sessile lesions associated with focal thickening of gallbladder wall at lesional attachment site
- Smooth fat plane separating adjacent organs
- Diffuse wall thickening with heterogeneous enhancement
- Diffuse wall thickening with strong, thick inner wall enhancement and weak enhancement of outer layer (2-layered pattern)
- Focal wall thickening with outer surface dimpling at tumor base
    - T3 disease
      - Apparent nodularity on serosal aspect, indicating serosal extension of tumor
      - Tumor perforates serosa (visceral peritoneum) &/or directly invades liver or other adjacent organ or structure (e.g., stomach; duodenum; colon; or pancreas, omentum, or extrahepatic bile ducts)
    - T4 disease
      - Tumor invades main portal vein or hepatic artery or invades multiple extrahepatic organs or structures
  - Nodal disease (N)
    - Lymphatic spread is present in > 50% of patients at initial diagnosis
    - Regional lymph nodes (N1) are limited to hepatic hilus and include nodes along common bile duct, hepatic artery, portal vein, and cystic duct
    - Celiac, periduodenal, peripancreatic, and superior mesenteric artery nodes are considered N2 disease (stage IVB)
- MR
  - MR with MRCP and contrast-enhanced arterial and portal phase 3D angiographic (MR angiography) images
    - Up to 100% sensitive for bile duct and vascular invasion
    - 67% sensitive for hepatic invasion and 56% for lymph node metastases
- PET/CT
  - Promising role in detection of unsuspected metastases, which may alter staging and therapy

Restaging

- CECT is mainstay for follow-up after tumor resection
- Attention to common areas of tumor recurrence including
  - Liver at gallbladder bed
  - Liver metastasis away from gallbladder bed
  - Peritoneal metastases

CLINICAL ISSUES

Presentation

- Early stage carcinoma is typically diagnosed incidentally because of inflammatory symptoms related to coexistent cholelithiasis or cholecystitis
  - 1% of patients undergoing cholecystectomy for cholelithiasis has incidental gallbladder carcinoma
- Majority of patients with gallbladder carcinoma present with advanced disease
  - Symptoms are typically indolent and include
    - Chronic abdominal pain

- Anorexia
- Weight loss
- Physical examination may demonstrate
  - Palpable mass
    - Resulting from gallbladder distension due to gallbladder neck mass or large tumor replacing gallbladder
  - Hepatomegaly
  - Jaundice
    - Due to obstruction of biliary tree
    - Development of jaundice suggests involvement of hilar structures and usually reflects unresectability and poor prognosis
- Tumor markers in diagnosis of gallbladder carcinoma
  - CEA concentration > 4 µg/L
    - 93% specific but only 50% sensitive
  - CA-19.9 > 20 U/mL
    - 79.2% specific and 79.4% sensitive
  - CA-125 > 11 U/mL
    - 90% specific and 64% sensitive

Cancer Natural History & Prognosis

- Most patients present when disease is at advanced stage
  - Prognosis remains poor, with curative resection rate ranging only between 10-30%
- 5-year survival rates of patients with gallbladder carcinoma depends on stage at diagnosis (adjusted from data reported according to AJCC tumor staging, 6th edition)
  - Stage 0 (81%)
  - Stage I (50%)
  - Stage II (> 29%)
  - Stage III (7-9%)
  - Stage IV (2-3%)

Treatment Options

- Major treatment alternatives
  - Simple cholecystectomy
    - For tumors confined to gallbladder wall with negative surgical margin
    - Include unsuspected gallbladder cancer discovered in gallbladder mucosa at pathologic examination
      - Percentage of patients diagnosed with gallbladder cancer after simple cholecystectomy for presumed gallbladder stone disease is 0.5-1.5%
      - Curable in > 80% of cases
      - Patients with tumors confined to mucosa have 5-year survival rates of nearly 100%
  - Radical (extended) cholecystectomy
    - Surgery includes
      - Tumor resection with wedge of liver segments 4b and 5 at least 3 cm in depth
      - Regional lymphadenectomy including cystic and portal nodes, lymphatic tissue in hepatoduodenal ligament and liver hilum, nodes around pancreatic head, duodenum, and celiac artery
      - Excision of extrahepatic bile ducts with biliary reconstruction
    - Long-term disease-free survival will occasionally be achieved

- Laparoscopic cholecystectomy is absolutely contraindicated when gallbladder cancer is known or suspected preoperatively
- Because peritoneal involvement is common, diagnostic laparotomy at time of surgery is advised
- Palliative treatment options for unresectable tumor may include
  - Relief of biliary obstruction by percutaneous transhepatic catheter drainage or endoscopically placed stents
  - Standard external beam radiation therapy may relieve biliary obstruction in some patients and may supplement bypass procedures
  - Palliative surgery may relieve bile duct obstruction in selected patients
  - Standard chemotherapy is usually not effective, though occasional patients may be palliated
- Treatment options by stage
  - Tumor incidentally discovered during laparoscopic cholecystectomy or on histologic examination of gallbladder after cholecystectomy
    - Stage 0 and I (Tis or T1a)
      - No further treatment is necessary
    - Stage I (T1b)
      - Negative surgical margin → no further treatment is necessary
      - Positive surgical margin → radical cholecystectomy ± bile duct resection and biliary reconstruction
    - Stage II (T2)
      - Radical cholecystectomy
  - Tumor preoperatively suspected or confirmed
    - T2, T3, T4 → diagnostic laparoscopy/laparotomy
      - Radical cholecystectomy if tumor is resectable
      - Palliative procedures if tumor is not resectable
      - Direct involvement of colon, duodenum, and liver is not absolute contraindication to curative surgery
    - M1
      - Palliative procedures

REPORTING CHECKLIST

T Staging

- Patients presenting with acute cholecystitis should be carefully evaluated for gallbladder masses
- Patients found to have gallbladder masses should be evaluated for
  - Extension to liver, duodenum, stomach, omentum, and pancreas
    - Involvement of ≥ 2 extrahepatic organs or structures is considered T4 disease
  - Submucosal extension along cystic duct into common bile duct
  - Portal vein or hepatic artery involvement is considered T4 disease

N Staging

- Hepatic hilar nodes including nodes along common bile duct, hepatic artery portal vein, and cystic duct are considered regional or N1 nodes

- Celiac, periduodenal, peripancreatic, and superior mesenteric artery nodes are considered N2 disease (stage IVB)

M Staging

- Liver metastases other than direct invasion are considered M1 disease

SELECTED REFERENCES

1. American Joint Committee on Cancer: AJCC Cancer Staging Manual. 7th ed. New York: Springer. 211-7, 2010
2. Wakai T et al: Mode of hepatic spread from gallbladder carcinoma: an immunohistochemical analysis of 42 hepatectomized specimens. Am J Surg Pathol. 34(1):65-74, 2010
3. Furlan A et al: Gallbladder carcinoma update: multimodality imaging evaluation, staging, and treatment options. AJR Am J Roentgenol. 191(5):1440-7, 2008
4. Gourgiotis S et al: Gallbladder cancer. Am J Surg. 196(2):252-64, 2008
5. Kim SJ et al: Accuracy of preoperative T-staging of gallbladder carcinoma using MDCT. AJR Am J Roentgenol. 190(1):74-80, 2008
6. Nakata T et al: Impact of tumor spread to the cystic duct on the prognosis of patients with gallbladder carcinoma. World J Surg. 31(1):155-61; discussion 162-3, 2007
7. Shukla PJ et al: Can we do better than 'incidental' gallbladder cancer? Hepatogastroenterology. 54(80):2184-5, 2007
8. Fong Y et al: Evidence-based gallbladder cancer staging: changing cancer staging by analysis of data from the National Cancer Database. Ann Surg. 243(6):767-71; discussion 771-4, 2006
9. Kalra N et al: MDCT in the staging of gallbladder carcinoma. AJR Am J Roentgenol. 186(3):758-62, 2006
10. Nishiyama Y et al: Dual-time-point 18F-FDG PET for the evaluation of gallbladder carcinoma. J Nucl Med. 2006 Apr;47(4):633-8. Erratum in: J Nucl Med. 47(8):1266, 2006
11. Jarnagin WR et al: Patterns of initial disease recurrence after resection of gallbladder carcinoma and hilar cholangiocarcinoma: implications for adjuvant therapeutic strategies. Cancer. 98(8):1689-700, 2003
12. Koh T et al: Differential diagnosis of gallbladder cancer using positron emission tomography with fluorine-18-labeled fluoro-deoxyglucose (FDG-PET). J Surg Oncol. 84(2):74-81, 2003
13. Yamaguchi R et al: Perineural invasion has a negative impact on survival of patients with gallbladder carcinoma. Br J Surg. 89(9):1130-6, 2002
14. Levy AD et al: Gallbladder carcinoma: radiologic-pathologic correlation. Radiographics. 21(2):295-314; questionnaire, 549-55, 2001

GALLBLADDER CARCINOMA

Stage I (T1 N0 M0)

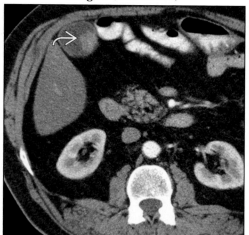

Stage II (T2 N0 M0)

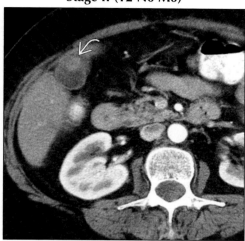

(Left) Axial CECT in a patient with vague right upper quadrant abdominal pain shows a sessile polypoid lesion ➤ within the gallbladder. *(Right)* Axial CECT in a 51-year-old woman who presented with left lower abdominal pain demonstrates an enhancing gallbladder mass ➤. This was found on histological examination to invade the perimuscular connective tissue without extension beyond the serosa, representing T2 disease.

Stage II (T2 N0 M0)

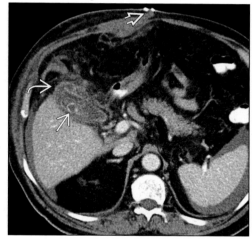

Stage II (T2 N0 M0)

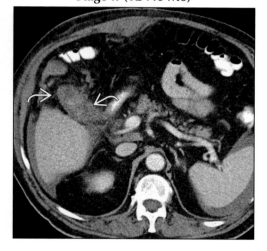

(Left) Axial CECT shows diffuse gallbladder wall thickening ➤ and a gallstone ➤ in this patient who presented with features of acute cholecystitis. During laparoscopic cholecystectomy, a gallbladder mass was found. Surgery was aborted, and the patient underwent staging CT and MR. Note the surgical clips ➤ from the aborted laparoscopic procedure. *(Right)* Axial CECT in the same patient shows diffuse gallbladder wall thickening ➤.

Stage II (T2 N0 M0)

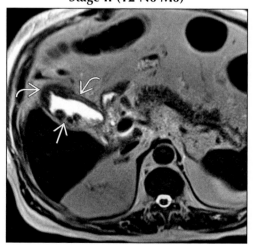

Stage II (T2 N0 M0)

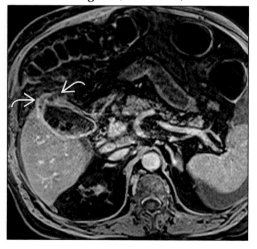

(Left) Axial T2WI MR in the same patient shows thickening ➤ of the anterior wall and fundus of the gallbladder without tumor extension beyond the wall into the surrounding fat. Multiple gallstones are also seen ➤. *(Right)* Axial T1WI C+ MR in the same patient shows gallbladder fundal wall asymmetric thickening ➤, which shows heterogeneous enhancement. The asymmetric pattern of wall thickening is difficult to differentiate from that due to other causes of wall thickening.

GALLBLADDER CARCINOMA

(Left) Axial CECT during the late arterial phase shows a polypoid gallbladder lesion ➡ with a small nodular extension ➡ on the outer contour of the gallbladder in this 37-year-old patient with familial polyposis syndrome. **(Right)** Axial CECT in the same patient during the venous phase shows the polypoid gallbladder lesion ➡ with a small nodular extension ➡ on the outer contour of the gallbladder without invasion into the liver. Adenocarcinoma with serosal penetration was confirmed during surgery.

Stage IIIA (T3 N0 M0)

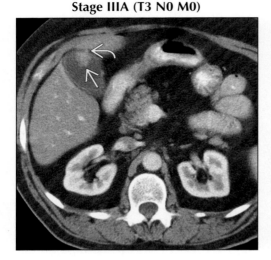

Stage IIIA (T3 N0 M0)

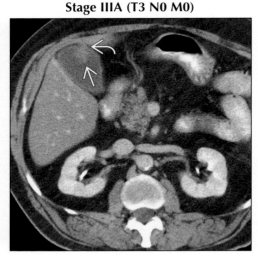

(Left) Axial CECT in a 65-year-old woman shows a heterogeneous gallbladder mass ➡ and heterogeneous, predominantly peripheral enhancement ➡ of the right lobe of the liver. Gallbladder carcinoma invading the liver tends to have a peripheral enhancing rim, which helps to differentiate it from hepatocellular carcinoma invading the gallbladder. **(Right)** Axial CECT in the same patient shows fundal tumor ➡ with involvement of the adjacent liver ➡. Gallstones ➡ are present.

Stage IIIA (T3 N0 M0)

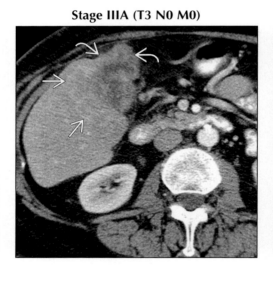

Stage IIIA (T3 N0 M0)

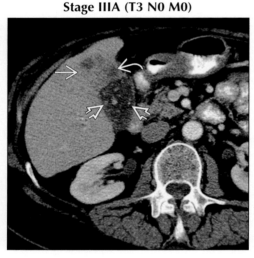

(Left) Axial CECT in a 50-year-old woman who presented with vague abdominal pain shows thickening of the wall of the gallbladder with tumor extending beyond the wall of the gallbladder ➡ and into the liver ➡. **(Right)** Coronal CECT in the same patient shows gallbladder wall thickening ➡ and a subtle area of tumor invasion into the liver ➡. During surgery, minimal invasion into the liver was found, making this T3 disease.

Stage IIIA (T3 N0 M0)

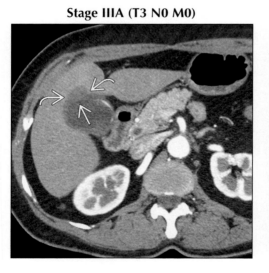

Stage IIIA (T3 N0 M0)

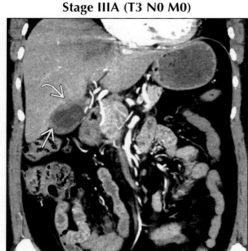

GALLBLADDER CARCINOMA

Stage IIIB (T3 N1 M0)

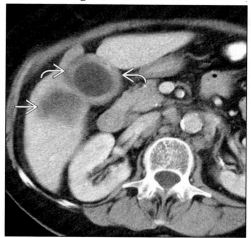

Stage IIIB (T3 N1 M0)

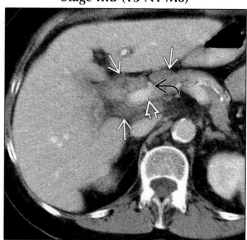

(Left) Axial CECT in a 70-year-old man who presented with elevated liver enzymes shows diffuse thickening of the gallbladder wall ➡ and tumor extension ➡ into segment 5 of the right lobe of the liver. Involvement of the liver constitutes T3 disease. (Right) Axial CECT in the same patient shows multiple enlarged lymph nodes ➡ encasing the portal vein ➡ and hepatic artery ➡, constituting N1 disease.

Stage IIIB (T3 N1 M0)

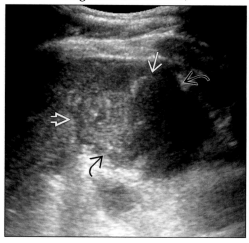

Stage IIIB (T3 N1 M0)

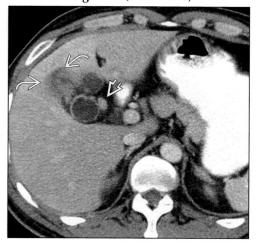

(Left) Longitudinal transabdominal ultrasound in 39-year-old man who presented with acute abdominal pain shows a mass ➡ replacing the gallbladder. The mass shows areas of increased echogenicity with shadowing ➡ due to trapped stones or tumoral calcifications. There is a poor interface with the liver ➡, suggesting liver invasion. (Right) Axial CECT in the same patient shows tumor invading the liver ➡ and an enlarged porta hepatis lymph node ➡.

Stage IIIB (T3 N1 M0)

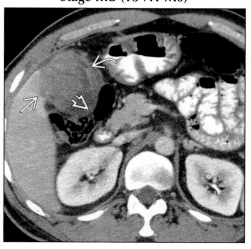

Stage IIIB (T3 N1 M0)

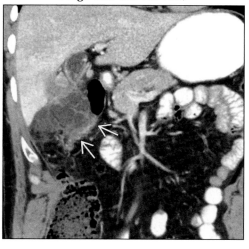

(Left) Axial CECT in the same patient shows the gallbladder mass ➡ invading the liver ➡ and the hepatic flexure of the colon ➡. (Right) Coronal CECT in the same patient confirms invasion of the wall of the hepatic flexure of the colon ➡. Coronal reformatted images are very helpful in demonstrating invasion of local structures.

GALLBLADDER CARCINOMA

(Left) Axial CECT shows a pericholecystic fluid collection ⇗ and diffuse enhancement of the cystic ⇒ and common hepatic ⇛ ducts in this 67-year-old man who presented with acute abdominal pain and clinical features of acute cholecystitis. *(Right)* Axial CECT in the same patient shows diffuse thickening and enhancement of the gallbladder wall ⇗ with mass-like focal wall thickening ⇛ that was found to perforate the serosa on histologic examination.

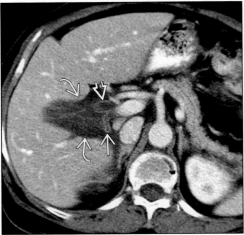
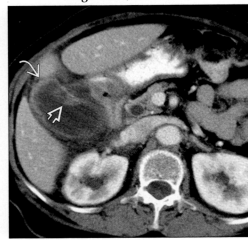

Stage IIIB (T3 N1 M0)   Stage IIIB (T3 N1 M0)

(Left) Axial CECT in the same patient during the portal venous phase shows diffuse persistent thickening of the gallbladder wall ⇗ and pericholecystic fat stranding ⇒. Acute cholecystitis was confirmed at surgery, which also showed adenocarcinoma at the site of focal wall thickening. *(Right)* Axial T1WI MR in the same patient 1 week after cholecystectomy shows a focal area of low signal intensity ⇗ within the liver at the gallbladder bed.

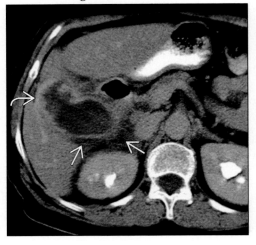
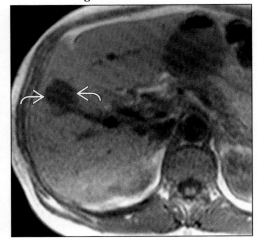

Stage IIIB (T3 N1 M0)   Stage IIIB (T3 N1 M0)

(Left) Axial T2WI FS MR in the same patient shows focal area of increased signal intensity ⇗ within the liver at the gallbladder bed following cholecystectomy. *(Right)* Axial T1WI C+ FS MR in the same patient again shows peripheral contrast enhancement ⇗ at the gallbladder bed. There is also an enlarged periportal lymph node ⇛. Wedge resection of the liver and lymphadenectomy was performed, confirming liver and periportal lymph node involvement.

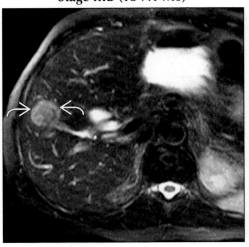
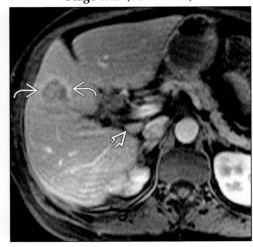

GALLBLADDER CARCINOMA

Stage IIIB (T3 N1 M0)

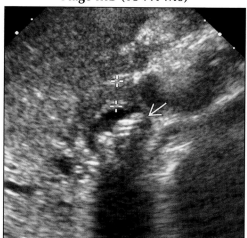

Stage IIIB (T3 N1 M0)

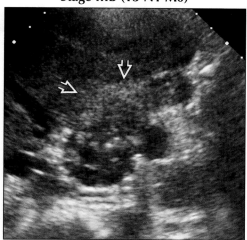

(Left) Transverse transabdominal ultrasound in a 49-year-old man who presented with vague abdominal pain shows diffuse gallbladder wall thickening (calipers) and multiple gallstones ➡. *(Right)* Longitudinal transabdominal ultrasound in the same patient shows a tumor invading into the liver ➡. Although ultrasound can show gallbladder carcinoma and hepatic invasion, its use in staging is limited by its inability to demonstrate involvement of viscus organs or vascular structures.

Stage IIIB (T3 N1 M0)

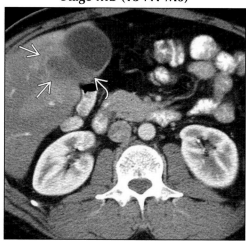

Stage IIIB (T3 N1 M0)

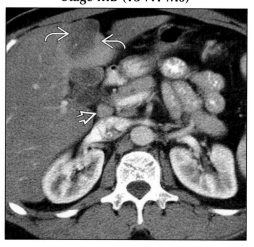

(Left) Axial CECT in the same patient shows a gallbladder mass ➡ invading into segment 5 of the right lobe of the liver ➡. *(Right)* Axial CECT in the same patient shows extension of the tumor to segment 4 of the left lobe of the liver ➡ and an enlarged porta hepatis lymph node ➡. Tumor extension to the liver constitutes T3 disease.

Stage IIIB (T3 N1 M0)

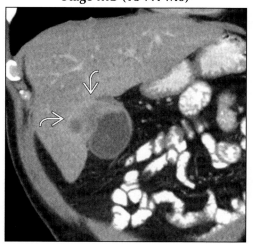

Stage IIIB (T3 N1 M0)

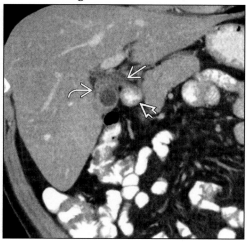

(Left) Axial CECT in the same patient shows tumor invading into the right lobe of the liver ➡. The depth of hepatic invasion does not affect local staging of gallbladder carcinoma. *(Right)* Coronal CECT in the same patient shows the tumor extending to the gallbladder neck ➡. The tumor also extends into the hepatoduodenal ligament ➡ to reach the duodenum ➡ without obvious invasion of the duodenal wall.

GALLBLADDER CARCINOMA

Stage IVA (T4 N0 M0)

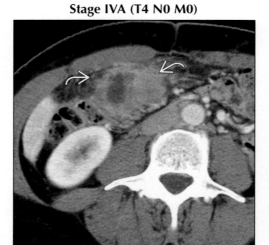

Stage IVA (T4 N0 M0)

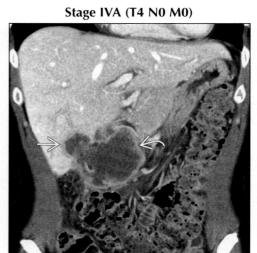

(Left) Axial CECT in a 30-year-old woman shows a heterogeneously enhancing mass ⟹ replacing the gallbladder. *(Right)* Coronal CECT in the same patient shows the gallbladder mass ⟹ invading into the liver parenchyma ⟹. Tumors arising from the gallbladder and invading the liver tend to exhibit a peripheral pattern of enhancement, which helps to differentiate them from primary hepatic tumors invading the gallbladder.

Stage IVA (T4 N0 M0)

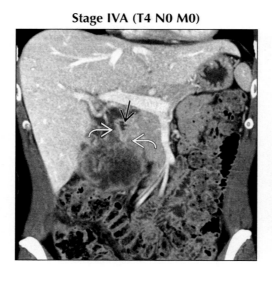

Stage IVA (T4 N0 M0)

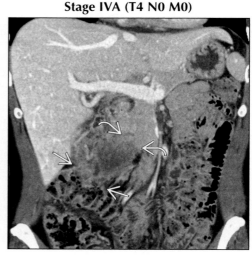

(Left) Coronal CECT in the same patient shows the tumor ⟹ infiltrating the wall of the duodenum ⟹. *(Right)* Coronal CECT in the same patient shows tumor invading the head of pancreas ⟹ and the hepatic flexure of the colon ⟹. Coronal reformatted images are very helpful in determining the local extent of the tumor and involvement of adjacent structures such as the colon and duodenum.

Stage IVA (T4 N0 M0)

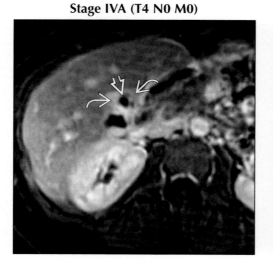

Stage IVA (T4 N0 M0)

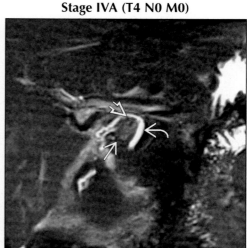

(Left) Axial T1WI C+ FS MR in the same patient shows tumor enhancement ⟹ around the cystic duct ⟹. *(Right)* Coronal T2WI MR HASTE in the same patient shows the common bile duct ⟹ stretched over the tumor ⟹ with wall irregularity ⟹, suggesting invasion of the extrahepatic bile duct. Biopsy of the gallbladder mass revealed squamous cell carcinoma.

Stage IVB (T3 N2 M0)

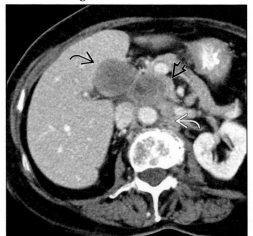

Stage IVB (T3 N2 M0)

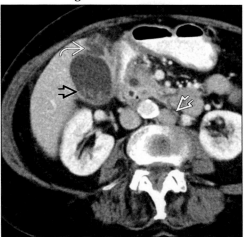

(Left) Axial CECT in a 69-year-old woman who presented with acute right upper quadrant abdominal pain and clinical features of acute cholecystitis shows extensive porta hepatis ⤴, as well as superior mesenteric ⮊ and periaortic ⮞ lymphadenopathy. *(Right)* Axial CECT in the same patient shows perforation of the gallbladder with a pericholecystic abscess ⮞. An enlarged periaortic lymph node ⮊ is also seen, as are multiple gallstones ⮊.

Stage IVB (T3 N2 M0)

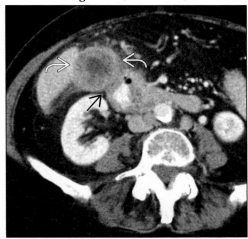

Stage IVB (T3 N2 M0)

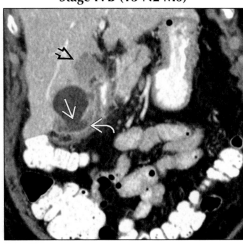

(Left) Axial CECT in the same patient shows circumferential gallbladder wall thickening ⮞. The thickened gallbladder abuts the duodenum ⮕ without obvious invasion. *(Right)* Coronal CECT in the same patient shows a defect in the gallbladder wall ⮞ and pericholecystic abscess ⮞, which explains the acute presentation. Coronal reformatted images are helpful in confirming gallbladder perforation. Invasion of the liver is also seen ⮊.

Stage IVB (T4 N2 M0)

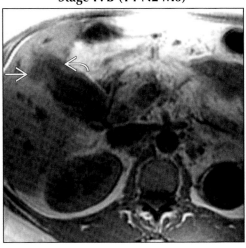

Stage IVB (T4 N2 M0)

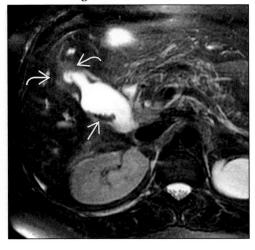

(Left) Axial T1WI MR in an elderly woman who presented with right upper quadrant abdominal pain shows a low signal intensity fundal mass ⮞ infiltrating into the adjacent liver parenchyma ⮞. *(Right)* Axial T2WI FS MR in the same patient shows slightly hyperintense fundal mass ⮞. Multiple layering gallstones ⮞ are also present.

GALLBLADDER CARCINOMA

Stage IVB (T4 N2 M0)

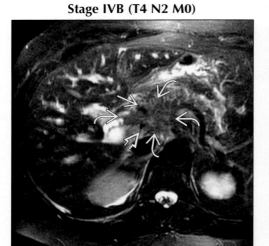

Stage IVB (T4 N2 M0)

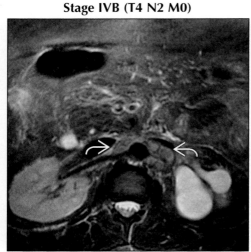

(Left) Axial T2WI FS MR in the same patient shows a large, poorly defined, slightly hyperintense mass ➡ that encases and narrows the hepatic artery ➡ and portal vein ➡. *(Right)* Axial T2WI FS MR in the same patient shows enlarged periaortic lymph nodes ➡. Enlargement of periaortic lymph nodes is considered N2 disease.

Stage IVB (T3 N1 M1)

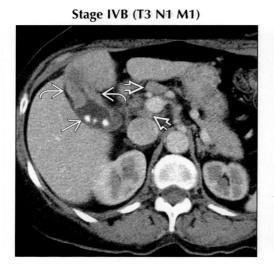

Stage IVB (T3 N1 M1)

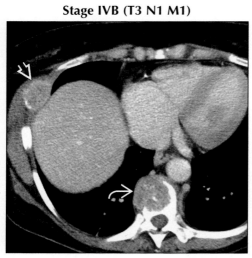

(Left) Axial CECT in a 54-year-old woman who presented with chest wall pain shows thickening of the wall of the gallbladder ➡ and multiple gallstones ➡. Enlarged periportal lymph nodes are also present ➡. *(Right)* Axial CECT in the same patient shows destructive bony metastatic lesions involving the right 8th rib ➡ and the T10 vertebral body ➡.

Stage IVB (T3 N1 M1)

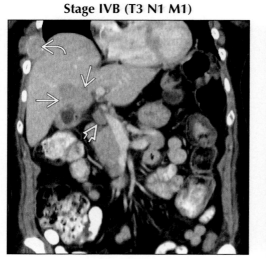

Stage IVB (T3 N1 M1)

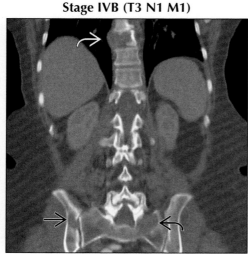

(Left) Coronal CECT in the same patient shows the gallbladder mass invading into the liver ➡, the 8th rib metastatic lesion ➡, and the periportal lymph node ➡. *(Right)* Coronal CECT in the same patient, bone window, shows multiple bony destructive lesions involving the T10 vertebral body ➡, left ala of the sacrum ➡, and right iliac bone ➡.

Stage IVB (T3 N2 M1)

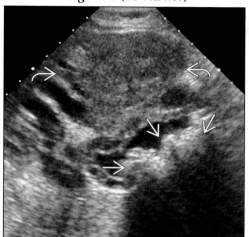

Stage IVB (T3 N2 M1)

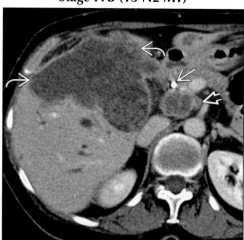

(Left) Transverse transabdominal ultrasound shows a large heterogeneous mass ➡ arising from the anterior wall of the gallbladder. Multiple gallstones with posterior shadowing ➡ are seen within the gallbladder lumen. (Right) Axial CECT in the same patient shows a large gallbladder mass ➡ invading into the liver. There is a large celiac lymph node ➡. A biliary stent ➡ has been placed because of biliary obstruction caused by hepatic duct involvement.

Stage IVB (T3 N2 M1)

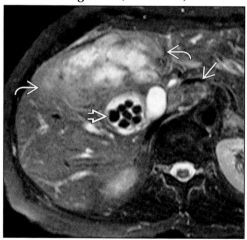

Stage IVB (T3 N2 M1)

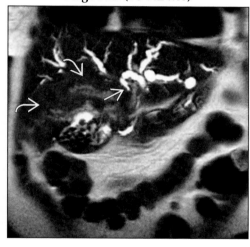

(Left) Axial T2WI FS MR shows a hyperintense tumor ➡ invading into the liver parenchyma. Enlarged celiac lymph node ➡ and multiple gallstones ➡ are also seen. (Right) Coronal T2 HASTE in the same patient shows large tumor ➡ invading into the liver and causing obstruction of the hepatic duct ➡ just below the confluence of the right and left ducts, causing dilatation of the intrahepatic bile ducts in the right and left lobes.

Stage IVB (T3 N2 M1)

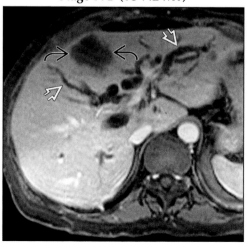

Stage IVB (T3 N2 M1)

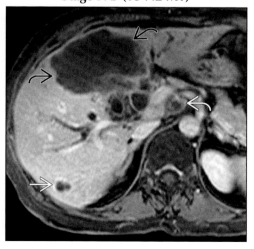

(Left) Axial T1WI C+ MR in the same patient shows tumor invading into the liver ➡ and intrahepatic biliary dilatation ➡. (Right) Axial T1WI C+ MR in the same patient shows tumor invading into the liver ➡ and an enlarged celiac lymph node ➡. In addition there is a right lobe peripherally enhancing lesion ➡ separate from the primary mass, representing a parenchymal metastatic liver lesion and M1 disease.

GALLBLADDER CARCINOMA

Stage IVB (T3 N2 M1)

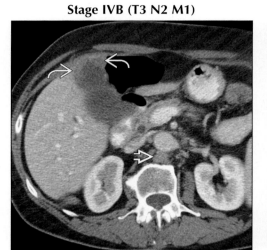

Stage IVB (T3 N2 M1)

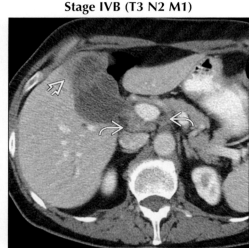

(Left) Axial CECT in a 47-year-old woman who presented with right upper quadrant abdominal pain shows thickening of the wall of the gallbladder ➡. Periaortic lymph node is present ➡. (Right) Axial CECT in the same patient shows gallbladder mass invading into the liver ➡ as well as enlarged periportal lymph nodes ➡.

Stage IVB (T3 N2 M1)

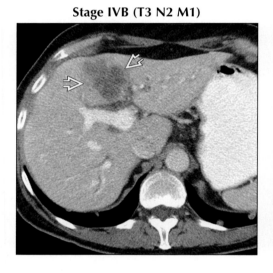

Stage IVB (T3 N2 M1)

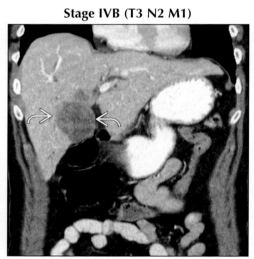

(Left) Axial CECT in the same patient shows tumor invading into the medial segment of the left lobe of the liver (segment 4) ➡. (Right) Coronal CECT in the same patient shows tumor invading into the medial segment of the left lobe ➡.

Stage IVB (T3 N2 M1)

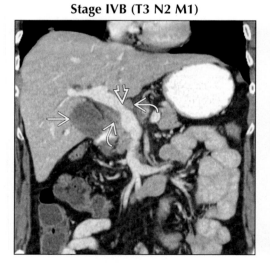

Stage IVB (T3 N2 M1)

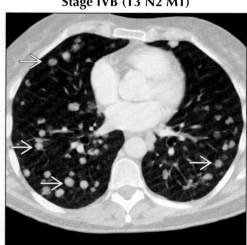

(Left) Coronal CECT in the same patient shows tumor invading into the liver ➡. There is also periportal adenopathy ➡ that causes narrowing of the portal vein ➡ without actual invasion. (Right) Axial CECT in the same patient, lung window, shows multiple bilateral pulmonary nodules ➡ due to widespread metastatic disease.

Stage IVB (T3 N2 M1)

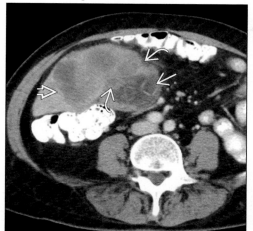

Stage IVB (T3 N2 M1)

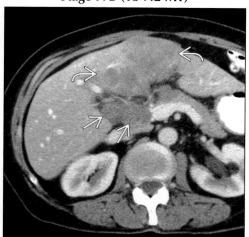

(Left) Axial CECT in a 69-year-old woman who presented with abdominal pain shows a large gallbladder mass ➜ invading into the liver ➜. Note large gallstones ➜. (Right) Axial CECT in the same patient shows deep invasion into the liver ➜ and large periportal lymph nodes ➜.

Stage IVB (T3 N2 M1)

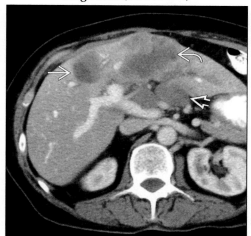

Stage IVB (T3 N2 M1)

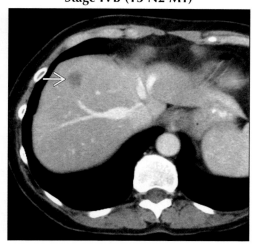

(Left) Axial CECT in the same patient shows liver invasion contiguous with the primary tumor ➜, as well as a liver mass ➜ separate from the primary tumor. Enlarged celiac node ➜ is present at the celiac trifurcation. (Right) Axial CECT in the same patient shows another hepatic lesion ➜ separate from the primary tumor. The presence of hepatic lesions separate from the primary tumor represents distal metastasis (M1 disease).

Stage IVB (T3 N2 M1)

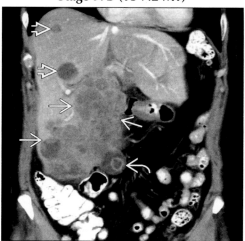

Stage IVB (T3 N2 M1)

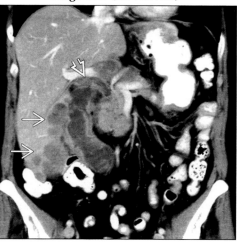

(Left) Coronal CECT in the same patient shows the extensive local involvement of both the right and left lobes of the liver from direct tumor invasion ➜. The gallbladder ➜ is visible at the lower edge of the liver. Metastatic liver lesions ➜ are present away from the primary tumor. (Right) Coronal CECT in the same patient shows tumor extending into the liver ➜ and along the bile duct ➜.

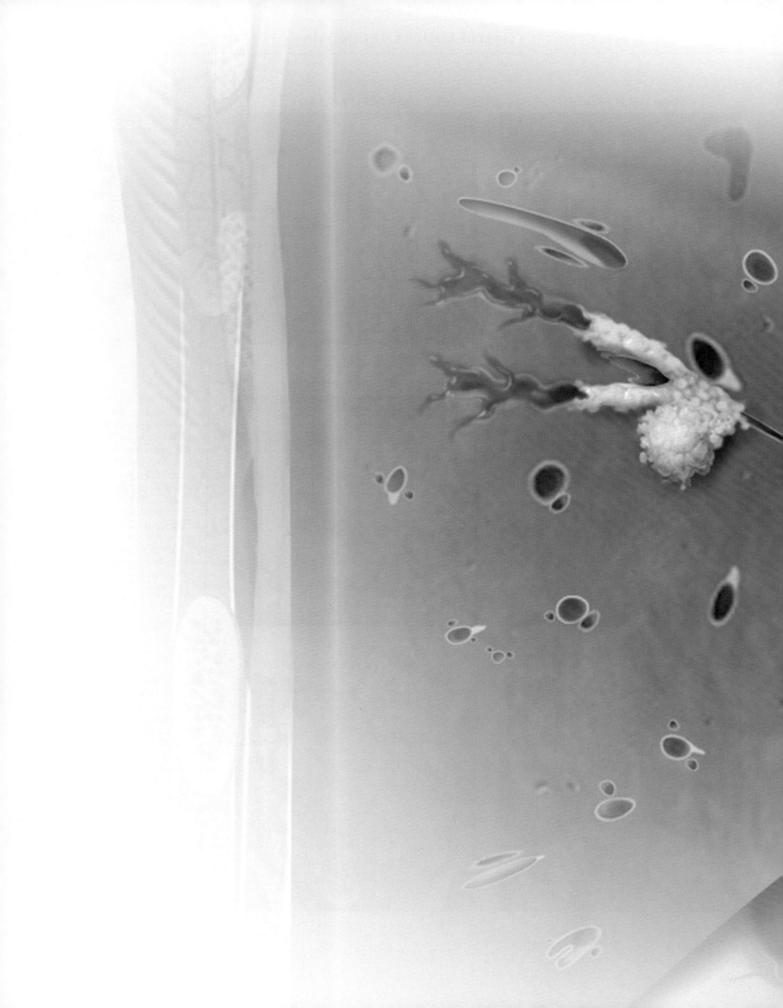

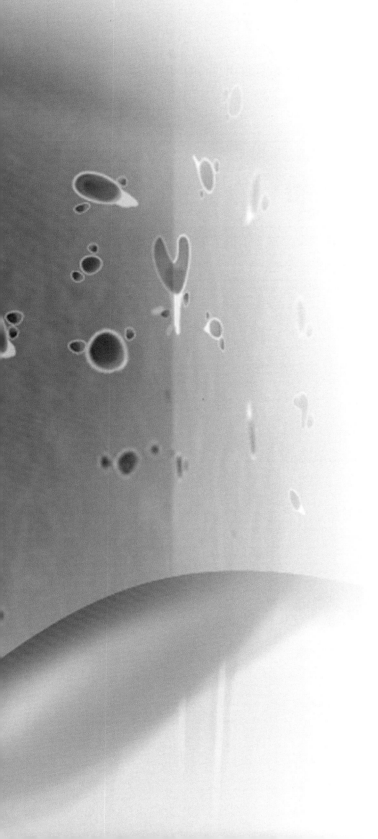

Intrahepatic Bile Duct Carcinoma

INTRAHEPATIC BILE DUCT CARCINOMA

(T) Primary Tumor

Adapted from 7th edition AJCC Staging Forms.

TNM	Definitions
TX	Primary tumor cannot be assessed
T0	No evidence of primary tumor
Tis	Carcinoma in situ (intraductal tumor)
T1	Solitary tumor without vascular invasion
T2a	Solitary tumor with vascular invasion
T2b	Multiple tumors, with or without vascular invasion
T3	Tumor perforating the visceral peritoneum or involving the local extrahepatic structures by direct invasion
T4	Tumor with periductal invasion

(N) Regional Lymph Nodes

NX	Regional lymph nodes cannot be assessed
N0	No regional lymph node metastasis
N1	Regional lymph node metastasis present

(M) Distant Metastasis

M0	No distant metastasis
M1	Distant metastasis present

AJCC Stages/Prognostic Groups

Adapted from 7th edition AJCC Staging Forms.

Stage	T	N	M
0	Tis	N0	M0
I	T1	N0	M0
II	T2	N0	M0
III	T3	N0	M0
IVA	T4	N0	M0
	Any T	N1	M0
IVB	Any T	Any N	M1

INTRAHEPATIC BILE DUCT CARCINOMA

T1

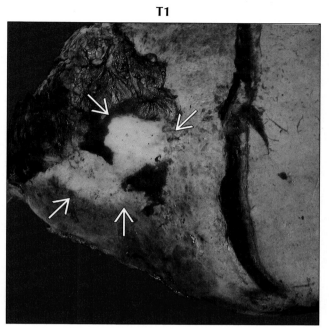

The cut surface of a partial hepatic lobectomy specimen shows a solitary gray-white tumor ➡ located in the subcapsular region with surrounding liver parenchyma.

T1

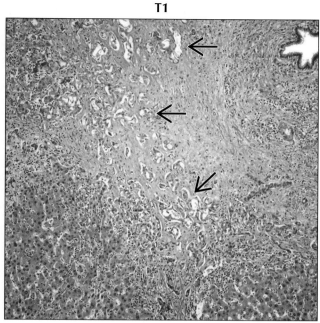

H&E stained section from a solitary intrahepatic bile duct carcinoma shows infiltrative neoplastic cells arranged in well-formed glands ➡ invading into and replacing the liver parenchyma with surrounding fibrosis. No vascular invasion was evident in the tumor. (Original magnification 100x.)

T1

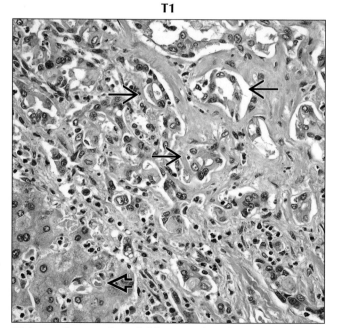

High magnification of a well-differentiated intrahepatic bile duct carcinoma shows well-formed glands ➡ infiltrating into markedly fibrotic stroma. Note the residual liver cells in the left lower aspect of the micrograph ➡. (Original magnification 400x.)

T1

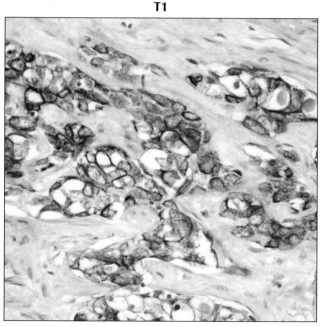

Immunohistochemical stain with antibody against cytokeratin (CK7) shows tumor cells staining positively (brown staining), supporting the diagnosis of cholangiocarcinoma. Immunohistochemical stains are useful to differentiate primary tumors from metastatic lesions such as colon cancer. (Original magnification 400x.)

INTRAHEPATIC BILE DUCT CARCINOMA

T2a

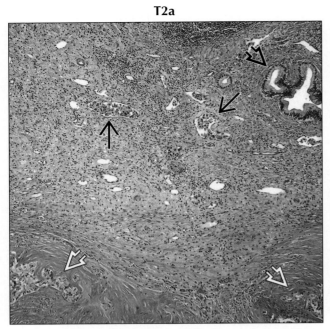

H&E stained section of an intrahepatic bile duct carcinoma with vascular invasion shows nests of infiltrative carcinoma with fibrosis ⇨. Malignant cells are present inside a few vessel lumens ➡. Note residual normal bile duct ⇨. (Original magnification 100x.)

T2a

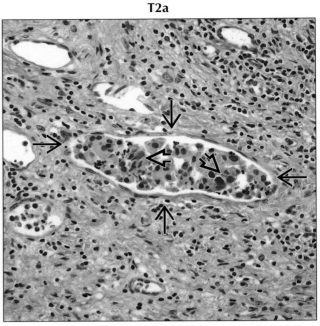

Higher magnification of the previous image shows malignant cells ⇨ inside a vessel lumen, which is lined by endothelial cells ➡. (Original magnification 400x.)

T3

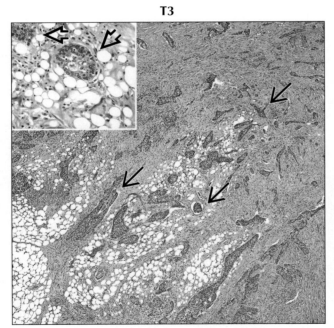

H&E stained section shows nests of intrahepatic bile duct carcinoma with surrounding fibrosis ➡ and extrahepatic extension. (Original magnification 100x.) The inset demonstrates neoplastic nests ⇨ that infiltrate into the fibrofatty soft tissue of the hepatic hilum. (Original magnification 300x.)

T3

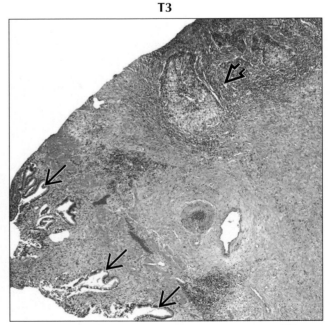

H&E stained section from the same specimen shows tumor ⇨ further extending to involve the wall of the gallbladder. Note the gallbladder mucosa ➡.

T1

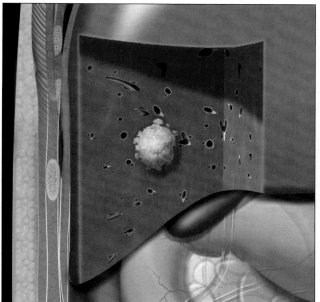

Graphic depicts the cut surface of the liver with a solitary tumor of the peripheral bile ducts. There is no vascular invasion at tumor stage T1.

T2a

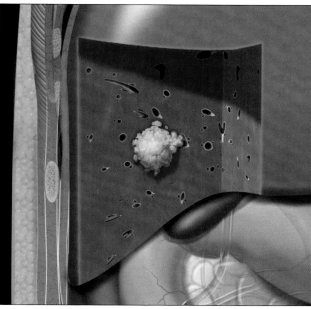

Graphic depicts cut surface of the liver with a solitary tumor of the intrahepatic bile ducts with small vessel invasion, a feature of tumor stage T2a.

T2a

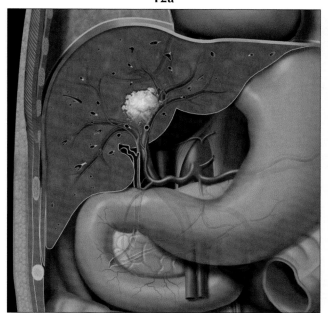

Graphic depicts cut surface of the liver with a solitary tumor of the intrahepatic bile ducts with major vessel invasion. Tumors of stage T2a can have small or large vessel invasion.

T2b

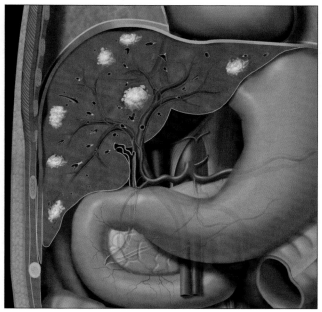

Graphic depicts the cut surface of the liver with multiple tumors of the peripheral biliary tree. The presence of multiple tumors constitutes T2b disease.

INTRAHEPATIC BILE DUCT CARCINOMA

T2b

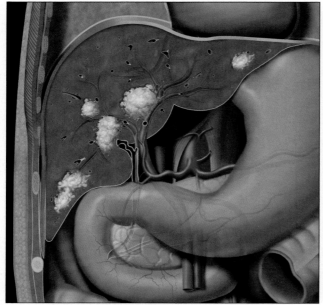

Graphic depicts the cut surface of the liver with multiple tumors of the peripheral biliary tree with small and large vessel invasion. The presence of multiple tumors constitutes stage T2b, with or without vascular invasion.

T3

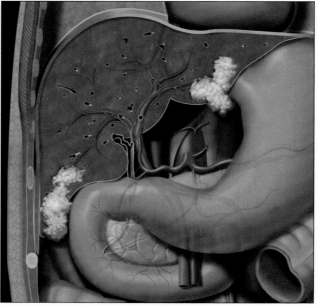

Graphic depicts the cut surface of the liver with tumors of the peripheral bile ducts invading the liver capsule and visceral peritoneum.

T3

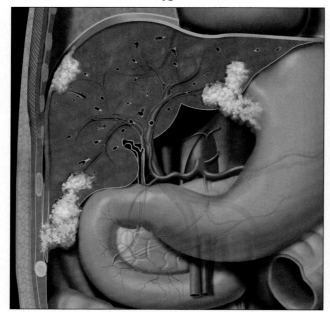

Graphic depicts the cut surface of the liver with tumors of the intrahepatic bile ducts directly invading adjacent structures. T3 tumors can invade adjacent bowel, the abdominal wall, &/or the diaphragm.

T4

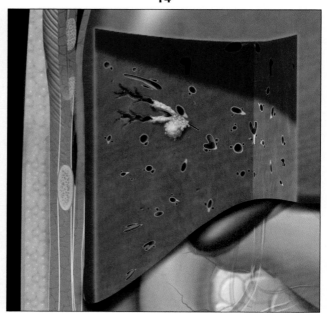

Graphic depicts the cut surface of the liver with tumor demonstrating periductal invasion, consistent with T4 disease. Periductal infiltration is defined as diffuse longitudinal growth along the intrahepatic bile ducts. There may or may not be a mass-forming component to the tumor.

INTRAHEPATIC BILE DUCT CARCINOMA

N1

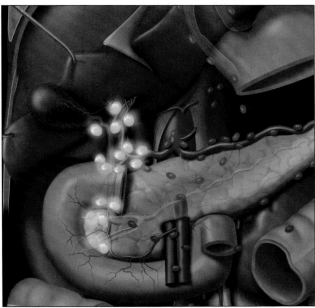

Graphic highlights the regional lymph nodes for tumors of the right hepatic lobe. These include hilar (common bile duct, hepatic artery, portal vein and cystic duct), periduodenal, and peripancreatic lymph nodes.

N1

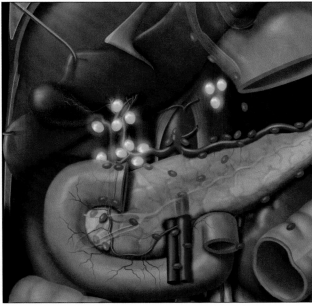

Graphic highlights the regional lymph nodes for tumors of the left hepatic lobe. These include hilar (common bile duct, hepatic artery, portal vein and cystic duct) and gastrohepatic lymph nodes. Inferior phrenic nodes are not depicted but are also considered regional lymph nodes.

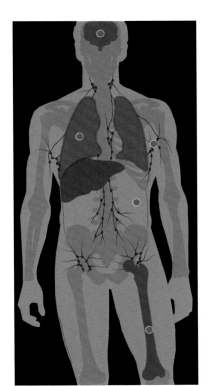

METASTASES, ORGAN FREQUENCY

Lymph nodes

Peritoneal cavity

Lung

Bone (mainly vertebrae)

Brain

The literature only offers isolated cases of cholangiocarcinoma with distant metastasis. The number is not sufficiently significant to quantify organ frequency.

INTRAHEPATIC BILE DUCT CARCINOMA

OVERVIEW

General Comments

- Tumor arising in intrahepatic bile ducts
  - Peripheral to 2nd order bile ducts
- 15-20% of primary liver malignancies
- 20% of cholangiocarcinomas are intrahepatic
- 80% of cholangiocarcinomas are extrahepatic
  - 70-80% are perihilar
  - 20-30% are distal bile duct

Classification

- Histologic types
  - Cholangiocarcinoma (CCA)
    - Tumor growth pattern
      - Mass-forming
      - Periductal infiltrating
      - Mixed
  - Combined hepatocellular cholangiocarcinoma

PATHOLOGY

Routes of Spread

- **Contiguous spread**
  - Intrahepatic tumor tends to grow centrally
  - Peripheral intrahepatic tumors can invade portal vein with tumor thrombus
  - Tendency toward perineural spread
- **Lymphatic spread**
  - 30-50% have nodal metastases at presentation
  - More common than with hepatoma
  - Reactive adenopathy is common in primary sclerosing cholangitis (PSC) and should be confirmed with histology
  - Intrahepatic lymphatic drainage has laterality
    - Segments 2-3 → drain along lesser curvature of stomach → celiac nodal basin
    - Segments 5-8 → hilar nodes → caval & paraaortic nodes
  - Regional lymph nodes
    - Tumors in segments 2-4 (left lobe)
      - Hilar
      - Gastrohepatic
      - Inferior phrenic
    - Tumors in segments 5-8 (right lobe)
      - Hilar: Nodes along common bile duct, hepatic artery, portal vein, cystic duct
      - Periduodenal
      - Peripancreatic
      - Inferior phrenic
  - Distant metastases
    - Celiac
    - Paraaortic
    - Caval
- **Hematogenous spread**
  - 10-20% have distant metastases at presentation
  - 50% have metastatic disease at autopsy
  - Liver, lung, bones, adrenal glands
  - Rare reported cases of metastases to
    - Central nervous system
    - Breast
    - Skeletal muscle
- **Peritoneal seeding**
  - 10-20% have peritoneal metastases at presentation

General Features

- Comments
  - 3% of gastrointestinal tumors
  - 2nd most common primary liver malignancy
    - 15-20% of primary liver tumors
- Genetics
  - Gene mutations suggest possible genetic link
    - Inactivation of tumor suppressor genes
    - Mutations in oncogenes
    - Chromosomal aneuploidy
  - No established clinical role for molecular profiling at this time
- Etiology
  - Risk factors
    - Age
    - Primary sclerosing cholangitis
    - Chronic ulcerative colitis
    - Hepatolithiasis
    - Caroli disease
    - Choledochal cysts
    - Tobacco abuse (in association with PSC)
    - Bile duct adenoma & biliary papillomatosis
    - Hepatobiliary flukes
    - Chronic typhoid carriers
    - Exposure to thorotrast
    - Familial polyposis
  - Additional risk factors in USA and Europe
    - Cirrhosis
    - Chronic hepatitis C infection
    - Alcohol abuse
- Epidemiology & cancer incidence
  - Incidence of 0.7 cases per 100,000 in USA
    - Incidence increasing in USA
    - 2,000-3,000 new cases in USA per year
  - Average age of diagnosis is 73 years
  - More than 2/3 diagnosed after age 65
  - Most common in Asia & southeast Asia
    - Diagnosed at younger age
    - Due to endemic hepatobiliary infections
- Associated diseases, abnormalities
  - Primary sclerosing cholangitis (PSC)
    - Common risk factor in western countries
    - Prevalence of CCA in this setting is 5-15%
    - Risk not associated with duration or severity of PSC or inflammatory bowel disease
  - Hepatobiliary flukes
    - *Opisthorchis viverrini* & *Clonorchis sinensis*
    - Endemic in east Asia
    - Ingested in undercooked fish
    - Infest biliary tree ± gallbladder
  - Choledochal cysts
    - 10-15% lifetime risk of carcinoma
    - Persistent risk even with cyst excision
  - Hepatolithiasis
    - Risk factor in parts of Asia
    - Up to 10% complicated by cholangiocarcinoma
    - In endemic areas, 70% of tumors manifest with hepatolithiasis

Gross Pathology & Surgical Features

- Patterns of tumor growth
  - Mass-forming (exophytic)
    - Most common pattern at intrahepatic location

INTRAHEPATIC BILE DUCT CARCINOMA

- 60% of intrahepatic tumors
  - Radial growth pattern invading into liver
  - Vascular invasion is less common than with hepatoma
  - Large white tumor with dense fibrosis
  - Not encapsulated
  - Well-defined gross tumor margins
- Periductal (infiltrating)
  - 20% of intrahepatic tumors
  - Sclerotic lesion with abundant fibrous tissue
  - Diffuse longitudinal growth along bile duct
  - Poorer prognosis
- Mixed (mass-forming and periductal)
  - 20% of intrahepatic tumors
- Intraductal (polypoid)
  - Usually papillary adenocarcinoma
  - Sometimes superficial mucosal growth pattern
  - Uncommon except in tumors arising in choledochal cysts
  - Better prognosis than other types

Microscopic Pathology

- H&E
  - 90% are adenocarcinomas
    - Most are well differentiated with glandular & tubular structures
    - Various degrees of coagulative necrosis
    - No reliable distinguishing histologic feature to differentiate from hepatic metastatic disease
  - Often markedly desmoplastic
    - Dense sparsely cellular fibrous stroma separates glandular elements
  - Tumor extends longitudinally and circumferentially in submucosal space
  - Mucin production is frequently present
    - Excludes hepatocellular carcinoma
  - No bile production
  - Vascular invasion less common than in hepatoma

IMAGING FINDINGS

Detection

- **Ultrasound**
  - Excellent for identifying biliary obstruction
  - Poor sensitivity and specificity for identifying a mass
    - Difficult to visualize intraductal or infiltrating lesions
    - Mass-forming tumors have variable echogenicity
    - Advanced when seen on US
  - Findings
    - Solid mass or diffusely abnormal echotexture
    - Mass with variable echogenicity
    - Hypovascular mass: Poor color Doppler signal
    - May be able to detect portal vein occlusion or infiltration
- **CT**
  - Findings
    - NECT
      - Hypodense mass
    - CECT
      - Early irregular thick rim and patchy central enhancement

- Progressive centripetal fill-in of tumor with contrast enhancement
- Delayed persistent enhancement greater than hepatic parenchyma
- Small lesions with less fibrosis may enhance intensely in arterial phase and persist on delayed phases
  - Overlying capsular retraction
  - Intrahepatic biliary dilation peripheral to mass
- **PET/CT**
  - Not superior to CT or MR/MRCP for detection of primary lesion
  - FDG accumulates in tumor cells but limited if large fibrotic component
  - Higher rate of tumor detection for nodular growth pattern than infiltrative
  - Some report better detection of intrahepatic tumor than perihilar or distal bile duct
  - Mucinous carcinoma → no FDG uptake
  - False-positive: Inflammatory/infectious mass, other malignancies
  - Efficacy of PET in setting of PSC is controversial
  - Focal FDG uptake and elevated CA-19.9 is more sensitive and specific
- **MR/MRCP**
  - Findings
    - T1WI
      - Hypointense to isointense mass
    - T2WI
      - Variable hyperintensity
      - Depends on fibrotic, mucinous, and necrotic components
    - Dynamic post-contrast imaging
      - Early peripheral enhancement with progressive centripetal fill-in
      - Persistent enhancement on delayed images
      - Small lesions with less fibrosis may enhance intensely in arterial phase and persist on delayed phases
    - DWI
      - Malignant lesions tend to have lower absolute diffusion coefficients
      - Lesion conspicuity is enhanced due to suppression of vascular high signal
    - MRCP
      - May have intrahepatic biliary dilation peripheral to mass
    - Overlying capsular retraction
  - Coagulative necrosis
    - Intermingled with fibrotic center
    - Hyperintense or hypointense on T2
    - No enhancement
  - Fibrotic component
    - More prominent centrally
    - Hypointense on T2
    - Delayed enhancement is persistent and heterogeneous
  - Mucinous carcinoma
    - Large amount of mucin with interspersed nests of tumor cells
    - Very hyperintense on T2
    - Hypointense on T1
    - No enhancement except in tumor periphery

INTRAHEPATIC BILE DUCT CARCINOMA

Staging

- Primary tumor may be staged by multiple modalities
- **Ultrasound**
  - Limited in detection of mass and vascular invasion
  - No role in staging
- **CT**
  - Multidetector CT allows rapid acquisition in multiple phases of contrast enhancement
    - Arterial phase
      - Used to determine arterial anatomy, invasion, encasement
    - Portal venous phase
      - Used to determine venous anatomy, invasion, encasement
    - Delayed (10-15 minutes)
      - Allows characterization of tumors with dominant fibrous component
  - Isotropic data allows multiplanar reformation
    - Minimum intensity projection
      - Visualization of biliary anatomy
      - Determine level of obstruction
      - Morphology of stricture
      - Presence of intraductal mass
    - Reconstruction of arterial and portal venous phases
      - Visualize vascular anatomy, tumor encasement, occlusion, or invasion
- **MR/MRCP**
  - Optimal initial examination for suspected cholangiocarcinoma
    - Liver and biliary anatomy
    - Tumor extent along bile ducts
    - Liver metastasis
    - Vascular invasion or encasement
  - Superior to CT for assessment of intraductal lesions
  - Comparable to conventional angiography for evaluation of vascular invasion
  - MR
    - Helpful for visualization of
      - Invasion of adjacent organs and vasculature
      - Satellite nodules
    - Dynamic 3D IV contrast-enhanced images
      - Multiphasic acquisition and improved spatial resolution
      - Vascular invasion
      - Direct invasion of adjacent structures
    - Tissue specific contrast agents
      - Iron oxide particles may improve tumor detection
      - Increase lesion-liver contrast and lesion conspicuity
  - MRCP
    - Navigator triggered isotropic 3D FSE
      - Improved signal to noise ratio and spatial resolution
      - Allows reformation and isolation of biliary tree
    - Advantages
      - Localizes level of obstruction
      - Morphology and longitudinal extent of strictures
      - Can evaluate biliary tree upstream to obstruction
    - Limitations
      - Not able to perform cytologic evaluation and bile sampling
      - Not able to relieve obstruction
      - Evaluation of intraductal lesions limited post stent placement
    - Ideally performed prior to biliary drainage
  - 3 tesla
    - Higher spatial resolution
    - Improved signal to noise ratio
- **Direct cholangiography (ERCP or PTC)**
  - Invasive
  - Useful for defining extent of infiltrating lesions
  - Allows bile duct sampling
    - Brush cytology has low reported accuracy
  - Allows stent placement to relieve obstruction
  - May not be able to evaluate bile ducts past the obstruction
- **Endoscopic ultrasound**
  - Can visualize distal extrahepatic bile duct, gallbladder, regional lymph nodes, and vasculature
  - Allows evaluation and US-guided FNA of regional lymph nodes
  - FNA of perihilar mass is not recommended due to risk of peritoneal seeding
- **Regional lymph nodes**
  - Anatomic and metabolic imaging has low sensitivity for lymph node metastasis
  - Fine needle aspiration biopsy may be performed with endoscopic ultrasound
    - 5-15% of those with negative CT have involved nodes with FNA at endoscopic ultrasound
- **Distant metastasis**
  - 10-20% have distant metastases at presentation
  - Usually occurs late in disease
  - Liver, lung, peritoneum
  - Satellite nodules in 10-20% → poor prognosis
  - CT is superior to MR for detection of subtle peritoneal seeding
  - Lymph nodes
    - Celiac
    - Paraaortic
    - Caval

CLINICAL ISSUES

Presentation

- Clinically silent until advanced stages
- Presents with symptoms of liver mass
  - Pain, cachexia, malaise
- Incidence is age-dependent
  - ↑ number of cases in 6th decade
  - Peak incidence in 9th decade
- Serum tumor markers
  - No specific tumor marker for cholangiocarcinoma
  - Can be used in conjunction with other diagnostic tests
  - CA-19.9
    - Elevated in up to 85% of patients
    - Elevated absolute level (> 100 U/mL) or change over time
    - Obstructive jaundice without malignancy can cause elevation but should not persist after decompression

INTRAHEPATIC BILE DUCT CARCINOMA

- Nonspecific, can also be elevated in
  - Pancreatic malignancy
  - Gastric malignancy
  - Severe hepatic injury
  - Lewis phenotype must be positive (10% of population is Lewis negative)
  - ○ CEA
    - Elevated in 30% of patients
    - Nonspecific, can be elevated in
      - Inflammatory bowel disease
      - Biliary obstruction
      - Severe hepatic injury
      - Other malignancies
  - ○ CA-125
    - Elevated in 40-50% of patients
    - May signify peritoneal involvement
    - Nonspecific, can be elevated in other GI and gynecologic malignancies

Treatment Options

- Major treatment alternatives
  - ○ Localized resectable tumor
    - Solitary mass or limited number of tumors confined to 1 lobe
    - Must allow complete resection with 1 cm margin of normal liver
    - Normal or minimally abnormal LFTs
    - No cirrhosis beyond Child-Pugh class A or chronic hepatitis
    - No tumor extension across interlobar planes
    - No tumor involvement of hepatic hilum
    - No tumor encroachment on IVC
    - 23% 5-year survival with partial hepatectomy in selected patients
    - Investigational options
      - Adjuvant chemoembolization
      - Arterial or systemic chemotherapy
      - Immunotherapy
  - ○ Localized unresectable tumor
    - Unresectable due to location or concomitant medical conditions
    - If small may be amenable to radiofrequency ablation, chemoembolization, cryosurgery, or percutaneous ethanol injection
    - Regional liver infusion of chemotherapy
    - Systemic chemotherapy has not been shown to have significant survival benefit
    - Surgery, chemotherapy, and radiation may be combined
  - ○ Advanced disease
    - No standard therapy
  - ○ Liver transplantation not typically an option due to high rate of recurrence
- Major treatment roadblocks
  - ○ Remnant liver volume
    - Remaining liver following resection needs to be sufficient to sustain hepatic function
    - Small remnant liver volume is associated with high morbidity due to liver failure
    - Minimum recommended volume of remnant liver is
      - Healthy liver: 25% of total pre-op liver volume
      - Chronic liver disease: 40% of total pre-op liver volume

- CT can estimate total liver volume pre-op and predict volume of post-op liver remnant
- Portal vein embolization may be considered if insufficient remnant liver volume precludes surgery
  - Coil embolization of affected liver lobe
  - Shunting of blood to future remnant liver induces hypertrophy
  - Improves functional reserve and decreases operative morbidity

REPORTING CHECKLIST

T Staging

- Solitary or multiple
- Vascular invasion
- Direct invasion of visceral peritoneum
- Direct invasion of extrahepatic structures
- Periductal invasion

N Staging

- Regional lymph nodes
  - ○ Left lobe tumor
    - Hilar, gastrohepatic, inferior phrenic
  - ○ Right lobe tumor
    - Hilar, periduodenal, peripancreatic, inf. phrenic

M Staging

- Hematogenous metastasis
- Peritoneal metastasis
- Lymphatic metastasis: Celiac, periaortic, pericaval

SELECTED REFERENCES

1. American Joint Committee on Cancer: AJCC Cancer Staging Manual. 7th ed. New York: Springer. 201-9, 2010
2. Moon CM et al: The role of (18)F-fluorodeoxyglucose positron emission tomography in the diagnosis, staging, and follow-up of cholangiocarcinoma. Surg Oncol. Epub ahead of print, 2009
3. Blechacz BR et al: Cholangiocarcinoma. Clin Liver Dis. 12(1):131-50, ix, 2008
4. Kim JY et al: Clinical role of 18F-FDG PET-CT in suspected and potentially operable cholangiocarcinoma: a prospective study compared with conventional imaging. Am J Gastroenterol. 103(5):1145-51, 2008
5. Sainani NI et al: Cholangiocarcinoma: current and novel imaging techniques. Radiographics. 28(5):1263-87, 2008
6. Walker SL et al: Diagnosing cholangiocarcinoma in primary sclerosing cholangitis: an "evidence based radiology" review. Abdom Imaging. 33(1):14-7, 2008
7. Lim JH et al: Early bile duct carcinoma: comparison of imaging features with pathologic findings. Radiology. 238(2):542-8, 2006
8. Han JK et al: Cholangiocarcinoma: pictorial essay of CT and cholangiographic findings. Radiographics. 22(1):173-87, 2002
9. Khan SA et al: Guidelines for the diagnosis and treatment of cholangiocarcinoma: consensus document. Gut. 51 Suppl 6:VI1-9, 2002
10. Maetani Y et al: MR imaging of intrahepatic cholangiocarcinoma with pathologic correlation. AJR Am J Roentgenol. 176(6):1499-507, 2001
11. Gores GJ: Early detection and treatment of cholangiocarcinoma. Liver Transpl. 6(6 Suppl 2):S30-4, 2000

INTRAHEPATIC BILE DUCT CARCINOMA

Stage I (T1 N0 M0)

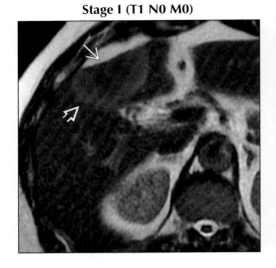

Stage I (T1 N0 M0)

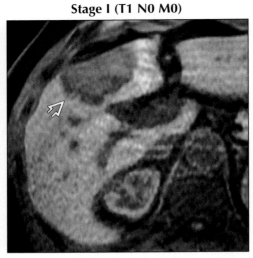

(Left) Axial T2WI MR shows a mass ➡ in the medial segment of the left hepatic lobe. Central low signal intensity ➡ and overlying capsular retraction corresponds to fibrosis typically induced by cholangiocarcinoma. (Right) Axial T1WI MR in the same patient shows the hypointense mass ➡.

Stage I (T1 N0 M0)

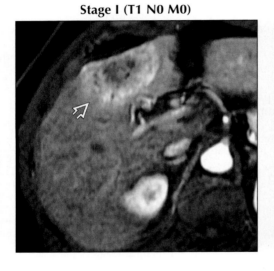

Stage I (T1 N0 M0)

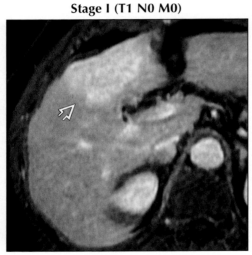

(Left) Axial T1WI C+ FS MR in the same patient shows thick irregular rim enhancement of the mass ➡ with patchy areas of central enhancement in the arterial phase. (Right) Axial T1 C+ FS MR in the same patient shows progressive delayed enhancement of the mass ➡. The central T2 hypointensity, delayed enhancement, and overlying capsular retraction are characteristic of this fibrous tumor.

Stage II (T2a N0 M0)

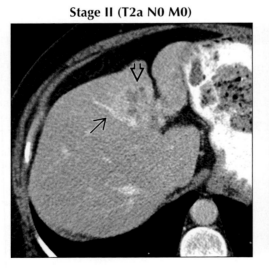

Stage II (T2a N0 M0)

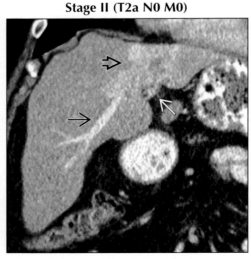

(Left) Axial CECT shows a mass ➡ in segment 4a with peripheral nodular and patchy central enhancement consistent with intrahepatic cholangiocarcinoma. The mass invades a branch of the middle hepatic vein ➡. (Right) Coronal CECT in the same patient shows the tumor ➡ encasing and narrowing the hepatic vein ➡, as well as spanning the fissure of the falciform ligament and involving the left portal vein ➡.

INTRAHEPATIC BILE DUCT CARCINOMA

Stage II (T2b N0 M0)

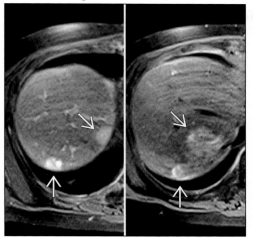

Stage II (T2b N0 M0)

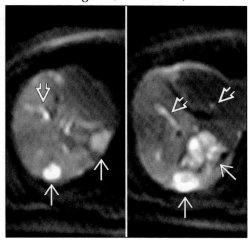

(Left) Axial T2WI FS MR shows multiple hyperintense masses ⮕ in the right hepatic lobe in this patient with multifocal cholangiocarcinoma. Additional masses are not shown. (Right) Axial DWI (b50) images in the same patient show multiple hyperintense masses ⮕. DWI with low b values can be helpful for improved lesion detection, as in this case. Additional small round and linear hyperintense areas in these images are bile ducts ⮕.

Stage II (T2b N0 M0)

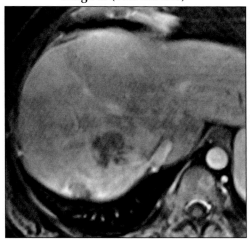

Stage II (T2b N0 M0)

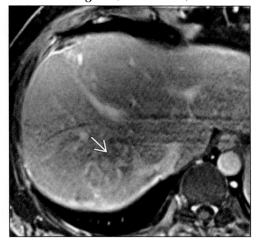

(Left) Axial T1WI C+ FS MR in the same patient obtained in the portal venous phase shows multiple hypovascular hepatic masses. There may be major vessel invasion considering the close proximity of the larger mass to the right hepatic vein; however, this does not affect the tumor stage. (Right) Axial T1WI C+ FS MR in the same patient obtained later shows the hepatic masses with progressively increasing enhancement ⮕, characteristic of cholangiocarcinoma.

Stage III (T3 N0 M0)

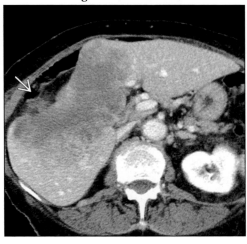

Stage III (T3 N0 M0)

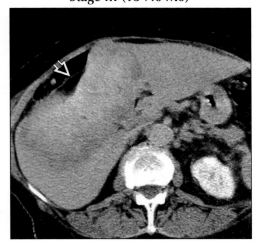

(Left) Axial CECT shows a large mass with early, irregular, thick rim enhancement and patchy areas of central enhancement. Tumor ⮕ perforating the visceral peritoneum and infiltrating the perihepatic fat constitutes tumor stage T3. (Right) Axial CECT in the same patient shows progressive centripetal fill-in of contrast enhancement within the mass. Overlying capsular retraction ⮕ and delayed enhancement is indicative of the fibrous nature of this tumor.

INTRAHEPATIC BILE DUCT CARCINOMA

Stage III (T3 N0 M0)

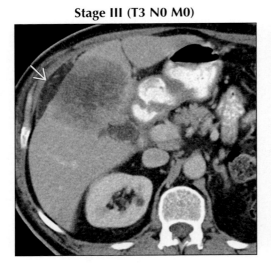

Stage III (T3 N0 M0)

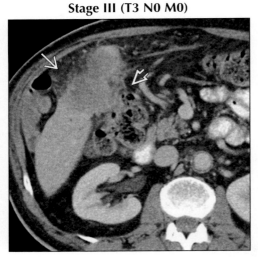

(Left) Axial CECT shows a large mass in the medial segment of the left hepatic lobe with irregular peripheral and central patchy enhancement. Note overlying capsular retraction and adjacent increased density and nodularity of the fat ➡. *(Right)* Axial CECT in the same patient shows extension of the mass beyond the liver capsule to invade the omentum ➡ and hepatic flexure of the colon ➡.

Stage III (T3 N0 M0)

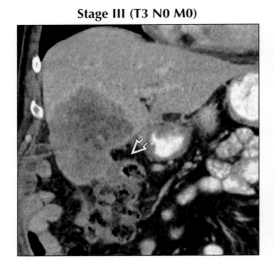

Stage III (T3 N0 M0)

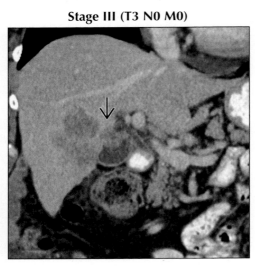

(Left) Coronal CECT in the same patient better demonstrates direct invasion of the hepatic flexure of the colon ➡. *(Right)* Coronal CECT in the same patient shows contiguous extension of the hepatic mass to invade the gallbladder ➡, again demonstrating the utility of multiplanar imaging.

Stage IVA (T4 N0 M0)

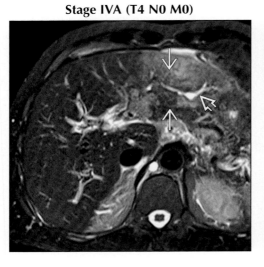

Stage IVA (T4 N0 M0)

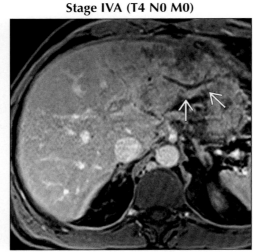

(Left) Axial T2WI FS MR shows diffuse hyperintensity in the left hepatic lobe. Lower signal encasing the dilated bile duct ➡ in this lobe corresponds to tumor ➡ infiltrating along the duct. The low signal of the tumor reflects its fibrotic nature. *(Right)* Axial T1WI C+ FS MR in the same patient shows enhancement of the periductal infiltrating tumor ➡. Tumor contrast enhancement was most evident in this delayed phase due to the fibrotic component.

Stage IVA (T2a N1 M0)

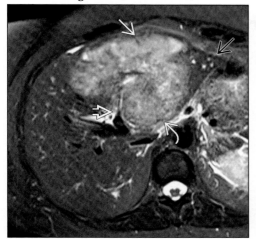

Stage IVA (T2a N1 M0)

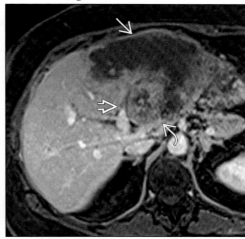

(Left) Axial T2WI FS MR shows a left hepatic lobe mass. Hyperintense areas ➡ anteriorly correspond to necrosis. Intermediate signal areas ⇒ correspond to viable tumor. Loss of the left portal vein flow void ➡ is compatible with occlusion. Biliary dilation ➡ peripheral to the mass is far more common with CCA than with metastases. (Right) Axial T1WI C+ FS MR shows lack of enhancement in areas of necrosis ⇒, enhancing viable tumor ⇒, and left portal vein obstruction ➡.

Stage IVA (T2a N1 M0)

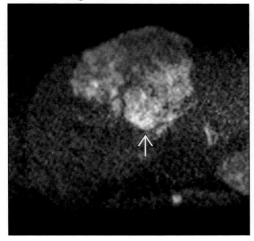

Stage IVA (T2a N1 M0)

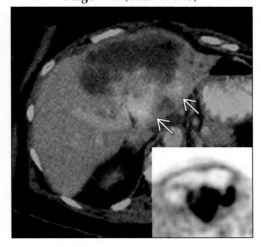

(Left) Axial DWI (b800) in the same patient shows hyperintensity in areas of viable tumor ➡. (Right) Axial fused PET/CT in the same patient shows FDG uptake in areas of viable tumor ⇒ corresponding to areas of contrast enhancement and hyperintensity on DWI. PET image (inset) shows avid FDG accumulation by viable tumor and absence in areas of necrosis.

Stage IVA (T2a N1 M0)

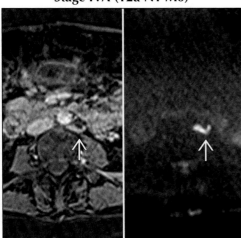

Stage IVA (T2a N1 M0)

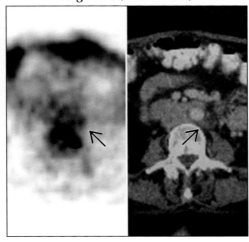

(Left) Axial T1WI C+ FS MR and DWI (b400) in the same patient show a left paraaortic lymph node ➡. This example highlights the utility of diffusion-weighted imaging for improved lesion detection. (Right) Axial PET and fused PET/CT in the same patient at the level of the same paraaortic lymph node ➡ show increased FDG uptake. Although small in size, this hypermetabolic lymph node is concerning for metastatic disease.

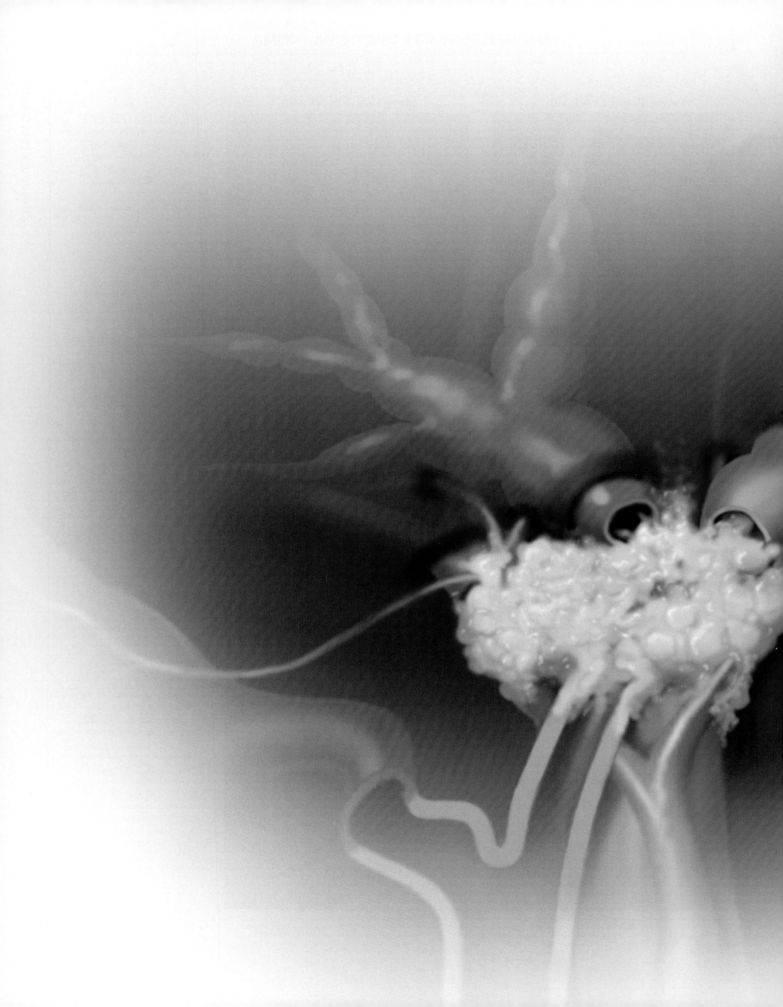

Perihilar Bile Duct Carcinoma

PERIHILAR BILE DUCT CARCINOMA

(T) Primary Tumor

Adapted from 7th edition AJCC Staging Forms.

TNM	Definitions
TX	Primary tumor cannot be assessed
T0	No evidence of primary tumor
Tis	Carcinoma in situ
T1	Tumor confined to the bile duct, with extension up to the muscle layer or fibrous tissue
T2a	Tumor invades beyond the wall of the bile duct to surrounding adipose tissue
T2b	Tumor invades adjacent hepatic parenchyma
T3	Tumor invades unilateral branches of the portal vein or hepatic artery
T4	Tumor invades main portal vein or its branches bilaterally; or the common hepatic artery; or the second-order biliary radicals bilaterally; or unilateral second-order biliary radicals with contralateral portal vein or hepatic artery involvement

(N) Regional Lymph Nodes

NX	Regional lymph nodes cannot be assessed
N0	No regional lymph node metastasis
N1	Regional lymph node metastasis (including nodes along the cystic duct, common bile duct, hepatic artery, and portal vein)
N2	Metastasis to periaortic, pericaval, superior mesenteric artery, &/or celiac artery lymph nodes

(M) Distant Metastasis

M0	No distant metastasis
M1	Distant metastasis

AJCC Stages/Prognostic Groups

Adapted from 7th edition AJCC Staging Forms.

Stage	T	N	M
0	Tis	N0	M0
I	T1	N0	M0
II	T2a, T2b	N0	M0
IIIA	T3	N0	M0
IIIB	T1, T2, T3	N1	M0
IVA	T4	N0, N1	M0
IVB	Any T	N2	M0
	Any T	Any N	M1

PERIHILAR BILE DUCT CARCINOMA

T1

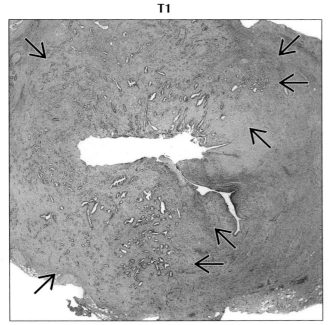

H&E stained section of a perihilar bile duct shows invasive carcinoma involving the duct wall. There is a patent central lumen with carcinoma ⇨ confined to the muscle and fibrous layer of the bile duct. (Original magnification 20x.)

T1

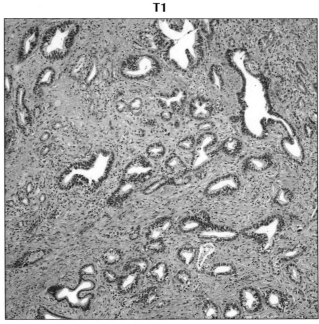

Higher magnification of the previous image again shows irregular glands of adenocarcinoma of various sizes and shapes infiltrating the muscle bundles and fibrous stroma of the wall of the perihilar bile duct. (Original magnification 200x.)

T2a

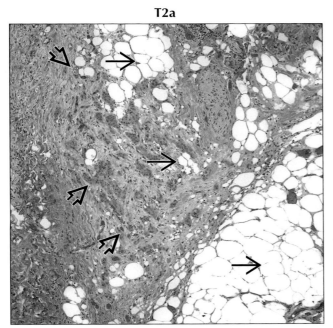

H&E stained section shows invasive carcinoma of the perihilar bile duct. The neoplastic cells are arranged in nests ⇨, are surrounded with fibrotic stroma, and infiltrate into the surrounding adipose tissue ⇨. (Original magnification 400x.)

T2b

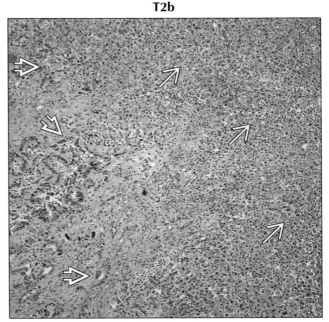

H&E stained section shows invasive carcinoma ⇨ of the perihilar bile duct that extends beyond the wall of the bile duct to involve the hepatic parenchyma ⇨. (Original magnification 100x.)

PERIHILAR BILE DUCT CARCINOMA

T1

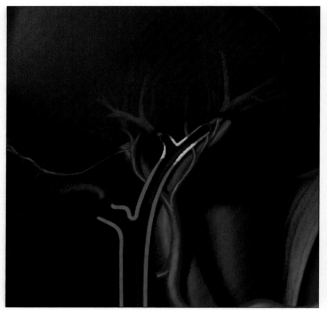

Graphic depicts the hepatic hilum with infiltrative tumor at the confluence of the right and left hepatic duct. Tumor confined to the bile duct wall is considered T1 disease.

T1

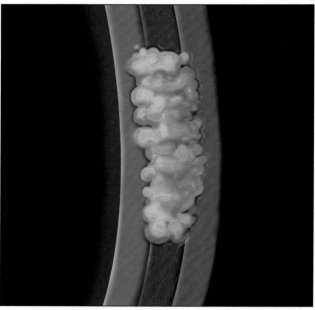

Graphic depicts the layers of the bile duct wall including the lamina propria, fibromuscular wall, and perifibromuscular connective tissue. T1 tumor is confined to the wall of the bile duct with invasion up to the muscle layer or fibrous tissue of the bile duct wall.

T2a

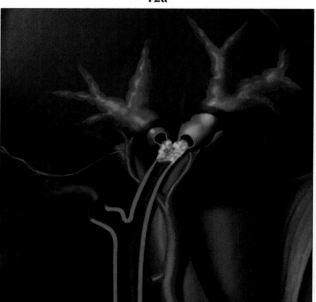

Graphic depicts the hepatic hilum with infiltrative tumor at the confluence of the right and left hepatic duct. Tumor extends beyond the wall of the bile duct, consistent with T2a disease.

T2a

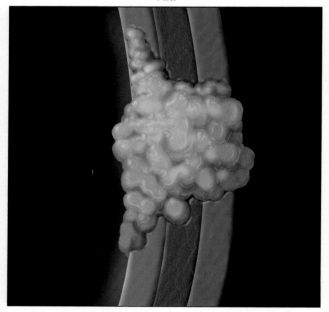

Graphic depicts the layers of the bile duct wall including the lamina propria, fibromuscular wall, and perifibromuscular connective tissue. T2a tumor invades beyond the bile duct wall into surrounding adipose tissue.

PERIHILAR BILE DUCT CARCINOMA

T2b

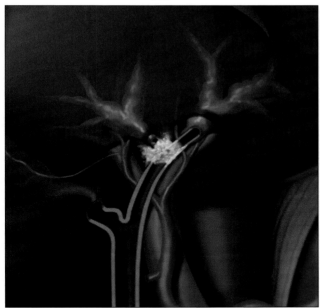

Graphic depicts the hepatic hilum with infiltrative tumor at the confluence of the right and left hepatic duct. Tumor extends to invade adjacent hepatic parenchyma, making this T2b disease.

T3

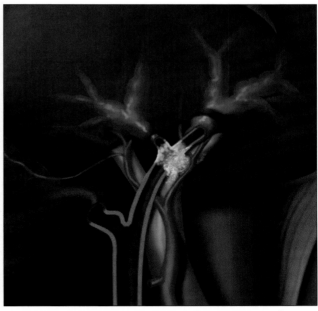

Graphic depicts the hepatic hilum with infiltrative tumor at the confluence of the right and left hepatic duct with an exophytic mass-forming component invading the left portal vein.

T3

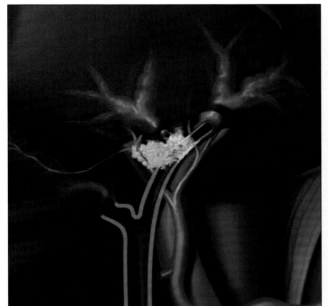

Graphic depicts the hepatic hilum with infiltrative tumor at the confluence of the right and left hepatic duct. There is an exophytic mass-forming component invading the right hepatic artery. Tumors of stage T3 can invade unilaterally the portal vein, hepatic artery, or both.

T3

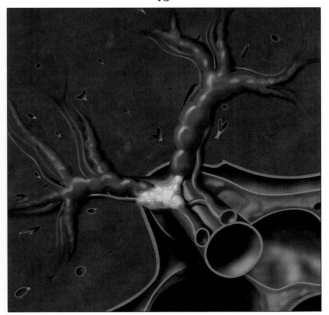

Axial graphic depicts the hepatic hilum with perihilar tumor encasing the right hepatic artery.

T4

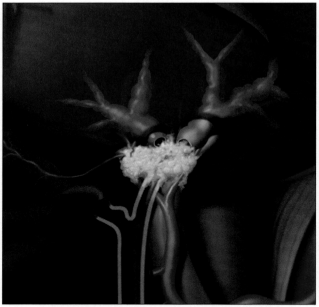

Graphic depicts the hepatic hilum with infiltrative tumor at the confluence of the right and left hepatic duct with an exophytic mass-forming component invading bilateral portal veins and hepatic arteries. Invasion of the common hepatic artery, main portal vein, or bilateral branches constitutes stage T4 tumor.

T4

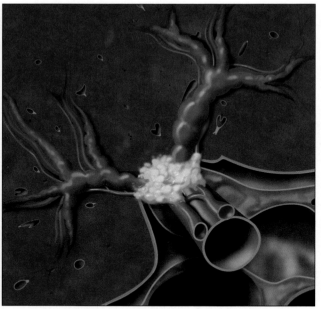

Axial graphic depicts the hepatic hilum with perihilar tumor encasing the right and left hepatic arteries.

T4

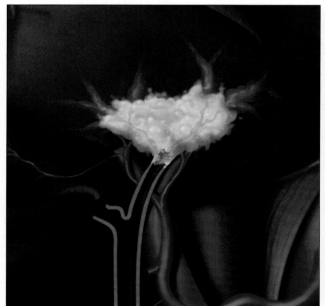

Graphic depicts the hepatic hilum with tumor at the confluence of the right and left hepatic duct with extension to the secondary biliary radicles on the right and left. Irrespective of vascular invasion, bilateral tumor extension to the secondary biliary radicles is stage T4.

T4

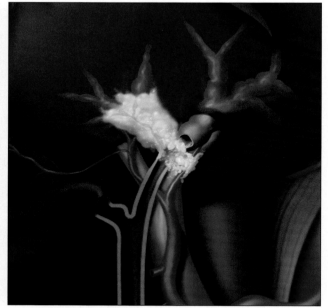

Graphic depicts the hepatic hilum with tumor at the confluence of the right and left hepatic duct with extension to the secondary biliary radicles on the right and invasion of the left portal vein and hepatic artery.

PERIHILAR BILE DUCT CARCINOMA

N1

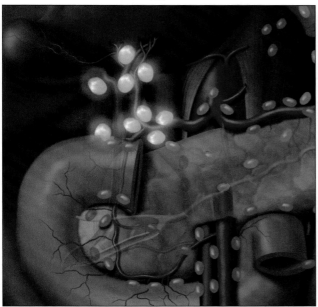

Graphic highlights N1 regional lymph nodes. These include nodes along the cystic duct, common bile duct, hepatic artery, and portal vein.

N2

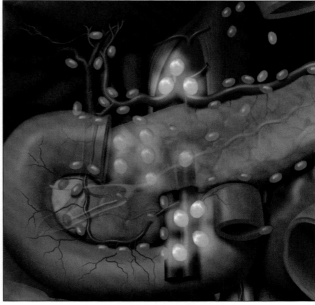

Graphic highlights N2 regional lymph nodes. These include periaortic, pericaval, superior mesenteric artery, and celiac artery lymph nodes.

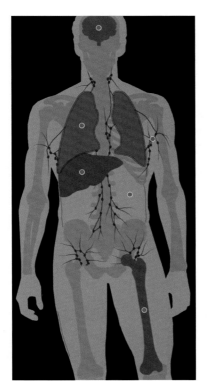

METASTASES, ORGAN FREQUENCY

Liver

Peritoneal cavity

Lymph nodes

Lung

Bones

Brain

The literature only offers isolated cases of cholangiocarcinoma with distant metastasis. The number is not sufficiently significant to quantify organ frequency.

PERIHILAR BILE DUCT CARCINOMA

OVERVIEW

General Comments
- Tumor arising in extrahepatic bile duct upstream to cystic duct origin
  - Klatskin tumor: Tumor at biliary confluence of right and left hepatic duct
- ~ 70% of cholangiocarcinomas (CCAs) are perihilar

Classification
- Histologic types
  - Adenocarcinoma
  - Adenocarcinoma, intestinal type
  - Clear cell adenocarcinoma
  - Mucinous carcinoma
  - Signet ring cell carcinoma
  - Squamous cell carcinoma
  - Adenosquamous carcinoma
  - Small cell (oat cell) carcinoma
  - Undifferentiated carcinoma
  - Papillomatosis
  - Papillary carcinoma, noninvasive
  - Papillary carcinoma, invasive
  - Carcinoma, not otherwise specified (NOS)

PATHOLOGY

Routes of Spread
- **Contiguous spread**
  - Predilection for longitudinal submucosal spread in duct wall
    - May have substantial extension of tumor beneath intact epithelial lining
      - Up to 2 cm proximally and 1 cm distally
    - Perihilar tumor tends to infiltrate into intrahepatic ducts
  - Spread along periductal tissues
    - Neural and perineural involvement
  - Direct invasion of adjacent structures
    - Invasion of hepatic parenchyma in 85%
    - Invasion of vasculature
      - Portal vein is common
      - Hepatic artery
    - Invasion of adjacent organs
      - Pancreas
      - Stomach, duodenum, or colon
      - Omentum and abdominal wall
- **Lymphatic spread**
  - Prevalence of 30-53%
  - ↑ prevalence of lymph node metastases with ↑ in primary tumor stage
  - Most commonly involves hepatoduodenal nodes
    - Hilar nodes
    - Pericholedochal nodes
  - N1 regional nodes
    - Cystic duct
    - Common bile duct
    - Hepatic artery
    - Portal vein
  - N2 regional nodes
    - Periaortic
    - Pericaval
    - Superior mesenteric artery

- Celiac artery
  - Incidence of N2 nodal metastases is 14-50% in patients with lymphatic spread
- **Hematogenous spread**
  - 10-20% have distant metastases at presentation
  - 50% have metastatic disease at autopsy
  - Liver is common site of metastases
  - Spread to other organs, especially extraabdominal, uncommon
- **Peritoneal spread**
  - 10-20% have peritoneal involvement

General Features
- Comments
  - 80% of cholangiocarcinomas are extrahepatic
    - 70-80% are perihilar
    - 20-30% are distal bile duct
- Genetics
  - Gene mutations suggest possible genetic link
    - Inactivation of tumor suppressor genes
    - Mutations in oncogenes
    - Chromosomal aneuploidy
  - No established clinical role for molecular profiling at this time
- Etiology
  - Risk factors
    - Age
    - Primary sclerosing cholangitis (PSC)
    - Chronic ulcerative colitis
    - Hepatolithiasis
    - Caroli disease
    - Choledochal cysts
    - Tobacco abuse (in association with PSC)
    - Bile duct adenoma & biliary papillomatosis
    - Hepatobiliary flukes
    - Chronic typhoid carriers
    - Exposure to thorotrast
    - Familial polyposis
  - Additional risk factors in USA and Europe
    - Cirrhosis
    - Chronic hepatitis C infection
    - Alcohol abuse
- Epidemiology & cancer incidence
  - Incidence is 1-2 per 100,000 in USA
  - Increasing incidence worldwide
- Associated diseases, abnormalities
  - Primary sclerosing cholangitis
    - Common risk factor in western countries
    - Prevalence of cholangiocarcinoma in this setting is 5-15%
    - Risk is not associated with duration or severity of PSC or inflammatory bowel disease
  - Hepatobiliary flukes
    - *Opisthorchis viverrini* and *Clonorchis sinensis*
    - Endemic in east Asia
    - Ingested in undercooked fish
    - Infest biliary tree ± gallbladder
  - Choledochal cysts
    - 10-15% lifetime risk of developing CCA
    - Malignant degeneration uncommon if excised early in life
    - 15-20% ↑ incidence if not treated until > 20 years of age
  - Hepatolithiasis
    - Risk factor in parts of Asia

PERIHILAR BILE DUCT CARCINOMA

- Up to 10% complicated by cholangiocarcinoma
- In endemic areas, 70% of tumors manifest with hepatolithiasis

Gross Pathology & Surgical Features

- Patterns of tumor growth
  - Mass-forming (exophytic)
    - Most common at intrahepatic location
    - Radial growth pattern invading into liver
  - Periductal (infiltrating)
    - Most common in perihilar tumors
    - Tendency to extend submucosally
    - Sclerotic lesion with abundant fibrous tissue
  - Mixed (mass-forming and periductal)
  - Intraductal (polypoid)
    - Usually papillary adenocarcinoma
    - Intraluminal polypoid mass
    - Uncommon except those tumors arising in choledochal cysts
- Macroscopic subtypes
  - Sclerosing
    - Majority of tumors
    - Perihilar > distal bile duct
    - Firm tumor → annular thickening of bile duct
    - Often diffuse infiltration & fibrosis of periductal tissues
  - Nodular
    - Firm, irregular nodule projecting into duct lumen
  - Papillary
    - 10% of cholangiocarcinomas
    - Distal bile duct > perihilar
    - Soft, friable tumor
    - May have little transmural invasion
    - Tends to be polypoid mass expanding duct
    - Can be quite large, but arising from well-defined stalk with majority of tumor mobile within duct

Microscopic Pathology

- H&E
  - 90% are adenocarcinomas
  - Usually well to moderately differentiated
  - Exhibit glandular or acinar structures
  - Cuboidal or low columnar cells resembling biliary epithelium
  - Intracytoplasmic mucin is common
  - Mitotic figures are rare
  - Dense sparsely cellular fibrous stroma
  - Tendency to invade lymphatics, blood vessels, perineural & periductal spaces, and portal tracts

IMAGING FINDINGS

Detection

- **Ultrasound**
  - Excellent for identifying biliary obstruction
  - Poor sensitivity & specificity for identifying mass
    - Difficult to see intraductal or infiltrating lesions
    - Mass-forming tumors have variable echogenicity
    - Advanced stage when seen on US
  - Findings
    - Segmental dilation with abrupt cut-off of right and left hepatic ducts at porta hepatis
    - Lobar atrophy results in crowding of dilated ducts
    - Hypovascular mass → poor color Doppler signal

- May detect portal vein occlusion or infiltration
- **CT**
  - Findings
    - NECT
      - Hypodense bile duct wall thickening
      - Mass at confluence of right & left hepatic ducts
    - CECT
      - Thickened bile duct wall continues to enhance on delayed images
      - Mass showing progressive and persistent enhancement on delayed images
  - Atrophy-hypertrophy complex
    - Bile duct dilation in an atrophic hepatic lobe with compensatory hypertrophy of contralateral lobe
  - Mass may not be visible; however, biliary dilation abruptly terminates at biliary confluence
  - No extrahepatic biliary dilation
  - Diffuse intrahepatic biliary ductal dilation
- **PET/CT**
  - FDG accumulates in tumor cells, but limited if large fibrotic component
  - Mucinous carcinoma → no FDG uptake
  - Higher rate of tumor detection for mass-forming growth pattern than infiltrative
  - Some report better detection of intrahepatic tumor than perihilar or distal bile duct
  - Efficacy of PET in setting of PSC is controversial
  - Focal FDG uptake & ↑ CA-19.9 is more sensitive & specific
- **MR/MRCP**
  - Findings
    - T1WI
      - Hypointense to isointense mass
    - T2WI
      - Bile duct wall thickening and obliteration of lumen at biliary confluence
      - Hyperintense to isointense mass
      - Signal intensity depends on fibrotic, mucinous, and necrotic components of tumor
      - Fat saturation improves conspicuity of hyperintense masses
    - Dynamic post-contrast images
      - Progressive and persistent enhancement on delayed images
    - DWI
      - Malignant lesions tend to have lower absolute diffusion coefficients
      - Lesion conspicuity is enhanced due to suppression of vascular high signal
    - MRCP
      - Abrupt occlusion of bile ducts at level of biliary confluence
      - Intrahepatic biliary dilation
      - No extrahepatic biliary dilation
      - Delineates level of obstruction, longitudinal extent, or multifocality of tumor
  - Atrophy-hypertrophy complex
    - Atrophy of 1 hepatic lobe with crowding of dilated bile ducts
    - Compensatory hypertrophy of contralateral lobe
    - Often indicates concomitant portal vein occlusion of atrophic lobe
  - Tissue-specific contrast agents
    - Iron oxide particles may improve tumor detection

PERIHILAR BILE DUCT CARCINOMA

- ■ Increase lesion-liver contrast & lesion conspicuity
  - ○ Primary sclerosing cholangitis
    - ■ Findings of superimposed CCA
      - – Progressive stricture formation (most common)
      - – Upstream bile duct dilation
      - – Polypoid intraductal mass

Staging

- • Primary tumor may be staged by multiple modalities
- • **Ultrasound**
  - ○ Limited in detection of mass and vascular invasion
  - ○ No role in staging
- • **CT**
  - ○ Multidetector CT allows rapid acquisition in multiple phases of contrast enhancement
    - ■ Arterial & portal venous phase
      - – Arterial & venous anatomy, invasion, encasement
    - ■ Delayed phase (10-15 minutes)
      - – Characterize tumors with dominant fibrous component
  - ○ Isotropic data allows multiplanar reformation
    - ■ Minimum intensity projection
      - – Visualization of biliary anatomy
      - – Determine level of obstruction
      - – Morphology of stricture
      - – Presence of intraductal mass
    - ■ Reconstruction of arterial & portal venous phases
      - – Visualize vascular anatomy, tumor encasement, occlusion, or invasion
  - ○ Criteria for vascular involvement
    - ■ Vessel occlusion or stenosis
    - ■ Vessel contour deformity associated with tumor contact
    - ■ > 50% perimeter contact with tumor
  - ○ Limited in defining longitudinal tumor extent
- • **PET/CT**
  - ○ Not superior to CT or MR/MRCP for detection of primary lesion
  - ○ Limitations for primary tumor
    - ■ Assessment of longitudinal tumor extent
    - ■ Evaluation of vascular invasion
    - ■ Detection of hepatic invasion
- • **MR/MRCP**
  - ○ Optimal initial examination for suspected CCA
    - ■ Liver and biliary anatomy
    - ■ Tumor extent along bile ducts
    - ■ Liver metastasis
    - ■ Vascular invasion or encasement
  - ○ Superior to CT for detection of intraductal lesions
  - ○ Comparable to conventional angiography for evaluation of vascular invasion
  - ○ MR
    - ■ Helpful for visualization of
      - – Exophytic component
      - – Invasion of adjacent organs & vasculature
      - – Satellite nodules
    - ■ In conjunction with MRCP, allows better estimation of longitudinal extent of tumor
    - ■ Dynamic 3D IV contrast-enhanced images
      - – Multiphasic acquisition and improved spatial resolution
      - – Vascular invasion
      - – Direct invasion of adjacent structures
  - ○ MRCP

- ■ Ideally performed prior to biliary drainage
- ■ Localizes level of obstruction
- ■ Defines morphology & longitudinal extent of strictures
- ■ Can evaluate biliary tree upstream to obstruction
- ■ Navigator triggered isotropic 3D FSE
  - – ↑ signal-to-noise ratio and spatial resolution
  - – Allows reformation and isolation of biliary tree
- ■ Limitations
  - – Not able to perform cytologic evaluation and bile duct sampling
  - – Not able to relieve obstruction
  - – Evaluation of intraductal lesions limited post stent placement
  - – Limited in periampullary region
  - ○ 3 tesla
    - ■ Higher spatial resolution
    - ■ Improved signal-to-noise ratio
- • **Direct cholangiography** (ERCP or percutaneous transhepatic cholangiography)
  - ○ Invasive
  - ○ Useful for defining extent of infiltrating lesions
  - ○ Allows bile duct sampling
    - ■ Brush cytology has low reported accuracy (9-24%)
    - ■ In patients with PSC, sensitivity is 60-73%
    - ■ Negative result does not exclude malignancy
  - ○ Allows stent placement to relieve obstruction
  - ○ May not be able to evaluate bile ducts past the obstruction
  - ○ Altered anatomy due to prior surgery may preclude ERCP
  - ○ Percutaneous transhepatic cholangiography is performed if
    - ■ Lumen obliterated by tissue
    - ■ Proximal lesion
    - ■ Biliary tree not well visualized with ERCP
- • **Endoscopic ultrasound**
  - ○ Invasive
  - ○ Can visualize distal extrahepatic bile duct, gallbladder, regional lymph nodes, and vasculature
  - ○ Assesses depth of intraductal lesions
  - ○ Localizes stricture for accurate FNA
    - ■ FNA of perihilar mass is not recommended due to risk of peritoneal seeding
- • **Bismuth-Corlette**
  - ○ Cholangiographic classification to delineate longitudinal extent of perihilar tumor
  - ○ MRCP may be used in place of conventional cholangiography except in setting of PSC
  - ○ Classification
    - ■ Type I: Involvement of common hepatic duct distal to confluence
    - ■ Type II: Involvement of biliary confluence
    - ■ Type IIIa: Involvement of biliary confluence and right hepatic duct
    - ■ Type IIIb: Involvement of biliary confluence and left hepatic duct
    - ■ Type IV: Involvement of right and left hepatic duct or multifocal tumor
- • **Regional lymph nodes**
  - ○ Anatomic imaging (CT & MR)
    - ■ Low sensitivity for lymph node metastasis
    - ■ Findings
      - – Size: ≥ 10 mm short axis

- Central necrosis
- ○ Metabolic imaging (PET/CT)
  - ■ Can be complementary to CT for nodal metastasis
  - ■ Sensitivity (32%), specificity (88%)
  - ■ Higher specificity and accuracy than CT alone
  - ■ Findings
    - Relative increased FDG uptake compared to normal nodes
- ○ Limitations of anatomic & metabolic imaging
  - ■ Differentiating reactive from malignant adenopathy
  - ■ Micrometastasis
- ○ Fine needle aspiration biopsy may be performed with endoscopic ultrasound
  - ■ 5-15% of those with negative CT have involved nodes with FNA at endoscopic ultrasound
- ○ Enlarged periportal lymph nodes are common in PSC, not necessarily indicative of metastasis
- **Metastatic disease**
  - ○ Common in liver
    - ■ Intrahepatic ductal extension
    - ■ Perineural
    - ■ Periductal lymphatics
  - ○ Extraabdominal sites are uncommon
    - ■ Peritoneal cavity, lung, brain, bone
  - ○ Metabolic imaging may be valuable in detection of unsuspected distant metastasis
    - ■ Sensitivity of PET is 65% & PET/CT is 56% (specificity 88-92%)
    - ■ May also be helpful for indeterminate lesions seen on conventional imaging

CLINICAL ISSUES

Presentation

- Age usually > 65 years (peak in 8th decade)
- Early symptoms are nonspecific (present in 30%)
  - ○ Abdominal pain, anorexia, weight loss
- Later symptoms of biliary obstruction
  - ○ Jaundice, pale stool, dark urine, pruritus
- Prolonged obstruction
  - ○ Decrease in fat-soluble vitamins
  - ○ Increase in prothrombin time
- Cholangitis is rare without biliary intervention
  - ○ Right upper quadrant pain, fever, chills
- Liver function tests → obstructive pattern
  - ○ ↑ alkaline phosphatase & bilirubin
  - ○ Aminotransferases are often normal, unless acute obstruction or cholangitis
- Serum tumor markers
  - ○ No specific tumor marker for cholangiocarcinoma
  - ○ Used in conjunction with other diagnostic tests
  - ○ CA-19.9
    - ■ ↑ in up to 85% of patients
    - ■ ↑ absolute level (> 100 U/mL) or change over time
    - ■ Obstructive jaundice without malignancy can cause ↑, but should not persist after decompression
    - ■ Nonspecific, can also be elevated in
      - Pancreatic malignancy
      - Gastric malignancy
      - Severe hepatic injury

- ■ Lewis phenotype must be positive (10% of population is Lewis negative)
- ○ CEA
  - ■ ↑ in 30% of patients
  - ■ Nonspecific, can be elevated in
    - Inflammatory bowel disease
    - Biliary obstruction
    - Severe hepatic injury
    - Other malignancies
- ○ CA-125
  - ■ ↑ in 40-50% of patients
  - ■ May signify peritoneal involvement
  - ■ Nonspecific, can be elevated in other GI and gynecologic malignancies

Cancer Natural History & Prognosis

- Most important stage-independent prognostic factor: Extent of resection & microscopic margin evaluation
- Factors negatively impacting survival
  - ○ High tumor grade
  - ○ Perineural invasion
  - ○ Vascular invasion
  - ○ Lobar atrophy
  - ○ Lymph node metastasis
- Hepatic parenchymal invasion has better prognosis than vascular invasion
- Papillary tumor has better prognosis

Treatment Options

- Major treatment alternatives
  - ○ Resection is only curative treatment option
    - ■ 20% resectable at diagnosis
    - ■ High operative mortality (5-10%)
    - ■ 5-year survival (9-18%)
  - ○ High local recurrence rates even with curative resection
  - ○ Goals of surgery
    - ■ Complete tumor excision
    - ■ Negative histologic margins
    - ■ Relief of biliary obstruction
    - ■ Re-establishment of biliary-enteric communication
  - ○ Localized resectable tumor
    - ■ Eligibility for resection depends on
      - Biliary and vascular anatomy
      - Location and extent of tumor
      - Hepatic parenchymal invasion
      - Relationship to vessels
    - ■ Extended hepatectomy improves negative margin rate and overall survival
      - Higher morbidity and mortality
    - ■ Resection strategy depends on Bismuth-Corlette (BC) classification of longitudinal tumor extent
      - BC types I, II, IIIa → extended right hepatectomy with resection of segment 4
      - BC type IIIb → left hepatectomy including segment 4
    - ■ Removal of caudate lobe is controversial
      - High % of resected specimens contain tumor
      - Most common site of hepatic recurrence
    - ■ Portal vein resection & reconstruction if gross invasion
    - ■ Must assess lymph node metastases at surgery
      - Important predictor of survival post-op

PERIHILAR BILE DUCT CARCINOMA

- External beam radiation has been used in conjunction with surgery
- Radiation therapy may improve local control
  - Unresectable tumor (e.g., Bismuth-Corlette type IV)
    - Includes majority of patients with bile duct cancer
    - Management directed at palliation
    - Relief of biliary obstruction
      - Surgical biliary-enteric anastomosis
      - Endoscopic stent
      - Percutaneous stent
    - Options under investigation
      - Radiation sensitizers
      - Chemotherapeutic agents
      - Photodynamic therapy
      - Transarterial embolization
      - Radiofrequency ablation (mass-forming lesion)
  - Liver transplantation
    - Considered for select cases following regimen of
      - High-dose external beam radiation
      - Chemotherapy
      - Brachytherapy
    - Must exclude stage III or greater disease and regional adenopathy
- Major treatment roadblocks
  - Findings precluding surgical resection
    - Longitudinal and radial tumor extent
      - Tumor invasion of right and left hepatic ducts to level of secondary biliary radicles
      - Multifocal tumor
      - Lobar atrophy with involvement of contralateral secondary biliary radicles
      - Invasion of secondary biliary radicles with contralateral vascular invasion
    - Vascular invasion
      - Lobar atrophy + contralateral vascular invasion
      - Main portal vein involvement
      - Common or proper hepatic artery encasement
      - Bilateral hepatic artery involvement
    - Remnant liver volume
      - Remaining liver following resection needs to be sufficient to sustain hepatic function
      - Small remnant liver volume is associated with high morbidity due to liver failure
      - Minimum recommended volume of remnant liver is 25% of total pre-op volume for healthy liver, 40% of total pre-op volume in chronic disease
    - Lymph node metastasis
    - Distant metastasis
    - Comorbidities
      - Significant liver disease, cirrhosis, cardiovascular or other systemic disease

REPORTING CHECKLIST

T Staging

- Level of obstruction
  - Secondary biliary radicles: Unilateral or bilateral
  - Ipsilateral or contralateral to vascular involvement
- Hepatic parenchymal invasion
- Portal vein involvement
  - Unilateral or bilateral branches
  - Main portal vein
- Hepatic artery involvement
  - Unilateral or bilateral branches
  - Common or proper hepatic artery

N Staging

- Size, shape, central necrosis
- N1 regional nodes
  - Cystic duct, common bile duct, hepatic artery, portal vein
- N2 regional nodes
  - Periaortic, pericaval, celiac, superior mesenteric

M Staging

- Hepatic satellite nodules
- Peritoneal involvement
- Distant adenopathy
- Lungs, bones, CNS

SELECTED REFERENCES

1. American Joint Committee on Cancer: AJCC Cancer Staging Manual. 7th ed. New York: Springer. 219-25, 2010
2. Moon CM et al: The role of (18)F-fluorodeoxyglucose positron emission tomography in the diagnosis, staging, and follow-up of cholangiocarcinoma. Surg Oncol. Epub ahead of print, 2009
3. Blechacz BR et al: Cholangiocarcinoma. Clin Liver Dis. 12(1):131-50, ix, 2008
4. Kim JY et al: Clinical role of 18F-FDG PET-CT in suspected and potentially operable cholangiocarcinoma: a prospective study compared with conventional imaging. Am J Gastroenterol. 103(5):1145-51, 2008
5. Li J et al: Preoperative assessment of hilar cholangiocarcinoma by dual-modality PET/CT. J Surg Oncol. 98(6):438-43, 2008
6. Park HS et al: Preoperative evaluation of bile duct cancer: MRI combined with MR cholangiopancreatography versus MDCT with direct cholangiography. AJR Am J Roentgenol. 190(2):396-405, 2008
7. Sainani NI et al: Cholangiocarcinoma: current and novel imaging techniques. Radiographics. 28(5):1263-87, 2008
8. Walker SL et al: Diagnosing cholangiocarcinoma in primary sclerosing cholangitis: an "evidence based radiology" review. Abdom Imaging. 33(1):14-7, 2008
9. Lee HY et al: Preoperative assessment of resectability of hepatic hilar cholangiocarcinoma: combined CT and cholangiography with revised criteria. Radiology. 239(1):113-21, 2006
10. Lim JH et al: Early bile duct carcinoma: comparison of imaging features with pathologic findings. Radiology. 238(2):542-8, 2006
11. Parikh AA et al: Operative considerations in resection of hilar cholangiocarcinoma. HPB (Oxford). 7(4):254-8, 2005
12. Gores GJ: Cholangiocarcinoma: current concepts and insights. Hepatology. 37(5):961-9, 2003
13. Han JK et al: Cholangiocarcinoma: pictorial essay of CT and cholangiographic findings. Radiographics. 22(1):173-87, 2002
14. Khan SA et al: Guidelines for the diagnosis and treatment of cholangiocarcinoma: consensus document. Gut. 51 Suppl 6:VI1-9, 2002
15. Gores GJ: Early detection and treatment of cholangiocarcinoma. Liver Transpl. 6(6 Suppl 2):S30-4, 2000
16. Jarnagin WR: Cholangiocarcinoma of the extrahepatic bile ducts. Semin Surg Oncol. 19(2):156-76, 2000

Stage II (T2a N0 M0)

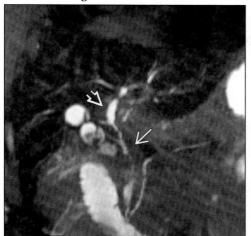

Stage II (T2a N0 M0)

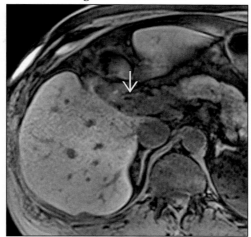

(Left) Coronal MRCP shows irregularity of the common hepatic and common bile duct ➡ with long segment narrowing. Note mild upstream biliary ductal dilation ➡. (Right) Axial T1WI MR in the same patient shows the thickened low signal wall of the common hepatic duct ➡.

Stage II (T2a N0 M0)

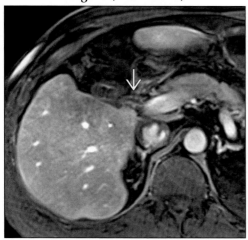

Stage II (T2a N0 M0)

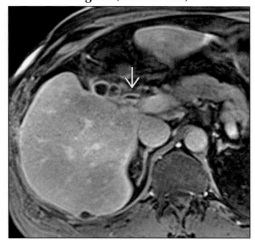

(Left) Axial T1WI C+ FS MR in the same patient shows common hepatic duct ➡ wall thickening with mild enhancement in the arterial phase. (Right) Axial T1 C+ FS MR in the same patient shows common hepatic duct ➡ wall thickening and progressive increase in enhancement in this delayed phase. The ill-defined duct wall suggests tumor invasion beyond the wall of the bile duct.

Stage II (T2a N0 M0)

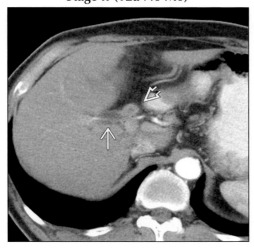

Stage II (T2a N0 M0)

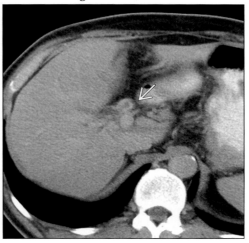

(Left) Axial CECT in the arterial phase shows circumferential wall thickening and enhancement at the confluence ➡ of the right and left hepatic ducts. Note normal imperceptible wall of the upstream right hepatic duct ➡. (Right) Axial CECT in the same patient obtained in the delayed phase shows persistent and progressive enhancement of the bile duct wall ➡, consistent with the fibrous stroma characteristic of cholangiocarcinoma.

PERIHILAR BILE DUCT CARCINOMA

(Left) *Coronal T2WI MR in the same patient shows hypointense wall thickening* ➡ *of the confluence and common hepatic duct with obliteration of the lumen. T2 hypointensity reflects the dominant fibrous component of this infiltrative tumor.* **(Right)** *ERCP in the same patient shows obstruction at the confluence* ➡ *of the hepatic ducts with upstream biliary duct dilation.*

Stage II (T2a N0 M0)

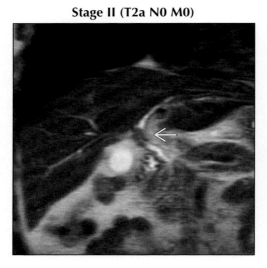

Stage II (T2a N0 M0)

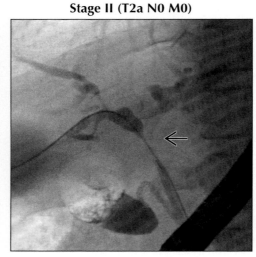

(Left) *Axial T2WI FS MR shows intrahepatic biliary ductal dilation* ➡ *abruptly terminating at a hypointense mass* ➡ *at the confluence of the right and left hepatic ducts. Note the left lobe cysts.* **(Right)** *Axial T1WI C+ FS MR in the same patient shows a hypovascular perihilar mass invading the adjacent hepatic parenchyma. Note hypoenhancement of the mass in the arterial phase* ➡ *with fill-in on the delayed phase* ➡.

Stage II (T2b N0 M0)

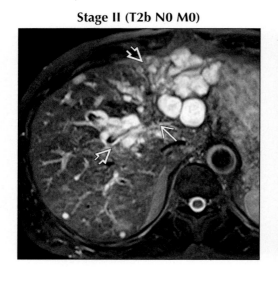

Stage II (T2b N0 M0)

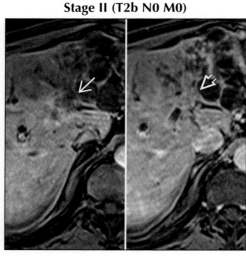

(Left) *Axial T2WI MR shows an exophytic hyperintense perihilar mass* ➡ *invading the gallbladder fossa* ➡. **(Right)** *Axial T2WI MR in the same patient shows extension of the hyperintense perihilar mass to encase the gallbladder* ➡.

Stage II (T2b N0 M0)

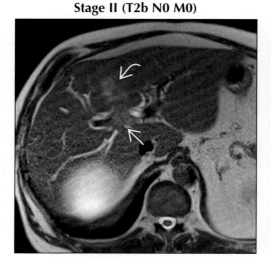

Stage II (T2b N0 M0)

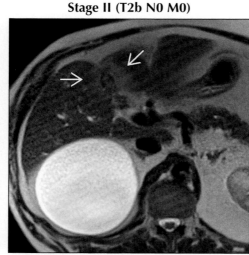

PERIHILAR BILE DUCT CARCINOMA

Stage IIIA (T3 N0 M0)

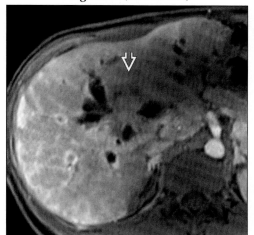

Stage IIIA (T3 N0 M0)

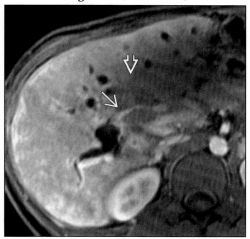

(Left) Axial T1WI C+ FS MR in the arterial phase shows a hilar mass ⇨ extending to the secondary biliary radicles in the right hepatic lobe. Progressive enhancement of the mass was present on delayed post-contrast images (not shown). *(Right)* Axial T1WI C+ FS MR in the same patient shows encasement of the right hepatic artery ➡ by the hypovascular mass ⇨. Replaced left hepatic artery is not shown.

Stage IIIA (T3 N0 M0)

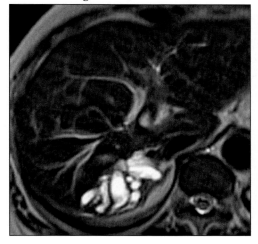

Stage IIIA (T3 N0 M0)

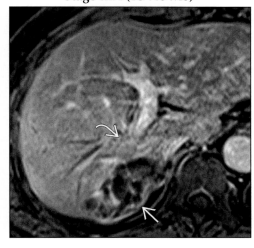

(Left) Axial T2WI MR in a different patient shows dilation and crowding of the bile ducts in the atrophic right hepatic lobe and compensatory hypertrophy of the left lobe. These findings suggest right portal vein occlusion by the perihilar mass (not shown). *(Right)* Axial T1WI C+ FS MR in the same patient shows obliteration and occlusion of the right portal vein ➡ by the perihilar mass (not shown) with resultant right lobe atrophy and crowding of the dilated biliary tree ⇨.

Stage IIIB (T2b N1 M0)

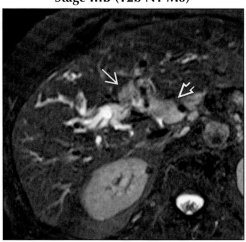

Stage IVA (T4 N0 M0)

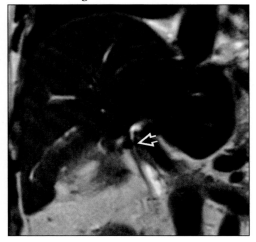

(Left) Axial T2WI FS MR at the level of the confluence of the right and left hepatic ducts shows a perihilar infiltrating mass with an hyperintense exophytic component ➡ invading the hepatic parenchyma. Regional lymph nodes ⇨ at the hepatic hilum characterize stage IIIB disease. *(Right)* Coronal T2WI MR shows hypointense wall thickening of the common hepatic duct. Minimal luminal patency is due to the biliary stent ⇨.

PERIHILAR BILE DUCT CARCINOMA

Stage IVA (T4 N0 M0)

Stage IVA (T4 N0 M0)

(Left) Axial T1WI C+ FS MR in the same patient shows wall thickening of the common hepatic duct ➡. Enhancement of the duct wall on this delayed post-contrast image is characteristic of the fibrotic nature of this malignancy. Note the portal vein ➡. *(Right)* Axial T1W C+ FS MR images in the same patient show diffuse wall thickening and multifocal stenoses ➡ of the intrahepatic bile ducts, consistent with multifocal tumor. Note bile duct dilation ➡ upstream to stenoses.

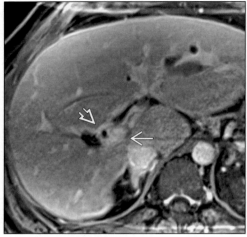

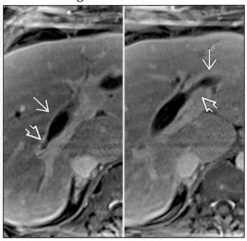

Stage IVA (T4 N0 M0)

Stage IVA (T4 N0 M0)

(Left) Axial CECT shows a hypovascular perihilar mass ➡ encasing the right and left portal veins ➡. Note intrahepatic biliary ductal dilation. *(Right)* Percutaneous biliary cholangiography in the same patient also shows the intrahepatic biliary ductal dilation, compatible with underlying primary sclerosing cholangitis (PSC).

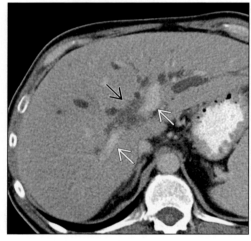

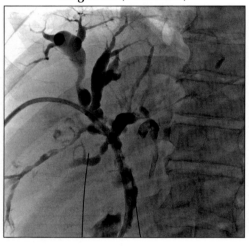

Stage IVA (T4 N0 M0)

Stage IVA (T4 N0 M0)

(Left) Coronal MRCP shows irregular dilation of the intrahepatic bile ducts. Alternating biliary stricture and dilation are characteristic of PSC. Diffuse intrahepatic biliary dilation is due to a perihilar mass. Common bile duct is normal in caliber ➡. *(Right)* Axial T2WI FS MR in the same patient shows a hyperintense infiltrative perihilar mass ➡ at the level of obstruction seen on MRCP. The exophytic component invades the hepatic parenchyma and right and left portal veins (flow voids) ➡.

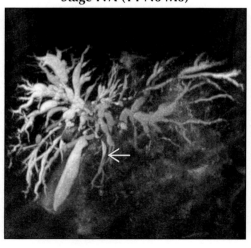

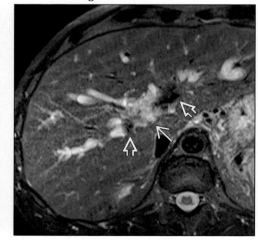

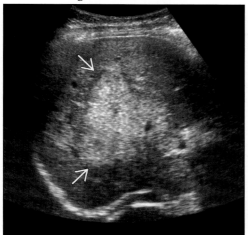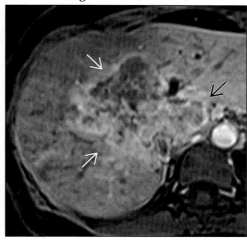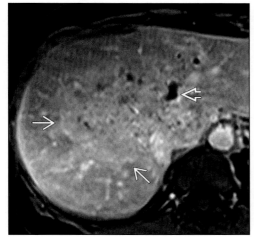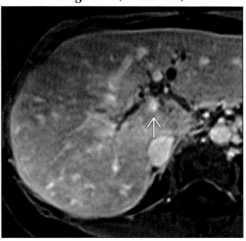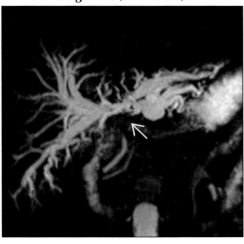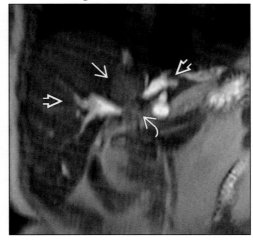

PERIHILAR BILE DUCT CARCINOMA

Stage IVA (T4 N0 M0)

Stage IVA (T4 N0 M0)

(Left) Transverse ultrasound in a patient with weight loss and increased bilirubin shows a large hyperechoic mass ➡ centrally in the liver. *(Right)* Axial T1WI C+ FS MR shows a large perihilar mass ➡ extending beyond the secondary biliary radicles in the right hepatic lobe. Note irregular peripheral and patchy central enhancement in the arterial phase, characteristic of cholangiocarcinoma. The caudate lobe ➡ is replaced by tumor.

Stage IVA (T4 N0 M0)

Stage IVA (T4 N0 M0)

(Left) Axial T1WI C+ FS MR in the same patient shows the perihilar mass ➡ with fill-in of contrast enhancement in the delayed phase. Note dilated intrahepatic bile ducts ➡. *(Right)* Axial T1WI C+ FS MR in the same patient shows encasement of the left portal vein ➡ by tumor. Involvement of the secondary biliary radicles in the right hepatic lobe and encasement of the left portal vein constitute T4 disease and also render this patient's disease nonresectable.

Stage IVA (T4 N0 M0)

Stage IVA (T4 N0 M0)

(Left) Coronal MRCP shows intrahepatic biliary ductal dilation to the level of the confluence ➡. The common hepatic duct is not visualized, and the downstream common bile duct is normal in caliber. *(Right)* Coronal T2WI MR in the same patient shows a hyperintense perihilar mass ➡ at the level of obstruction with a large exophytic component ➡. Dilated intrahepatic bile ducts ➡ abruptly terminate at the mass.

PERIHILAR BILE DUCT CARCINOMA

Stage IVA (T4 N0 M0)

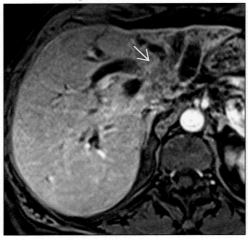

Stage IVA (T4 N0 M0)

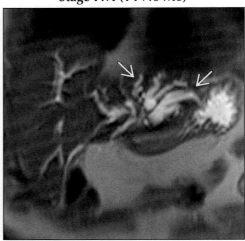

(Left) Axial T1WI C+ FS MR in the same patient obtained in the late arterial phase shows a hypovascular perihilar mass ➡. Intrahepatic biliary dilation to the level of the secondary biliary radicles corresponds to T4, nonresectable disease. *(Right)* Coronal T2WI MR in the same patient demonstrates the atrophy-hypertrophy complex. There is left hepatic lobe atrophy with crowding of the left lobe bile ducts ➡ due to left portal vein occlusion (not shown).

Stage IVB (T3 N2 M0)

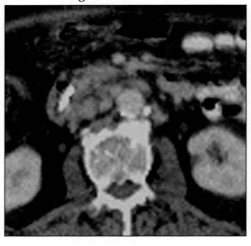

Stage IVB (T4 N2 M0)

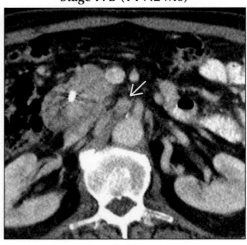

(Left) Axial fused PET/CT shows hypermetabolic interaortocaval adenopathy. Although small in size, these lymph nodes demonstrate increased FDG accumulation, consistent with N2 lymph node metastases. *(Right)* Axial CECT shows an enlarged lymph node ➡ adjacent to the superior mesenteric artery, consistent with N2 nodal metastasis. Note the common bile duct stent.

Stage IVB (T4 N0 M1)

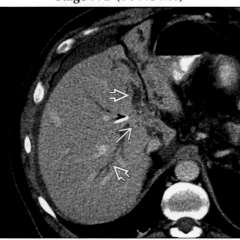

Stage IVB (T4 N0 M1)

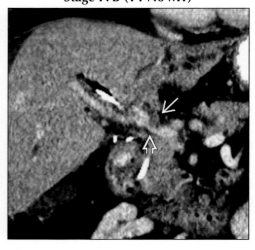

(Left) Axial CECT in the delayed phase shows intrahepatic biliary duct dilation ➡ abruptly terminating at a perihilar mass ➡. Bile duct stent and minimal ascites are also present. *(Right)* Coronal CECT shows extension of hypodense perihilar tumor ➡ to invade the main portal vein ➡. Stent is present in the common duct.

PERIHILAR BILE DUCT CARCINOMA

Stage IVB (T4 N0 M1)

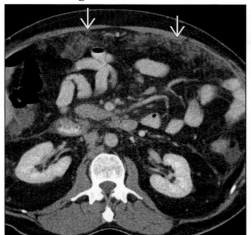

Stage IVB (T4 N0 M1)

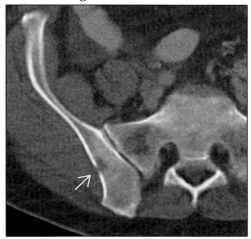

(Left) Axial CECT in the same patient shows soft tissue infiltration ➡ of the greater omentum, consistent with peritoneal metastatic disease. *(Right)* Axial CECT in the same patient shows a lytic lesion ➡ in the right iliac bone with cortical destruction, consistent with osseous metastatic disease.

Recurrence

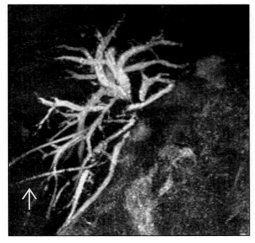

Recurrence

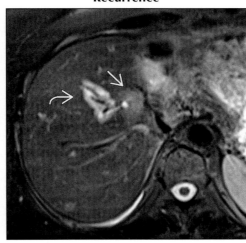

(Left) Coronal MRCP in a patient with history of perihilar cholangiocarcinoma status post left hepatic lobectomy shows diffuse dilation of the right intrahepatic biliary tree despite the presence of 2 drains ➡. *(Right)* Axial T2WI FS MR in the same patient obtained at the level of biliary obstruction shows a hyperintense perihilar mass ➡ and intrahepatic biliary ductal dilation ➡.

Recurrence

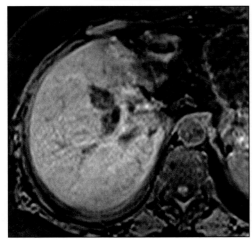

Recurrence

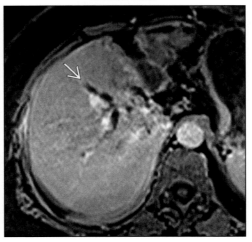

(Left) Axial T1WI MR in the same patient at the level of the perihilar mass shows slight hypointensity; otherwise the abnormality is difficult to visualize. *(Right)* Axial delayed T1WI C+ FS MR in the same patient emphasizes the occasional difficulty in visualizing bile duct carcinoma on post-contrast imaging. Optimal MR protocols employ a variety of sequences, including T2WI and DWI. Note the dilated intrahepatic bile duct ➡.

Recurrence

Recurrence

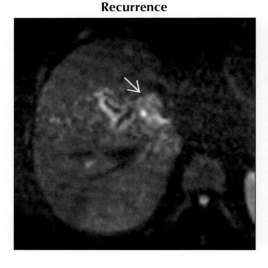
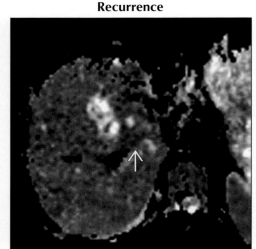

(Left) Axial diffusion-weighted image (b400) in the same patient shows a hyperintense perihilar lesion ➡ at the level of the biliary obstruction. *(Right)* ADC map shows diffusion restriction within the perihilar lesion ➡ suggesting cellularity. The DWI and ADC map in this case help to improve conspicuity of the recurrent mass and to confirm that the signal abnormality on T2WI is due to a malignant solid mass.

Bismuth-Corlette Type I

Bismuth-Corlette Type I

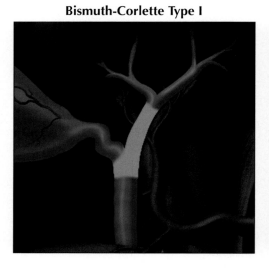
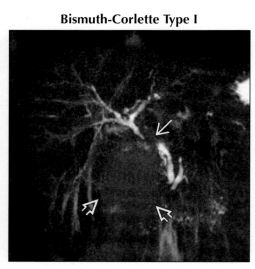

(Left) Graphic depicts tumor involving the common hepatic duct distal to the biliary confluence. *(Right)* Coronal MRCP shows occlusion of the common hepatic duct ➡ due to infiltrative tumor with upstream biliary dilation. The gallbladder ⊳ is distended due to occlusion of the cystic duct.

Bismuth-Corlette Type II

Bismuth-Corlette Type II

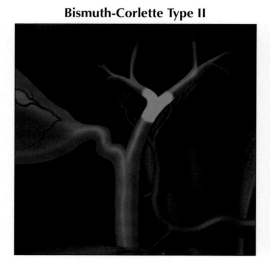
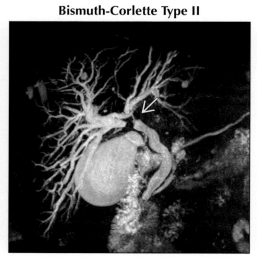

(Left) Graphic depicts tumor confined to the biliary confluence. *(Right)* Coronal MRCP shows complete occlusion at the confluence ➡ of the right and left hepatic ducts with resulting intrahepatic biliary ductal dilation.

PERIHILAR BILE DUCT CARCINOMA

Bismuth-Corlette Type IIIa

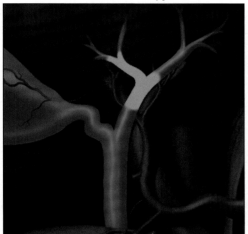

Bismuth-Corlette Type IIIa

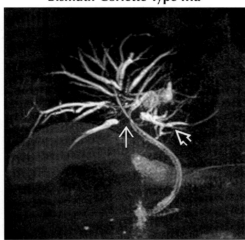

(Left) Graphic depicts tumor involving the biliary confluence and the right hepatic duct to the level of the secondary biliary radicles. *(Right)* Coronal MRCP shows tumor at the confluence ⮕ of the right and left ⮞ hepatic ducts, resulting in diffuse intrahepatic biliary dilation despite bilateral biliary stents. The branches of the right hepatic duct abruptly terminate upstream to the confluence, indicating intrahepatic extension of tumor on the right.

Bismuth-Corlette Type IIIb

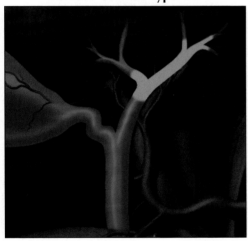

Bismuth-Corlette Type IIIb

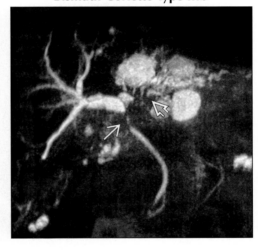

(Left) Graphic depicts tumor involving the biliary confluence and the left hepatic duct to the level of the secondary biliary radicles. *(Right)* Coronal MRCP shows obliteration of the hepatic duct confluence with abrupt termination ⮕ of the right and common hepatic ducts indicating perihilar tumor. Left hepatic ducts ⮞ terminate upstream to the confluence indicative of intrahepatic tumor infiltration. Note multiple simple cysts in the left lobe.

Bismuth-Corlette Type IV

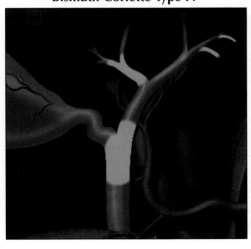

Bismuth-Corlette Type IV

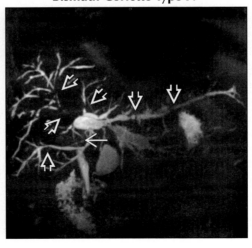

(Left) Graphic depicts multifocal tumor involving the common hepatic duct, biliary confluence, and intrahepatic bile ducts. Contiguous tumor involvement of the confluence and both hepatic ducts is also classified as type IV. *(Right)* Coronal MRCP shows multifocal strictures ⮞ and occlusion involving the right and left intrahepatic bile ducts, as well as the common hepatic duct ⮕.

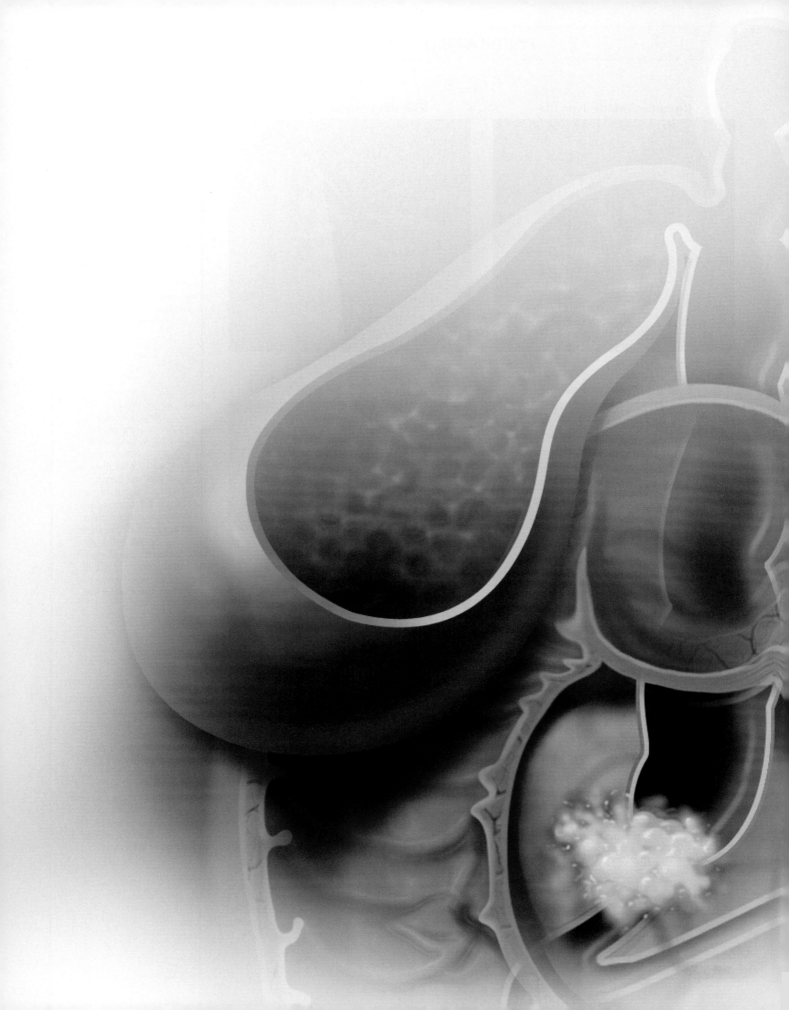

Distal Bile Duct Carcinoma

DISTAL BILE DUCT CARCINOMA

(T) Primary Tumor

Adapted from 7th edition AJCC Staging Forms.

TNM	Definitions
TX	Primary tumor cannot be assessed
T0	No evidence of primary tumor
Tis	Carcinoma in situ
T1	Tumor confined to the bile duct histologically
T2	Tumor invades beyond the wall of the bile duct
T3	Tumor invades the gallbladder, pancreas, duodenum, or other adjacent organs without involvement of the celiac axis or the superior mesenteric artery
T4	Tumor involves the celiac axis or the superior mesenteric artery

(N) Regional Lymph Nodes

NX	Regional lymph nodes cannot be assessed
N0	No regional lymph node metastasis
N1	Regional lymph node metastasis

(M) Distant Metastasis

M0	No distant metastasis
M1	Distant metastasis

AJCC Stages/Prognostic Groups

Adapted from 7th edition AJCC Staging Forms.

Stage	T	N	M
0	Tis	N0	M0
IA	T1	N0	M0
IB	T2	N0	M0
IIA	T3	N0	M0
IIB	T1	N1	M0
	T2	N1	M0
	T3	N1	M0
III	T4	Any N	M0
IV	Any T	Any N	M1

DISTAL BILE DUCT CARCINOMA

Tis

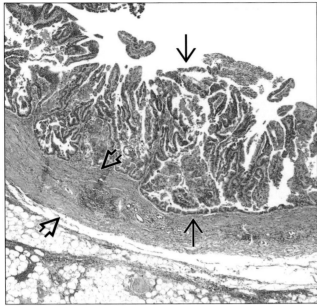

H&E stained section from a distal bile duct shows intraluminal papillary neoplasm (between ⇨) with carcinoma in situ that does not invade into the wall of the bile duct (between ⇔). The duct lumen is at the top of the image. (Original magnification 40x.)

Tis

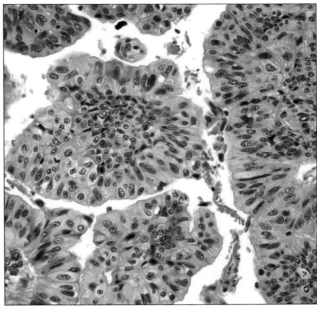

Higher magnification of the previous image shows a close-up view of the papillary structures. The epithelial lining is composed of low columnar to cuboidal-shaped cells with variable nuclei showing high nuclear to cytoplasmic ratio, open chromatin pattern, and prominent nucleoli. (Original magnification 400x.)

T1

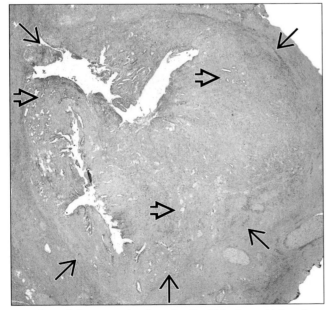

H&E shows full cross section from the distal bile duct with invasive bile duct carcinoma. The invasive neoplastic glands ⇨ infiltrate into the muscle and fibrous tissue of the wall of the duct ⇨ without extension beyond the wall to periductal tissue. (Original magnification 20x.)

T3

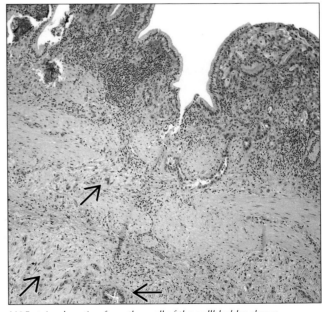

H&E stained section from the wall of the gallbladder shows invasive carcinoma of the distal bile duct with the neoplastic cells arranged in glands or singly ⇨ invading into the muscle layer of the gallbladder wall (left lower) toward the gallbladder mucosa and lumen (right upper). (Original magnification 100x.)

DISTAL BILE DUCT CARCINOMA

T1

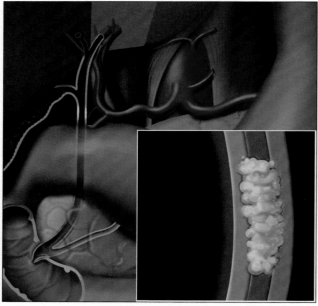

Graphic depicts infiltrative tumor confined to the wall of the bile duct histologically. Inset depicts the layers of the bile duct wall, including the lamina propria, fibromuscular wall, and perifibromuscular connective tissue. Muscle fibers are most prominent in the distal segment and sparse or absent proximally.

T2

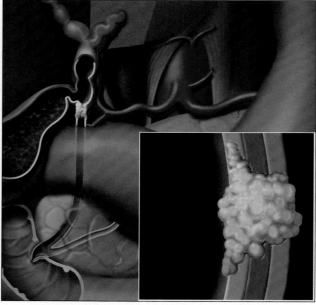

Graphic depicts tumor in the common bile duct extending beyond the bile duct wall. Inset depicts tumor infiltration of the perimural adventitial adipose tissue (extrahepatic ducts lack a serosa).

T3

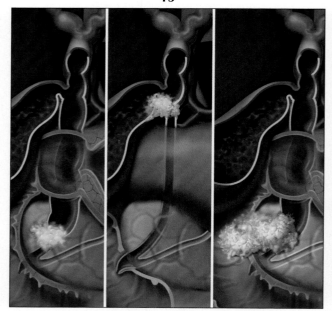

Graphic depicts tumors arising from the common bile duct with invasion of adjacent structures. T3 stage tumors may invade the pancreas (left), gallbladder (middle), duodenum (right), or other adjacent organs.

T4

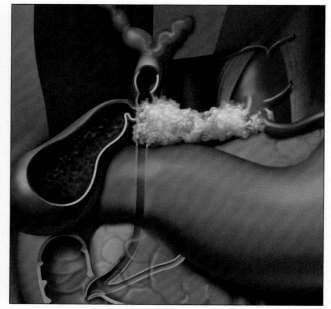

Graphic depicts tumor arising from the common bile duct extending to involve the celiac axis. Involvement of the celiac axis or superior mesenteric artery constitute T4 disease.

N1

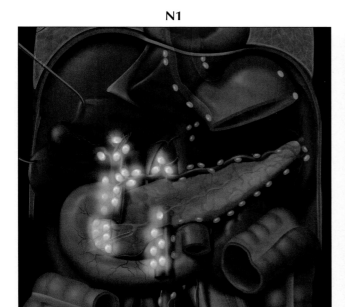

Graphic highlights regional lymph nodes, which include those along the common bile duct, hepatic artery, celiac trunk, posterior and anterior pancreaticoduodenal arteries, superior mesenteric vein, and right lateral wall of the superior mesenteric artery. These are identical to the regional nodes for cancer of the pancreatic head.

M1

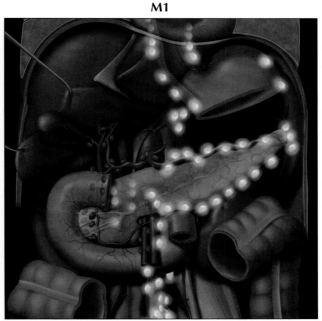

Graphic highlights lymph nodes constituting metastatic disease. These nodes include but are not limited to paraaortic, paracaval, and nodes along the left lateral aspect of the superior mesenteric artery and along the pancreatic body and tail.

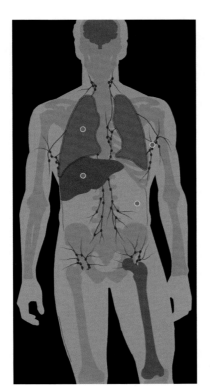

METASTASES, ORGAN FREQUENCY

Liver

Peritoneal cavity

Lung

Lymph nodes

The literature offers only isolated cases of cholangiocarcinoma with distant metastasis. The number is not sufficiently significant to quantify organ frequency.

DISTAL BILE DUCT CARCINOMA

OVERVIEW

General Comments
- Tumor arising in common bile duct
  - Between ampulla of Vater and cystic duct-common hepatic duct junction
  - Tumors arising in congenital choledochal cysts
- 80% of cholangiocarcinomas are extrahepatic
  - 20-30% are distal bile duct carcinomas
  - ~ 70% are perihilar carcinomas

Classification
- Histologic types
  - Carcinoma in situ
  - Adenocarcinoma (most common)
    - Intestinal type
    - Mucinous
    - Clear cell
  - Signet ring cell
  - Squamous cell
  - Adenosquamous
  - Small cell (oat cell)
  - Undifferentiated
  - Papillary carcinoma, noninvasive
  - Papillary carcinoma, invasive
  - Carcinoma, not otherwise specified

PATHOLOGY

Routes of Spread
- **Contiguous spread**
  - Predilection for longitudinal submucosal spread in duct wall
    - May have substantial extension of tumor beneath intact epithelial lining
      - Up to 2 cm proximally and 1 cm distally
  - Spread along periductal tissues
    - Neural & perineural involvement
  - Direct invasion of adjacent organs
    - Pancreas
    - Stomach, duodenum, or colon
    - Omentum & abdominal wall
- **Lymphatic spread**
  - Regional lymph nodes
    - Common bile duct
    - Hepatic artery and celiac trunk
    - Posterior and anterior pancreaticoduodenal
    - Superior mesenteric vein
    - Right lateral wall of superior mesenteric artery
  - Sentinel nodes → porta hepatis
  - Spread 1st to pericholedochal nodes in hepatoduodenal ligament → posterior pancreaticoduodenal nodes → periportal nodes → common hepatic nodes
  - Peripancreatic lymph nodes along body & tail are considered distant metastases
  - Ideally, resection specimen should include histologic examination of at least 12 lymph nodes
    - Fewer than 12 lymph nodes resected and all negative → assign pN0
- **Hematogenous spread**
  - Uncommon, occurs late in disease
  - Liver and lungs

- Peritoneal seeding
  - 10-20% have peritoneal involvement

General Features
- Genetics
  - Gene mutations suggest possible genetic link
    - Inactivation of tumor suppressor genes
    - Mutations in oncogenes
    - Chromosomal aneuploidy
  - No established clinical role for molecular profiling at this time
- Etiology
  - Risk factors
    - Age
    - Primary sclerosing cholangitis (PSC)
    - Chronic ulcerative colitis
    - Hepatolithiasis
    - Caroli disease
    - Choledochal cysts
    - Tobacco abuse (in association with PSC)
    - Bile duct adenoma & biliary papillomatosis
    - Hepatobiliary flukes
    - Chronic typhoid carriers
    - Exposure to thorotrast
    - Familial polyposis
  - Additional risk factors in USA and Europe
    - Cirrhosis
    - Chronic hepatitis C infection
    - Alcohol abuse
- Associated diseases, abnormalities
  - Primary sclerosing cholangitis
    - Common risk factor in western countries
    - Prevalence of cholangiocarcinoma (CCA) in this setting is 5-15%
    - Risk is not associated with duration or severity of PSC or inflammatory bowel disease (IBD)
  - Hepatobiliary flukes
    - *Opisthorchis viverrini* and *Clonorchis sinensis*
    - Endemic in east Asia
    - Ingested in undercooked fish
    - Infest biliary tree ± gallbladder
  - Choledochal cysts
    - 10-15% lifetime risk of carcinoma
    - Malignant degeneration uncommon if excised early in life
    - 15-20% ↑ incidence if not treated until > 20 years
  - Hepatolithiasis
    - Risk factor in parts of Asia
    - Up to 10% complicated by CCA
    - In endemic areas, 70% of tumors manifest with hepatolithiasis

Gross Pathology & Surgical Features
- Patterns of tumor growth
  - Mass-forming (exophytic)
    - Most common at intrahepatic location
    - Radial growth pattern invading adjacent structures
  - Periductal (infiltrating)
    - Most common in perihilar tumors
    - Sclerotic lesion with abundant fibrous tissue
    - Diffuse longitudinal growth along bile duct
  - Mixed (mass-forming and periductal)
  - Intraductal (polypoid)
    - Usually papillary adenocarcinoma

DISTAL BILE DUCT CARCINOMA

- Demonstrates extensive superficial spreading
- Uncommon except those tumors arising in choledochal cysts
- Macroscopic subtypes
  - Sclerosing
    - Majority of tumors
    - Perihilar > distal bile duct
    - Firm tumor causing annular thickening of bile duct
    - Diffuse infiltration & fibrosis of periductal tissues
  - Nodular
    - Firm, irregular nodule projecting into duct lumen
  - Papillary
    - 10% of cholangiocarcinomas
    - Distal bile duct > perihilar
    - Soft, friable tumor
    - May have little transmural invasion
    - Tends to be polypoid mass that expands duct
    - Can be quite large, but arising from well-defined stalk with majority of tumor mobile within duct

Microscopic Pathology

- H&E
  - 90% are adenocarcinomas
  - Usually well to moderately differentiated
  - Exhibit glandular or acinar structures
  - Cuboidal or low columnar cells resembling biliary epithelium
  - Intracytoplasmic mucin is common
  - Mitotic figures are rare
  - Dense, sparsely cellular, fibrous stroma
  - Tendency to invade lymphatics, blood vessels, perineural & periductal spaces, and portal tracts

IMAGING FINDINGS

Detection

- **Ultrasound**
  - Excellent for identifying biliary obstruction
  - Difficult to visualize intraductal or infiltrating lesions
  - Common bile duct often obscured by overlying bowel gas
  - Only finding may be intrahepatic & upstream extrahepatic biliary duct dilation
- **CT**
  - NECT
    - Hypodense intraductal polypoid mass or exophytic mass
    - Only finding may be biliary dilation with abrupt termination
  - CECT
    - Mass-like
      - Early heterogeneous enhancement
      - Progressive persistent enhancement
    - Infiltrative
      - Duct wall thickening and enhancement with obliteration of lumen
      - Upstream biliary dilation
    - Polypoid
      - Distension of duct by intraluminal mass
      - Heterogeneous mass enhancement
      - Intense enhancement of surrounding duct wall may be reactive or due to tumor infiltration

- **PET/CT**
  - Inferior to MR/MRCP for primary lesion detection
  - FDG accumulates in tumor cells, but limited if large fibrotic component
  - Several reports indicate poorer detection of infiltrative tumor than intraductal tumor
  - Efficacy of PET in setting of PSC is controversial
  - Focal FDG uptake and ↑ CA-19.9 is more sensitive and specific
- **MR/MRCP**
  - Mass-like
    - Exophytic mass arising from common bile duct
    - Difficult to differentiate from pancreatic mass
  - Infiltrative (periductal)
    - Bile duct wall thickening extending for variable length longitudinally
  - Polypoid (intraductal)
    - Intraductal mass expanding common bile duct
    - Filling defect in bright bile on MRCP and T2WI
    - Enhancement of surrounding bile duct wall may be reactive or due to tumor infiltration
  - T1WI
    - Hypointense to isointense
  - T2WI
    - Variable, usually slightly hyperintense
  - Dynamic post-contrast imaging
    - Early mild or heterogeneous enhancement
    - Progressive persistent enhancement in delayed phase
  - MRCP
    - Delineates level of obstruction
    - Delineates longitudinal tumor extent
    - Upstream biliary dilation
    - Mass is seen as filling defect in bright bile
  - Primary sclerosing cholangitis
    - Findings of superimposed CCA
      - Progressive stricture formation (most common)
      - Upstream bile duct dilation
      - Polypoid intraductal mass

Staging

- **Primary tumor**
  - Staging goals
    - Delineate longitudinal tumor spread
    - Assess vascular involvement
    - Assess involvement of adjacent structures
- Ultrasound
  - No role in staging
- CT
  - Multidetector CT allows rapid acquisition in multiple phases of contrast enhancement
    - Arterial & portal venous phase
      - Arterial & venous anatomy, invasion, encasement
      - Identify invasion of adjacent structures
    - Delayed (10-15 minutes)
      - Allows characterization of tumors with dominant fibrous component
  - Isotropic data allows multiplanar reformation
    - Minimum intensity projection
      - Visualization of biliary anatomy
      - Determine level of obstruction
      - Morphology of stricture
      - Presence of intraductal mass
    - Reconstruction of arterial & portal venous phases

DISTAL BILE DUCT CARCINOMA

- Visualize vascular anatomy, tumor encasement, occlusion, or invasion
  - ○ Criteria for vascular involvement
    - Vessel occlusion or stenosis
    - Vessel contour deformity associated with tumor contact
    - \> 50% perimeter contact with tumor
  - ○ Limited in defining longitudinal tumor extent
- PET/CT
  - ○ Not superior to CT or MR/MRCP for detection of primary lesion
  - ○ Limitations for primary tumor
    - Assessment of longitudinal tumor extent
    - Evaluation of vascular invasion
- MR/MRCP
  - ○ Optimal initial examination for suspected CCA
    - Liver and biliary anatomy
    - Tumor extent along bile ducts
    - Liver metastasis
    - Vascular invasion or encasement
  - ○ Superior to CT for assessment of intraductal lesions
  - ○ Comparable to conventional angiography for the evaluation of vascular invasion
  - ○ MR
    - Helpful for visualization of
      - Exophytic component
      - Invasion of adjacent organs and vasculature
      - Satellite nodules
    - In conjunction with MRCP, allows better estimation of longitudinal extent of tumor
    - Dynamic 3D IV contrast-enhanced images
      - Multiphasic acquisition and improved spatial resolution
      - Vascular invasion
      - Direct invasion of adjacent structures
  - ○ MRCP
    - Ideally performed prior to biliary drainage
    - Localizes level of obstruction
    - Defines morphology and longitudinal extent of strictures
    - Can evaluate biliary tree upstream to obstruction
    - Navigator triggered isotropic 3D FSE
      - Improved signal-to-noise ratio & spatial resolution
      - Allows reformation & isolation of biliary tree
    - Limitations
      - Not able to perform cytologic evaluation & bile duct sampling
      - Not able to relieve obstruction
      - Evaluation of intraductal lesions limited post stent placement
      - Limited in periampullary region
  - ○ 3 tesla
    - Higher spatial resolution
    - Improved signal-to-noise ratio
- Direct cholangiography (ERCP or PTC)
  - ○ Invasive
  - ○ Useful for defining extent of infiltrating lesions
  - ○ Allows bile duct sampling
    - Brush cytology has low reported accuracy (9-24%)
    - In patients with PSC, sensitivity is 60%
    - Negative result does not exclude malignancy
  - ○ Allows stent placement to relieve obstruction

- ○ May not be able to evaluate bile ducts upstream to obstruction
- ○ Altered anatomy (prior surgery) may preclude ERCP
- ○ PTC performed if
  - Lumen obliterated by tissue
  - Proximal lesion
  - Biliary tree not well visualized with ERCP
- Endoscopic ultrasound
  - ○ Invasive
  - ○ Can visualize distal extrahepatic bile duct, gallbladder, regional lymph nodes, and vasculature
  - ○ Localizes stricture for accurate FNA
  - ○ Assesses depth of intraductal lesions
  - ○ Allows evaluation & guided FNA of regional nodes
- **Regional lymph nodes**
  - ○ Anatomic imaging (CT & MR)
    - Anatomic imaging has low sensitivity for lymph node metastasis
    - Findings
      - Size ≥ 10 mm short axis
      - Central necrosis
  - ○ Metabolic imaging (PET/CT)
    - Sensitivity (32%), specificity (88%)
    - Higher specificity and accuracy than CT alone
    - Findings
      - Relative increased FDG uptake compared to normal nodes
  - ○ Limitations of anatomic & metabolic imaging
    - Differentiating reactive from malignant adenopathy
    - Micrometastasis
  - ○ Fine needle aspiration biopsy may be performed with endoscopic ultrasound
    - 5-15% of those with negative CT have involved nodes with FNA at endoscopic ultrasound
  - ○ Enlarged periportal lymph nodes are common in PSC, not necessarily indicative of metastasis
- **Metastatic disease**
  - ○ Occurs late in disease course
  - ○ Most commonly involves liver, lung, & peritoneum
  - ○ Metabolic imaging may be valuable in detection of unsuspected distant metastasis
    - Sensitivity of PET is 65% & PET/CT is 56% (specificity 88-92%)
    - May also be helpful for indeterminate lesions seen on conventional imaging

CLINICAL ISSUES

Presentation

- Age usually > 65 years (peak is 8th decade)
- Symptoms of biliary obstruction
  - ○ Jaundice, pale stool, dark urine, pruritus
- Prolonged obstruction
  - ○ Decrease in fat-soluble vitamins
  - ○ Increase in prothrombin time
- Cholangitis is rare without biliary intervention
  - ○ Right upper quadrant pain, fever, chills
- Liver function tests show obstructive pattern
  - ○ ↑ alkaline phosphatase & bilirubin
  - ○ Aminotransferases are often normal, unless acute obstruction or cholangitis
- Serum tumor markers

DISTAL BILE DUCT CARCINOMA

- ○ No specific tumor marker for CCA
- ○ Used in conjunction with other diagnostic tests
- ○ CA-19.9
  - ▪ ↑ in up to 85% of patients
  - ▪ ↑ absolute level (> 100 U/mL) or change over time
  - ▪ Obstructive jaundice without malignancy can cause elevation, but should not persist after decompression
  - ▪ Nonspecific, can also be elevated in
    - – Pancreatic malignancy
    - – Gastric malignancy
    - – Severe hepatic injury
  - ▪ Lewis phenotype must be positive (10% of population is Lewis negative)
- ○ CEA
  - ▪ ↑ in 30% of patients
  - ▪ Nonspecific, can be elevated in
    - – Inflammatory bowel disease
    - – Biliary obstruction
    - – Severe hepatic injury
    - – Other malignancies
  - ▪ CA-125
    - – ↑ in 40-50% of patients
    - – May signify peritoneal involvement
    - – Nonspecific, can be elevated in other GI and gynecologic malignancies

Cancer Natural History & Prognosis

- • Adverse pathologic prognostic factors
  - ○ Histologic type
  - ○ Histologic grade
  - ○ Vascular invasion
  - ○ Lymphatic invasion
  - ○ Perineural invasion
- • Other prognostic indicators
  - ○ Tumor size
  - ○ Positive resection margins
    - ▪ Most important stage-independent prognostic factor
  - ○ Lymph node metastasis
  - ○ Poorly differentiated histology
  - ○ Invasion of pancreas by tumor
    - ▪ Reflects extent of local & regional disease
  - ○ Pre-treatment CEA and CA-19.9 levels
- • Papillary carcinomas have better outcomes

Treatment Options

- • Major treatment alternatives
  - ○ < 10% curable by surgery
  - ○ Localized resectable tumor
    - ▪ 25-30% of distal bile duct tumors are candidates for total resection
    - ▪ 25% 5-year survival for distal CBD tumor
    - ▪ Resectability depends on tumor location, relationship to vessels, & extension to adjacent structures
    - ▪ Must assess lymph node metastases at surgery
    - ▪ High operative mortality (5-10%)
    - ▪ Low curability
    - ▪ External beam radiation has been used in conjunction with surgery
    - ▪ Radiation therapy is reported to improve local control
  - ○ Unresectable tumor
    - ▪ Includes majority of patients with bile duct cancer

- ▪ Management directed at palliation
- ▪ Relief of biliary obstruction by surgical biliary-enteric anastomosis, endoscopic, or percutaneous stent
- ▪ Options under investigation
  - – Radiation sensitizers
  - – Chemotherapeutic agents
  - – Photodynamic therapy

REPORTING CHECKLIST

T Staging

- • Invasion beyond bile duct wall
- • Invasion of adjacent organs
- • Involvement of celiac or superior mesenteric artery

N Staging

- • Size, shape, central necrosis
- • Regional lymph nodes
  - ○ Common bile duct
  - ○ Hepatic artery
  - ○ Celiac trunk
  - ○ Posterior & anterior pancreaticoduodenal
  - ○ Superior mesenteric vein
  - ○ Right lateral wall of superior mesenteric artery

M Staging

- • Liver, lungs, peritoneum

SELECTED REFERENCES

1. American Joint Committee on Cancer: AJCC Cancer Staging Manual. 7th ed. New York: Springer. 227-33, 2010
2. Moon CM et al: The role of (18)F-fluorodeoxyglucose positron emission tomography in the diagnosis, staging, and follow-up of cholangiocarcinoma. Surg Oncol. Epub ahead of print, 2009
3. National Institutes of Health: Extrahepatic bile duct cancer treatment. http://www.cancer.gov/cancertopics/pdq/treatment/bileduct/HealthProfessional/page2. Accessed May 2009
4. Blechacz BR et al: Cholangiocarcinoma. Clin Liver Dis. 12(1):131-50, ix, 2008
5. Kim JY et al: Clinical role of 18F-FDG PET-CT in suspected and potentially operable cholangiocarcinoma: a prospective study compared with conventional imaging. Am J Gastroenterol. 103(5):1145-51, 2008
6. Park HS et al: Preoperative evaluation of bile duct cancer: MRI combined with MR cholangiopancreatography versus MDCT with direct cholangiography. AJR Am J Roentgenol. 190(2):396-405, 2008
7. Sainani NI et al: Cholangiocarcinoma: current and novel imaging techniques. Radiographics. 28(5):1263-87, 2008
8. Walker SL et al: Diagnosing cholangiocarcinoma in primary sclerosing cholangitis: an "evidence based radiology" review. Abdom Imaging. 33(1):14-7, 2008
9. Lim JH et al: Early bile duct carcinoma: comparison of imaging features with pathologic findings. Radiology. 238(2):542-8, 2006
10. Han JK et al: Cholangiocarcinoma: pictorial essay of CT and cholangiographic findings. Radiographics. 22(1):173-87, 2002
11. Khan SA et al: Guidelines for the diagnosis and treatment of cholangiocarcinoma: consensus document. Gut. 51 Suppl 6:VI1-9, 2002
12. Jarnagin WR: Cholangiocarcinoma of the extrahepatic bile ducts. Semin Surg Oncol. 19(2):156-76, 2000

DISTAL BILE DUCT CARCINOMA

Stage IA (T1 N0 M0)

Stage IA (T1 N0 M0)

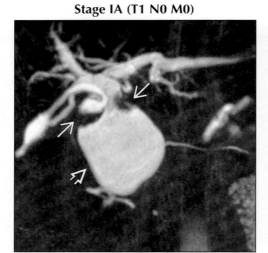

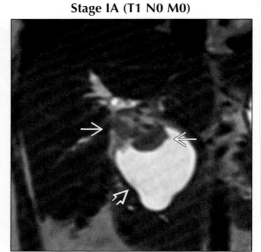

(Left) Coronal MRCP MIP shows fusiform dilation of the common bile duct ⇒ *with focal concentric narrowing* ⇒. *(Right) Coronal T2WI MR in the same patient shows fusiform dilation of the common bile duct* ⇒ *with focal concentric wall thickening and a polypoid intraductal mass* ⇒.

Stage IA (T1 N0 M0)

Stage IA (T1 N0 M0)

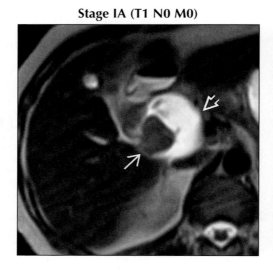

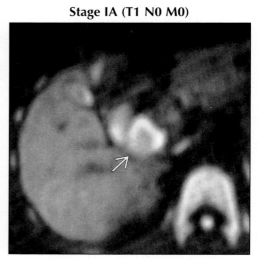

(Left) Axial T2WI MR in the same patient shows fusiform dilation of the common bile duct ⇒ *with a polypoid intraductal mass* ⇒. *(Right) Axial DWI in the same patient shows hyperintensity in the intraductal mass* ⇒, *indicative of restricted water diffusion and tumor cellularity.*

Stage IA (T1 N0 M0)

Stage IA (T1 N0 M0)

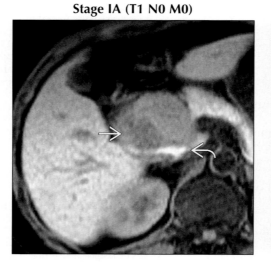

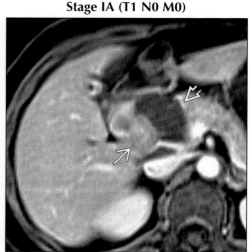

(Left) Axial T1WI MR in the same patient shows hypointensity of the intraductal mass ⇒. *Note the hyperintense layering debris* ⇒ *within the dilated common bile duct. (Right) Axial T1WI C+ FS MR in the same patient shows enhancement of the polypoid intraductal mass, consistent with a type 1 choledochal cyst* ⇒ *complicated by cholangiocarcinoma* ⇒. *The polypoid intraductal growth pattern is uncommon except in tumors arising in choledochal cysts.*

DISTAL BILE DUCT CARCINOMA

Stage IA (T1 N0 M0)

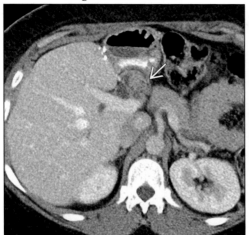

Stage IA (T1 N0 M0)

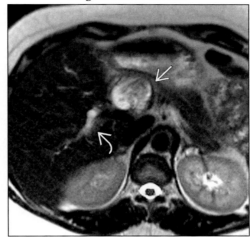

(Left) Axial CECT shows fusiform dilation of the extrahepatic duct ➡ with intraluminal hyperdensity. (Right) Axial T2WI MR in the same patient shows fusiform dilation of the extrahepatic bile duct ➡ and mild intrahepatic biliary dilation ➡. There is an irregular polypoid intraluminal filling defect in the bright bile. This mass corresponds to that seen on the CT.

Stage IA (T1 N0 M0)

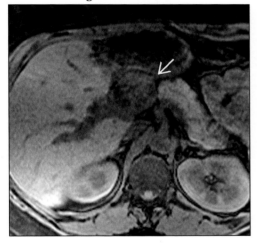

Stage IA (T1 N0 M0)

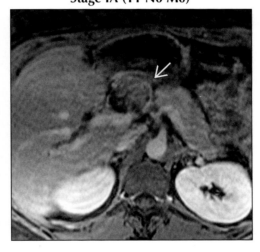

(Left) Axial T1WI FS MR in the same patient shows an intermediate signal intensity intraluminal mass in the dilated common duct ➡. (Right) Axial T1 C+ FS MR at the same level shows enhancement of the intraluminal filling defect ➡, confirming the presence of a solid polypoid bile duct mass that is consistent with cholangiocarcinoma.

Stage IA (T1 N0 M0)

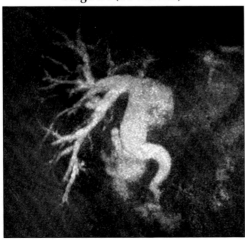

Stage IA (T1 N0 M0)

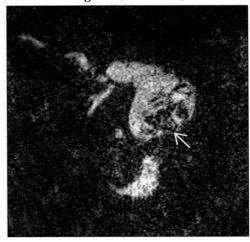

(Left) Coronal MRCP MIP in the same patient shows fusiform dilation of the extrahepatic and intrahepatic biliary tree, consistent with a choledochal cyst. MIP images provide an excellent overview of the entire biliary tree but should be interepreted with caution since an intraluminal filling defect may be difficult to see, as in this case. (Right) Coronal MRCP shows the intraluminal mass ➡, which in the setting of a choledochal cyst is concerning for polypoid cholangiocarcinoma.

DISTAL BILE DUCT CARCINOMA

Stage IB (T2 N0 M0)

Stage IB (T2 N0 M0)

(Left) Axial CECT shows thickening and hyperenhancement of the common bile duct ➡. An ill-defined outer duct wall is concerning for invasion beyond the wall of the duct. *(Right)* Coronal CECT in the same patient shows segmental wall thickening and hyperenhancement of the common bile duct ➡. Ill-defined outer duct wall is suggestive of invasion beyond the wall of the duct. Note the upstream intrahepatic biliary ductal dilation.

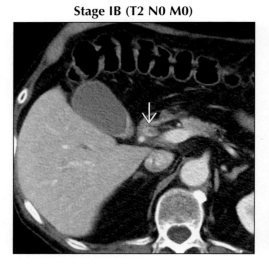

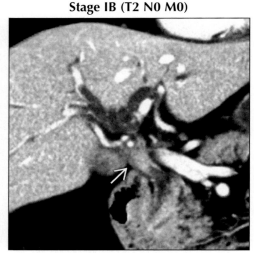

Stage IB (T2 N0 M0)

Stage IB (T2 N0 M0)

(Left) Axial and coronal CECT show abrupt termination of biliary dilation and soft tissue enhancement ➡ in the common bile duct just past the insertion of the cystic duct. *(Right)* ERCP in the same patient shows dilated beaded intrahepatic bile ducts, consistent with primary sclerosing cholangitis. The extrahepatic biliary tree is dilated with abrupt termination ➡ in the proximal common bile duct, characteristic of a malignant stricture.

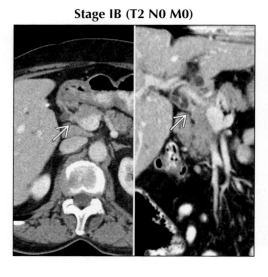

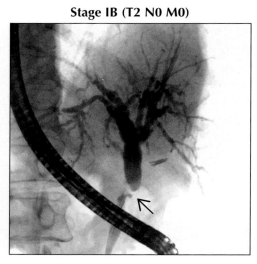

Stage IB (T2 N0 M0)

Stage IB (T2 N0 M0)

(Left) Contiguous coronal CECT images show common bile duct wall thickening ➡ for a length of 1.5 cm. There is upstream biliary dilation ➡ and distention of the gallbladder. The downstream common bile duct ➡ is normal in caliber. *(Right)* ERCP in the same patient shows segmental stenosis of the common bile duct corresponding to the area of wall thickening on CECT. Brushings revealed atypical cells.

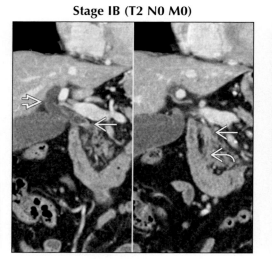

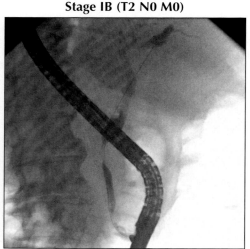

DISTAL BILE DUCT CARCINOMA

Stage IIB (T3 N1 M0)

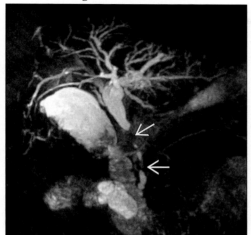

Stage IIB (T3 N1 M0)

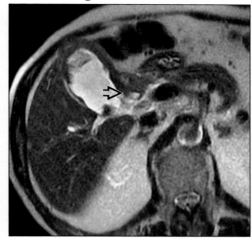

(Left) Coronal MRCP MIP shows irregularity and occlusion of the common hepatic and common bile ducts ➡ with upstream extrahepatic and intrahepatic biliary ductal dilation. The gallbladder is also distended due to a tumor at the level of the cystic duct insertion. (Right) Axial T2WI MR shows a hypointense mass ➡ encasing the common hepatic duct. Note the distension and wall thickening of the gallbladder due to cystic duct occlusion.

Stage IIB (T3 N1 M0)

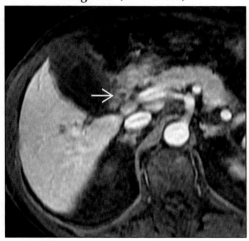

Stage IIB (T3 N1 M0)

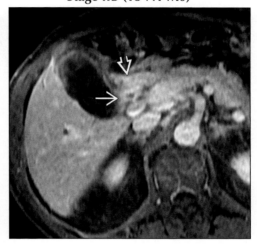

(Left) Axial T1WI C+ FS MR in the same patient in the arterial phase shows common hepatic duct wall thickening ➡. The mass enhances poorly in the early phase, as would be expected for a fibrous tumor. (Right) Axial T1WI C+ FS MR in the same patient in the delayed phase shows increased enhancement of the thickened common hepatic duct wall ➡ and the exophytic mass ➡. There is invasion of the adjacent duodenum and gallbladder.

Stage IIB (T3 N1 M0)

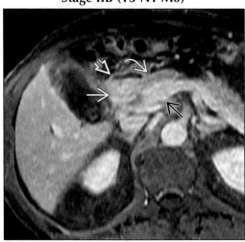

Stage IIB (T3 N1 M0)

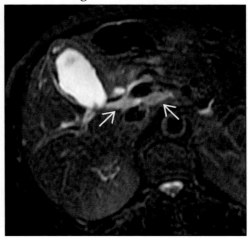

(Left) Axial T1WI C+ FS MR in the delayed phase at a slighly more caudal level shows the mass ➡ obliterating the common hepatic duct. Invasion of the pancreas is evident due to avid enhancement of the mass and poor enhancement of the pancreas ➡ in the delayed phase. Again note invasion of the duodenum ➡ and portal vein ➡. (Right) Axial T2WI FS MR shows portocaval lymphadenopathy ➡. Fat saturation in this image highlights the characteristic hyperintensity of lymph nodes on T2WI.

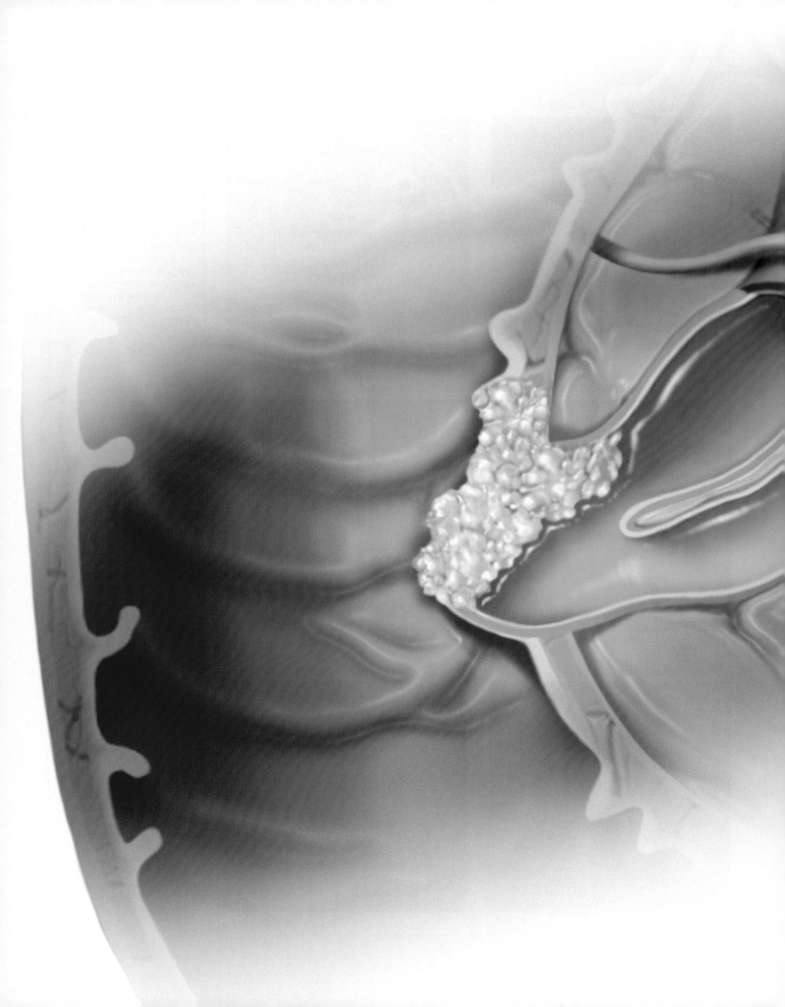

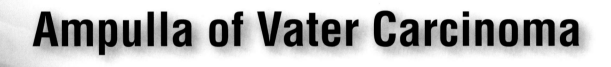

Ampulla of Vater Carcinoma

AMPULLA OF VATER CARCINOMA

(T) Primary Tumor

Adapted from 7th edition AJCC Staging Forms.

TNM	Definitions
TX	Primary tumor cannot be assessed
T0	No evidence of primary tumor
Tis	Carcinoma in situ
T1	Tumor limited to the ampulla of Vater or sphincter of Oddi
T2	Tumor invades duodenal wall
T3	Tumor invades pancreas
T4	Tumor invades peripancreatic soft tissues or other adjacent organs or structures other than pancreas

(N) Regional Lymph Nodes

NX	Regional lymph nodes cannot be assessed
N0	No regional lymph node metastasis
N1	Regional lymph node metastasis

(M) Distant Metastasis

M0	No distant metastasis
M1	Distant metastasis

AJCC Stages/Prognostic Groups

Adapted from 7th edition AJCC Staging Forms.

Stage	T	N	M
0	Tis	N0	M0
IA	T1	N0	M0
IB	T2	N0	M0
IIA	T3	N0	M0
IIB	T1	N1	M0
	T2	N1	M0
	T3	N1	M0
III	T4	Any N	M0
IV	Any T	Any N	M1

AMPULLA OF VATER CARCINOMA

Tis

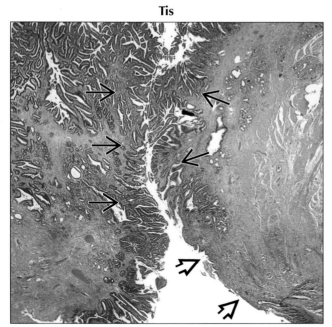

H&E stained section of the ampulla of Vater shows the epithelium of the common bile duct (CBD) thrown into folds and involved by carcinoma in situ ➡. A small portion of normal surface duodenal epithelium ➡ is seen. (Original magnification 20x.)

Tis

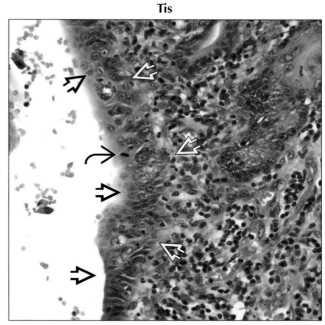

Higher magnification shows dysplastic surface epithelium lining CBD. Cells ➡ are crowded and elongated with hyperchromatic nuclei showing increased nuclear to cytoplasmic ratio. A mitotic figure ➡ is present. Dysplastic cells do not invade the basement membrane ➡. (Original magnification 500x.)

T1

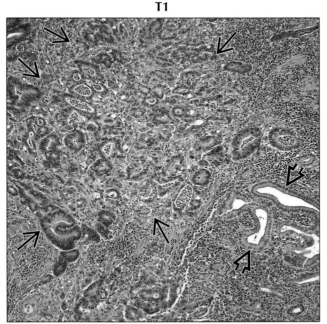

H&E stained section of ampulla of Vater shows an invasive adenocarcinoma ➡ in close proximity to uninvolved glands of common bile duct lined by cuboidal to low columnar epithelium ➡. (Original magnification 100x.)

T1

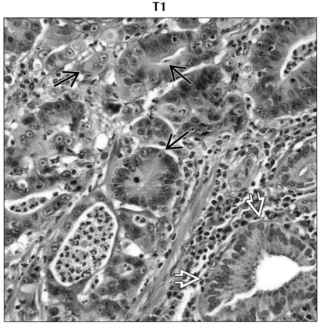

Higher magnification shows invasive adenocarcinoma ➡ arranged in glands and single cells. The neoplastic cells show enlarged nuclei with increased nuclear to cytoplasmic ratio and prominent nucleoli. Nonneoplastic epithelium of the CBD ➡ is seen. (Original magnification 500x.)

AMPULLA OF VATER CARCINOMA

T2

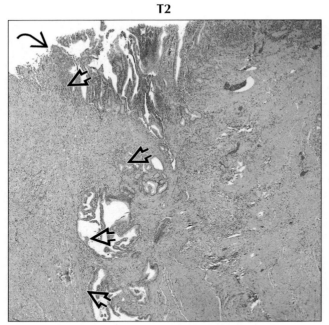

H&E stained section of the ampulla of Vater shows invasive adenocarcinoma ⊳ arising from the surface epithelium ⇗ and extending to involve the muscle wall of the duodenum. (Original magnification 40x.)

T2

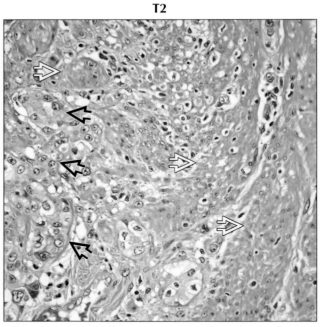

Higher magnification of the previous image shows the neoplastic glands and cells ⊳ infiltrating through the muscle bundles ⊳ of the duodenal wall. (Original magnification 400x.)

T3

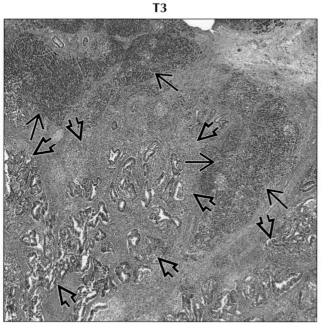

H&E stained section shows invasive adenocarcinoma of the ampulla of Vater infiltrating into the pancreas. The neoplastic glands of ampullary adenocarcinoma ⊳ invade into the pancreatic tissue, dissecting between pancreatic lobules ⇗. (Original magnification 40x.)

T4

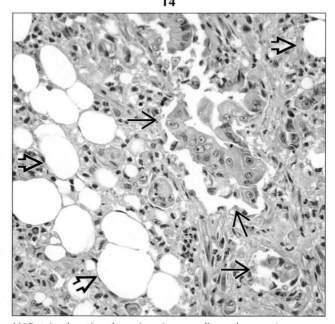

H&E stained section shows invasive ampullary adenocarcinoma invading peripancreatic fibrofatty tissue. The neoplastic cells and glands ⇒ infiltrate peripancreatic soft tissue, which is composed predominantly of fat cells ⊳. (Original magnification 400x.)

T1

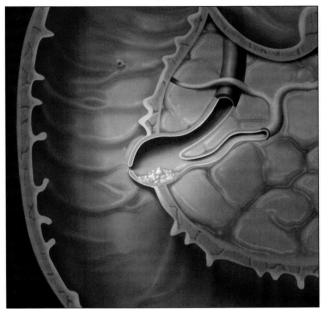

Graphic illustrates tumor limited to the ampulla of Vater, where the common bile duct merges with the pancreatic duct or, in patients where the ducts do not merge, to the distal 1 cm of the common bile duct.

T1

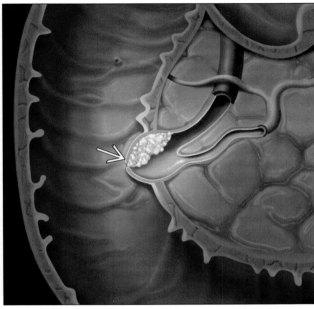

Graphic illustrates tumor involving the sphincter of Oddi ➡️, the muscular valve that controls the flow of biliary and pancreatic secretion through the ampulla of Vater.

T2

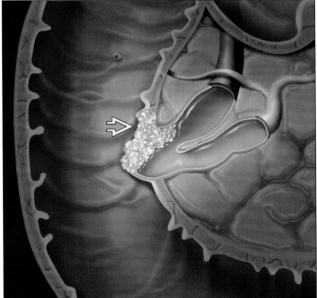

Sagittal graphic shows ampullary tumor involving the duodenal wall ➡️, consistent with T2 disease.

T2

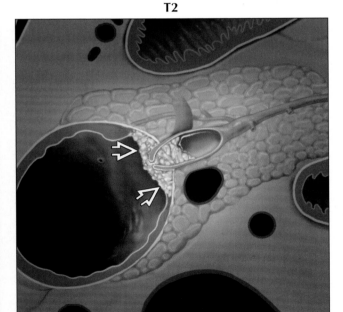

Axial graphic shows ampullary tumor involving the duodenal wall ➡️, consistent with T2 disease.

AMPULLA OF VATER CARCINOMA

T3

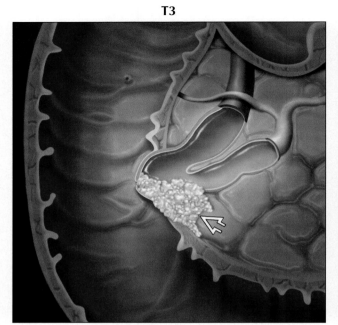

Sagittal graphic shows ampullary tumor invading the pancreas ⇨, consistent with T3 disease.

T3

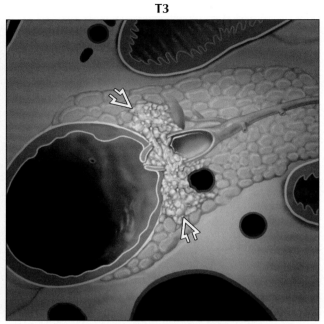

Axial graphic shows ampullary tumor invading the pancreas ⇨, consistent with T3 disease.

T4

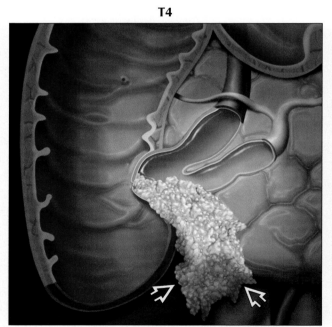

Sagittal graphic shows ampullary tumor invading through the pancreas into the peripancreatic tissues ⇨, consistent with T4 disease.

T4

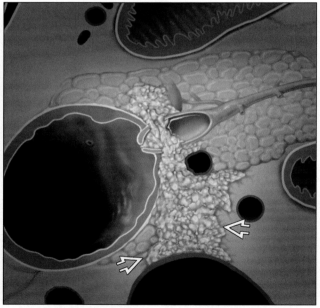

Axial graphic shows ampullary tumor invading through the pancreas into the peripancreatic tissues ⇨, consistent with T4 disease.

N1

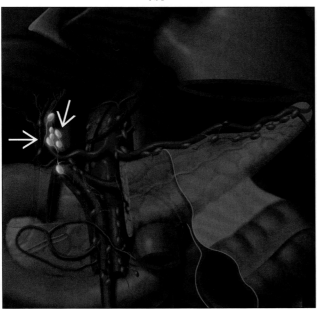

Nodes along the hepatic ➡ and celiac arteries are considered regional nodes (N1).

N1 and M1

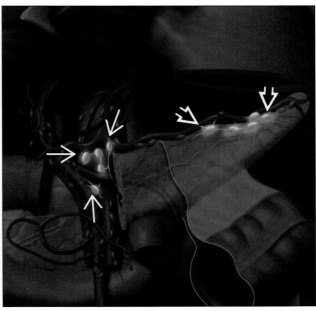

Peripancreatic nodes ➡ are considered regional nodes (N1), whereas nodes along the tail of the pancreas ➡ are considered distal metastases (M1).

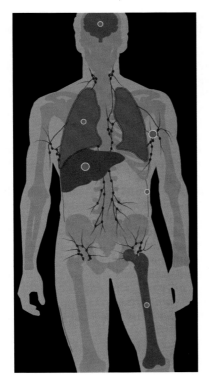

METASTASES, ORGAN FREQUENCY

Liver	23-30%
Distant lymph nodes	24%
Peritoneum	7-9%
Lung	9%
Bone	5-6%

AMPULLA OF VATER CARCINOMA

OVERVIEW

General Comments
- Malignant tumor arising from glandular epithelium of ampulla of Vater (confluence of pancreatic and common bile duct)
  - In about 40% of individuals, ampulla constitutes distal 1-1.5 cm of common bile duct since pancreatic duct opens separately into duodenum

Classification
- Adenocarcinoma is most common type
  - Histologic types
    - Carcinoma in situ
    - Adenocarcinoma, not otherwise specified (NOS)
    - Adenocarcinoma, intestinal type
    - Adenocarcinoma, pancreatobiliary type
    - Mucinous adenocarcinoma
    - Clear cell adenocarcinoma
    - Signet ring cell carcinoma
    - Adenosquamous carcinoma
    - Squamous cell carcinoma
    - Small cell (oat cell) carcinoma
    - Undifferentiated carcinoma
      - Spindle and giant cell types
      - Small cell types
    - Papillomatosis
    - Papillary carcinoma, noninvasive
    - Papillary carcinoma, invasive
    - Carcinoma, NOS
- Malignant mesenchymal tumors, although rare, include
  - Embryonal rhabdomyosarcoma
  - Leiomyosarcoma
  - Malignant fibrous histiocytoma

PATHOLOGY

Routes of Spread
- Local spread
  - Spread to duodenum and pancreas is common
  - Can also spread along common bile duct
- Lymphatic spread
  - Ampullary cancer mainly spreads to posterior pancreaticoduodenal nodes, then to inferior pancreaticoduodenal node group, and finally to paraaortic nodes
  - Nodal metastases present at diagnosis in 35%
    - Incidence of lymph node metastasis increases with advanced T disease
      - T1-T2 (8-22%)
      - T3-T4 (60-69%)
    - Rate of lymph node metastasis is low in tumors not extending beyond sphincter of Oddi
- Distant metastases
  - Rare at presentation
  - Common sites are liver, distant lymph nodes, peritoneum, lungs, and bones

General Features
- Comments

- Ampullary and duodenal cancers share same molecular development, and clinical outcomes of both are better than those of bile duct and pancreatic cancer
- Genetics
  - Associated with familial adenomatous polyposis (FAP) syndrome
    - FAP patients have ↑ risk of both benign and malignant ampullary tumors
  - Associated with neurofibromatosis
- Etiology
  - Evidence supporting adenoma-carcinoma sequence of neoplastic lesions in ampulla of Vater
    - May arise from villous adenoma or villoglandular polyp
      - Incidence of adenoma surrounding ampullary carcinoma (82-91%)
- Epidemiology & cancer incidence
  - Relatively uncommon tumor that accounts for approximately 0.2% of gastrointestinal tract malignancies
  - Estimated incidence of 6 per 1,000,000 persons per year
  - 2nd most common periampullary neoplasm following pancreatic carcinoma
    - Approximately 15-25% of all periampullary carcinomas
      - Pancreatic carcinoma is most common (50-70%)
  - Peak incidence is in 7th and 8th decades of life
  - Slight male to female preponderance

Gross Pathology & Surgical Features
- Tumors may appear as
  - Polypoid lesions protruding within common bile duct or duodenum
  - Infiltrating mass obstructing bile duct

Microscopic Pathology
- Carcinomas originating in periampullary region can arise from 1 of 4 epithelial types
  - Terminal common bile duct
  - Duodenal mucosa
  - Pancreatic duct
  - Ampulla of Vater
- In general, true ampullary cancers produce sialomucins, whereas periampullary tumors secrete sulfated mucins
- Ampullary tumors are usually poorly differentiated
  - Differentiation is based on % glands
    - Well differentiated (> 95%)
    - Moderately differentiated (50-95%)
    - Poorly differentiated (5-49%)
    - Undifferentiated (< 5%)
- Adenomatous areas are found frequently within or in the vicinity of carcinoma of ampulla of Vater
- 2 major morphological types
  - Intestinal (arising from covering intestinal mucosa of papilla)
    - Resembles primary adenocarcinomas of colon and rectum
    - Large elongated tubules
    - Has more favorable clinical outcome
  - Pancreaticobiliary (derived from ductal epithelium that penetrates duodenal muscularis propria)

- Similar to adenocarcinoma of pancreas or distal bile duct
- Smaller glands/tubules with desmoplastic stroma
- Has less favorable clinical outcome
- Less common subtypes are signet ring, mucinous, medullary, or mixed

IMAGING FINDINGS

Detection
- General imaging features
  - Direct signs: 2 predominant patterns
    - Nodular type: Discrete nodular mass, with irregular filling defect at ampulla
    - Periductal thickening type: Irregular periductal thickening
  - Indirect signs
    - Intrahepatic and extrahepatic biliary dilatation
    - Pancreatic ductal dilatation, unless patient has pancreatic divisum
    - Gallbladder distension and cholecystolithiasis
    - Intrahepatic and extrahepatic bile ducts stones
- Ultrasound
  - Ampullary mass is seen in ~ 27% of patients with ampullary carcinoma
  - Indirect signs are seen in ~ 93% of patients with ampullary carcinoma
- CT
  - Diagnosis of ampullary carcinoma depends on visualization of ampullary soft tissue mass and filling defect in 2nd part of duodenum
    - Ampullary mass is seen in ~ 30-85% of patients
    - Indirect signs are seen in ~ 95% of patients
  - Difficult to distinguish ampullary carcinoma from other periampullary carcinomas, such as pancreatic head carcinoma and cholangiocarcinoma of lower common bile duct
  - Fatty infiltration of pancreas improves visualization of ampullary tumors
- MRCP
  - Ampullary mass is seen in ~ 24% of patients with ampullary carcinoma
  - Indirect signs are seen in ~ 93% of patients with ampullary carcinoma
- MR
  - 2 patterns can be seen on MR
    - Nodular type: Usually hypointense on T2-weighted images
    - Periductal thickening type: Periductal low signal with delayed contrast enhancement
- ERCP and endoscopic ultrasound (EUS)
  - EUS is superior to CT in terms of tumor visualization
  - Allows direct tumor visualization and possibility of obtaining multiple biopsy specimens
- Intraductal ultrasound (IDUS)
  - IDUS is superior to EUS and CT in terms of tumor visualization
- PET/CT
  - Can be helpful in tumor detection in patients with suspected ampullary lesions not seen on CT
  - Sensitivity and accuracy are 88% and 74%, respectively
  - Range of SUVmax is 2.3-7.7

Staging
- Ultrasound
  - US is not suitable for local tumor staging
  - Potentially useful in detection of liver metastases, ascites, and regional lymphadenopathy
- CT and MR
  - Not reliable in demonstrating duodenal or pancreatic invasion except in large tumors
  - Useful for evaluation of regional adenopathy, liver and peritoneal metastases
- Endoscopic ultrasound
  - Has better sensitivity and specificity compared to CECT in evaluation of pancreatic and duodenal invasion and evaluation of regional lymph nodes
  - IDUS improves accuracy of EUS in loconodal staging of ampullary tumors
  - Not useful in evaluation of hepatic or peritoneal metastases
  - Major disadvantage is limited availability

CLINICAL ISSUES

Presentation
- Symptoms occur early in course of disease
  - Abdominal pain
  - Jaundice
  - Weight loss
- May present as recurrent pancreatitis

Cancer Natural History & Prognosis
- Ampullary cancer has best resectability rate and best prognosis among periampullary cancers
  - Earlier presentation because of anatomic location of ampullary tumors
    - Tumor stage at presentation
      - Stage IA (17%)
      - Stage IB (20%)
      - Stage IIA (20%)
      - Stage IIB (38%)
      - Stage III (3%)
      - Stage IV (1%)
  - Difference in biological aggressiveness compared with pancreatic adenocarcinoma
    - Frequently manifests as polypoid or papillary form
      - Papillary or polypoid tumors tend to have better prognosis than infiltrative tumors
    - Extraluminal extension is relatively infrequent
    - Undifferentiated histologic type is less common in ampullary carcinoma than in others
    - Lymphatic spread and perineural invasion are also infrequent in ampullary carcinoma
- Improved 5-year survival compared to other periampullary tumors
  - Stage 0 (48.9%)
  - Stage IA (39.7%)
  - Stage IB (43.7%)
  - Stage IIA (33%)
  - Stage IIB (26.4%)
  - Stage III (16.1%)
  - Stage IV (3.7%)
- Poor prognostic factors include

- ○ High stage
- ○ Tumor size ≥ 2.5 cm
- ○ Deep tumor infiltration
- ○ Perineural invasion
- ○ Angiolymphatic invasion
- ○ Invasion of muscle of sphincter of Oddi
- ○ Nodal metastases
- ○ Pancreaticobiliary, signet ring, or poorly differentiated histology
- ○ Positive surgical margins

Treatment Options
- Major treatment alternatives
  - ○ Standard surgical approach is pancreaticoduodenal resection (Whipple procedure)
    - ▪ Involves en bloc resection of gastric antrum and duodenum; a segment of 1st portion of jejunum, gallbladder, and distal common bile duct; head and often neck of pancreas; and adjacent regional lymph nodes
    - ▪ Preoperative biliary drainage may be indicated in patients with biliary obstruction presenting with jaundice
    - ▪ Relatively high resection rate, ~ 80% of cases
      - - Attributed to early presentation of disease
  - ○ Limited surgical resection
    - ▪ Indications for limited surgery are adenoma or cancer in adenoma with low possibility of invasion of sphincter of Oddi
  - ○ Transduodenal local resection is comparable mode of operation for low-risk group patients
  - ○ Adjuvant chemotherapy and radiotherapy
    - ▪ Recommended for resected ampullary carcinoma with adverse prognostic features including
      - - Size > 2 cm
      - - Positive lymph nodes
      - - Positive surgical margins
      - - Poor differentiation
      - - Neurovascular invasion
  - ○ Palliative procedures in unresectable tumors include
    - ▪ Percutaneous biliary drainage
    - ▪ Biliary stenting
    - ▪ Biliodigestive anastomosis ± gastroenterostomy
      - - Biliodigestive anastomosis includes hepatico-/choledocho-duodenostomy, hepatico-jejunostomy, and cholecystogastrostomy
- Treatment options by stage
  - ○ Resectable tumor
    - ▪ Pancreaticoduodenal resection (Whipple procedure)
  - ○ Unresectable tumor
    - ▪ Palliative procedures
    - ▪ Palliative chemotherapy based on pancreatic cancer type regimens
    - ▪ Resection of solitary liver metastases should be considered in appropriately selected patients

REPORTING CHECKLIST

T Staging
- Evaluate for local invasion of duodenum and pancreas

N Staging
- Regional nodes include peripancreatic nodes, which include nodes along hepatic artery and portal vein

M Staging
- Mainly to liver and lungs

SELECTED REFERENCES

1. American Joint Committee on Cancer: AJCC Cancer Staging Manual. 7th ed. New York: Springer. 235-40, 2010
2. Artifon EL et al: Prospective evaluation of EUS versus CT scan for staging of ampullary cancer. Gastrointest Endosc. 70(2):290-6, 2009
3. Na, SJ et al: Usefulness of 18F-FDG PET/CT in the diagnosis of locoregional periampullary cancer. Society of Nuclear Medicine Annual Meeting Abstracts 50(2_MeetingAbstracts): 1761, 2009
4. Chen WX et al: Multiple imaging techniques in the diagnosis of ampullary carcinoma. Hepatobiliary Pancreat Dis Int. 7(6):649-53, 2008
5. Kondo S et al: Guidelines for the management of biliary tract and ampullary carcinomas: surgical treatment. J Hepatobiliary Pancreat Surg. 15(1):41-54, 2008
6. O'Connell JB et al: Survival after resection of ampullary carcinoma: a national population-based study. Ann Surg Oncol. 15(7):1820-7, 2008
7. Tsukada K et al: Diagnosis of biliary tract and ampullary carcinomas. J Hepatobiliary Pancreat Surg. 15(1):31-40, 2008
8. Hsu HP et al: Predictors for patterns of failure after pancreaticoduodenectomy in ampullary cancer. Ann Surg Oncol. 14(1):50-60, 2007
9. Todoroki T et al: Patterns and predictors of failure after curative resections of carcinoma of the ampulla of Vater. Ann Surg Oncol. 10(10):1176-83, 2003
10. Kim JH et al: Differential diagnosis of periampullary carcinomas at MR imaging. Radiographics. 22(6):1335-52, 2002
11. Takashima M et al: Carcinoma of the ampulla of Vater associated with or without adenoma: a clinicopathologic analysis of 198 cases with reference to p53 and Ki-67 immunohistochemical expressions. Mod Pathol. 13(12):1300-7, 2000
12. Menzel J et al: Polypoid tumors of the major duodenal papilla: preoperative staging with intraductal US, EUS, and CT--a prospective, histopathologically controlled study. Gastrointest Endosc. 49(3 Pt 1):349-57, 1999

Stage IA (T1 N0 M0)

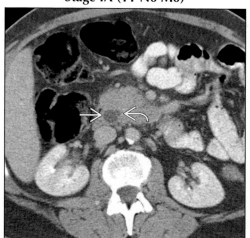

Stage IA (T1 N0 M0)

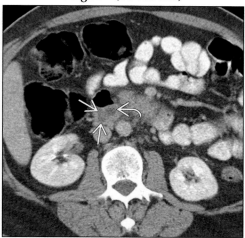

(Left) Axial CECT in a 57-year-old man who presented with jaundice shows dilatation of the distal common bile duct ➡ and pancreatic duct ➡. *(Right)* Axial CECT in the same patient shows dilatation of the proximal ampulla ➡ and a hypoattenuating mass ➡ arising from the ampulla.

Stage IA (T1 N0 M0)

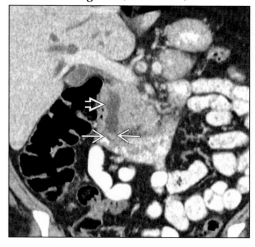

Stage IA (T1 N0 M0)

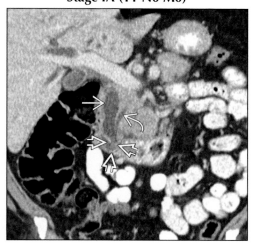

(Left) Coronal CECT in the same patient shows dilatation of the common bile duct ➡ and a soft tissue mass ➡ at the ampulla of Vater. *(Right)* Coronal CECT in the same patient shows common bile duct ➡ and pancreatic duct dilatation ➡ and a soft tissue ampullary mass ➡ protruding into the duodenal lumen. Ampullary carcinomas have better prognosis than pancreatic ductal tumors because of earlier detection due to obstruction of the common bile duct.

Stage IA (T1 N0 M0)

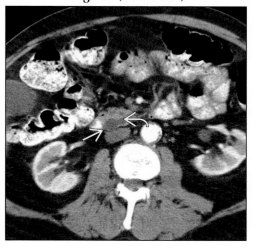

Stage IA (T1 N0 M0)

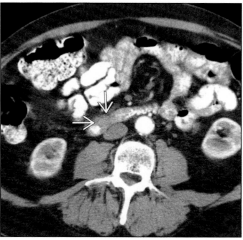

(Left) Axial CECT in a 54-year-old man who presented with vague abdominal pain shows dilatation of the common bile ➡ and pancreatic ➡ ducts. *(Right)* Axial CECT in the same patient shows a small ampullary mass ➡. Tumor localized to the ampulla without invasion of the duodenum or pancreas is T1 disease.

AMPULLA OF VATER CARCINOMA

Stage IA (T1 N0 M0)

Stage IA (T1 N0 M0)

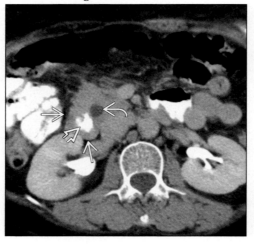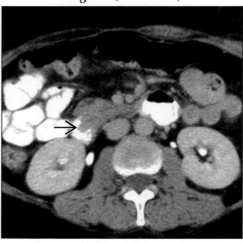

(Left) Axial CECT in a 53-year-old man who presented with right upper quadrant abdominal pain shows dilatation of the common bile duct ➡. Note incidental annular pancreas with pancreatic tissue ➡ surrounding the 2nd part of the duodenum ➡. *(Right)* Axial CECT in the same patient shows a large major papilla ➡ protruding into the duodenal lumen. The appearance is nonspecific and can be seen following stone passage.

Stage IA (T1 N0 M0)

Stage IA (T1 N0 M0)

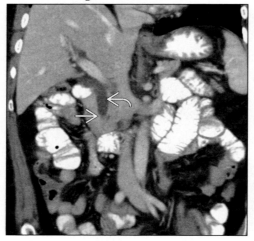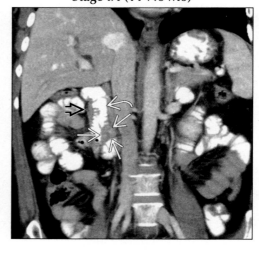

(Left) Coronal CECT in the same patient shows dilatation of the common bile duct ➡ with abrupt transition ➡ at the level of the ampulla. *(Right)* Coronal CECT in the same patient shows the large papilla ➡. Endoscopic ultrasound and biopsy confirmed ampullary tumor. Note the pancreatic tissue ➡ encircling the 2nd part of the duodenum ➡.

Stage IA (T1 N0 M0)

Stage IA (T1 N0 M0)

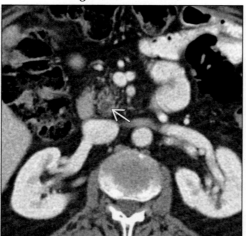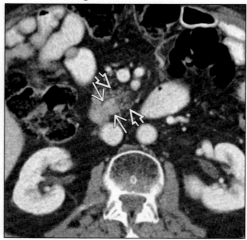

(Left) Axial CECT in a 70-year-old man who underwent CECT for follow-up of gastric carcinoma shows mild dilatation of the distal common bile duct ➡. *(Right)* Axial CECT in the same patient shows a small ampullary soft tissue mass ➡. Detection of small ampullary lesions is difficult on imaging; however, in this patient tumor detection was facilitated by the fatty infiltration of the pancreas ➡.

Stage IA (T1 N0 M0)

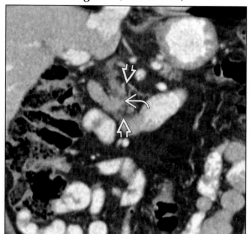

Stage IA (T1 N0 M0)

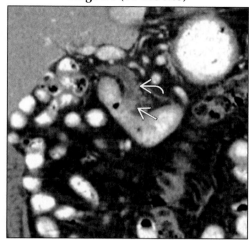

(Left) Coronal CECT in the same patient shows the small ampullary mass ➡ surrounded by the lower attenuation, fat-infiltrated pancreatic head ⇨. *(Right)* Coronal CECT in the same patient shows the ampullary tumor ➡ and mild common bile duct dilatation ➡.

Stage IA (T1 N0 M0)

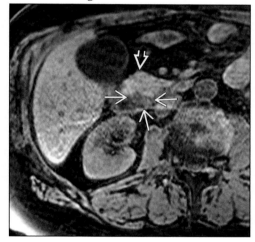

Stage IA (T1 N0 M0)

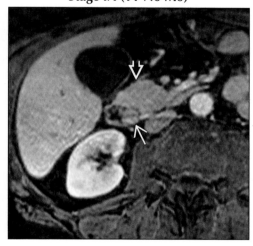

(Left) Axial T2WI FS MR in a 42-year-old man with history of familial polyposis syndrome shows a low signal intensity ampullary lesion ➡. The lesion is hypointense relative to the usually high signal intensity pancreatic head ⇨. *(Right)* Axial T1WI C+ FS MR in the same patient shows the ampullary mass ➡ enhancing to a lesser extent than the pancreatic head ⇨. The ampullary mass is surrounded by a relatively hypointense rim without evidence of invasion.

Stage IA (T1 N0 M0)

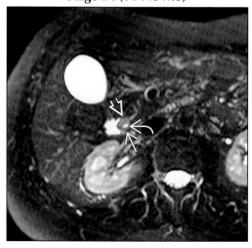

Stage IA (T1 N0 M0)

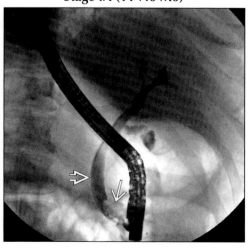

(Left) Axial T2WI FS MR in the same patient shows a bulging papilla ➡ with thickening of the wall of the ampulla ⇨ and narrowing of the bile duct ➡. *(Right)* ERCP in the same patient shows an ampullary lesion ➡ as a filling defect in the distal common bile duct. The bile duct ⇨ is slightly dilated.

AMPULLA OF VATER CARCINOMA

Stage IB (T2 N0 M0)

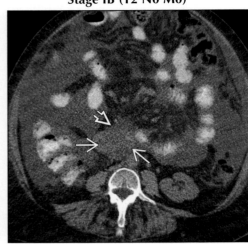

Stage IB (T2 N0 M0)

(Left) Axial CECT in a 72-year-old woman with ascites ➡ due to advanced hepatic cirrhosis shows dilatation of the distal common bile duct ➡. *(Right)* Axial CECT in the same patient shows a mass ➡ at the region of the ampulla of Vater with invasion of the duodenum ➡.

Stage IB (T2 N0 M0)

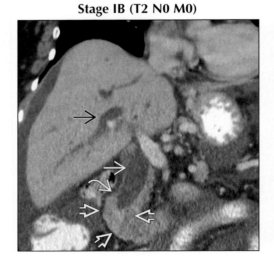

Stage IB (T2 N0 M0)

(Left) Coronal CECT in the same patient shows dilatation of the common bile duct ➡, intrahepatic biliary dilatation ➡, and an ampullary mass ➡ invading the wall of the duodenum ➡. *(Right)* Sagittal CECT in the same patient shows the ampullary mass ➡ with duodenal invasion ➡.

Stage IB (T2 N0 M0)

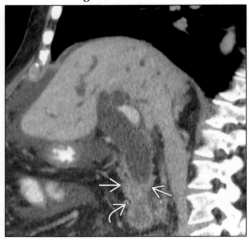

Stage IB (T2 N0 M0)

(Left) Axial PET/CT in the same patient shows a hypermetabolic mass ➡ arising from the ampulla of Vater and protruding into the duodenal lumen. *(Right)* Coronal PET/CT in the same patient shows tumor of the ampulla of Vater ➡ involving the duodenal wall ➡. No other sites of metastatic disease were found.

Stage IB (T2 N0 M0)

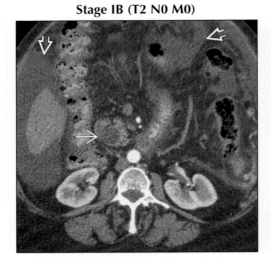
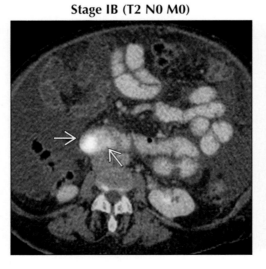
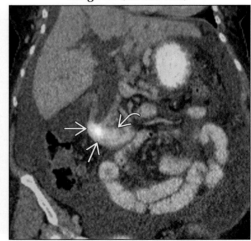

AMPULLA OF VATER CARCINOMA

Stage IB (T2 N0 M0)

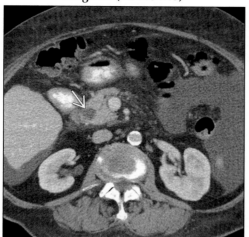

Stage IB (T2 N0 M0)

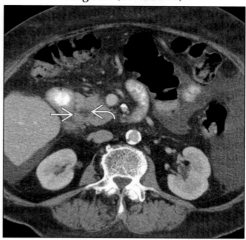

(Left) Axial CECT shows dilatation of the distal common bile duct ➡ in a 70-year-old woman with a history of hepatic cirrhosis who was undergoing CECT to screen for hepatocellular carcinoma. *(Right)* Axial CECT in the same patient shows the common bile duct ➡ with a soft tissue intraluminal component ➡.

Stage IB (T2 N0 M0)

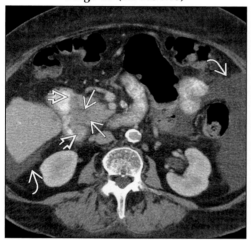

Stage IB (T2 N0 M0)

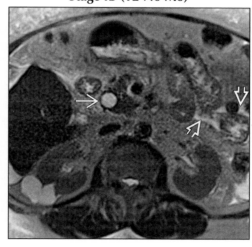

(Left) Axial CECT in the same patient shows an ampullary mass ➡ with invasion of the adjacent duodenum ➡. Note also the presence of ascites ➡ due to poor hepatic function. *(Right)* Axial T2WI MR in the same patient shows dilatation of the distal common bile duct ➡. There is also mesenteric edema ➡ resulting from poor hepatic function.

Stage IB (T2 N0 M0)

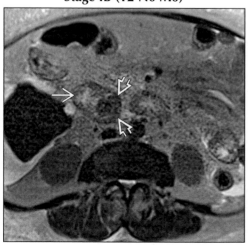

Stage IB (T2 N0 M0)

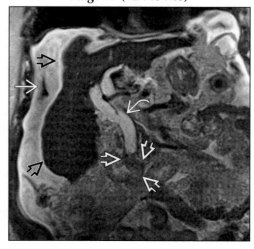

(Left) Axial T2WI MR in the same patient shows the sizable ampullary mass ➡ projecting into the duodenal lumen ➡. *(Right)* Coronal T2WI MR HASTE shows common bile duct dilatation ➡ and a relatively hypointense ampullary mass ➡. Note the cirrhotic liver morphology ➡ and ascites ➡.

Stage IB (T2 N0 M0)

Stage IB (T2 N0 M0)

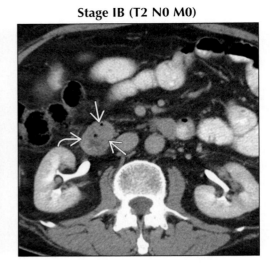

(Left) Axial CECT in a 62-year-old man who presented with painless jaundice shows dilatation of the common bile ➡ and pancreatic ⬈ ducts, as well as distension of the gallbladder ⬈. *(Right)* Axial CECT in the same patient shows an ampullary mass ➡ projecting into the duodenal lumen ⬈. No regional adenopathy is seen.

Stage IB (T2 N0 M0)

Stage IB (T2 N0 M0)

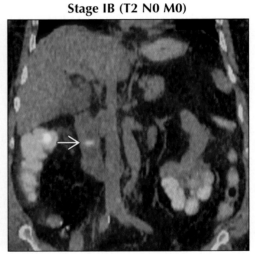

(Left) Axial PET/CT in the same patient shows increased metabolic activity of the ampullary mass ➡. *(Right)* Coronal PET/CT in the same patient shows the ampullary mass ➡ with increased metabolic activity. During surgery microinvasion of the duodenal wall was found, making this a T2 tumor.

Stage IB (T2 N0 M0)

Stage IB (T2 N0 M0)

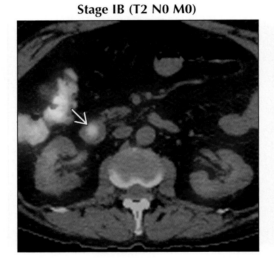

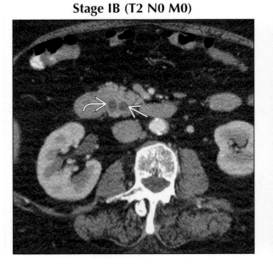

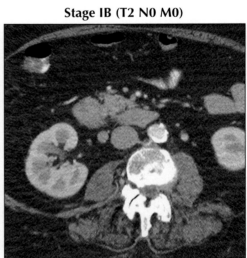

(Left) Axial CECT in an 80-year-old woman who presented with painless jaundice shows dilatation of the common bile duct ⬈ and pancreatic duct ➡. *(Right)* Axial CECT in the same patient shows abrupt termination of the ducts at the level of the ampulla. No definite mass is appreciated on the axial images.

AMPULLA OF VATER CARCINOMA

Stage IB (T2 N0 M0)

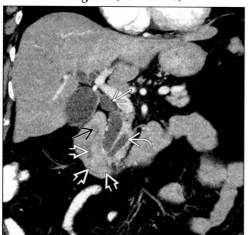

Stage IB (T2 N0 M0)

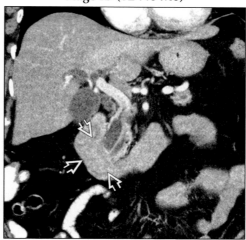

(Left) Coronal CECT in the same patient shows dilatation of the common bile ➡ and pancreatic ➡ ducts and an ampullary mass ➡ invading the wall of the duodenum ➡. (Right) Coronal CECT in the same patient shows ampullary mass ➡ filling the duodenal lumen. Coronal, sagittal, and curved reformats can be helpful in delineation of ampullary tumors not readily appreciated on axial images.

Stage IIA (T3 N0 M0)

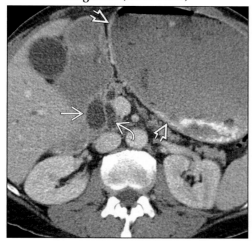

Stage IIA (T3 N0 M0)

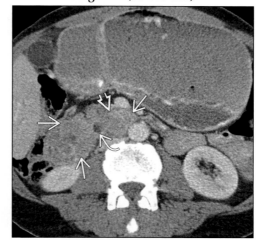

(Left) Axial CECT in a 69-year-old woman who presented with jaundice and vomiting shows dilatation of the common bile duct ➡ and pancreatic duct ➡. The stomach ➡ is markedly distended. (Right) Axial CECT in the same patient shows dilatation of the distal common bile duct ➡ and an ampullary tumor ➡ that involves the uncinate process of the pancreas ➡.

Stage IIA (T3 N0 M0)

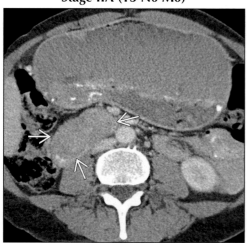

Stage IIA (T3 N0 M0)

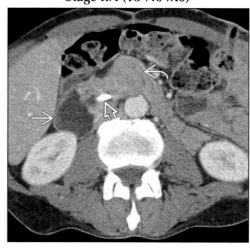

(Left) Axial CECT in the same patient shows a large tumor ➡ filling the duodenum and causing gastric outlet obstruction, resulting in marked dilatation of the stomach and repeated vomiting. (Right) Axial CECT in the same patient after placement of a biliary stent ➡ shows duodenal dilatation ➡ due to obstruction and tumor involving the pancreatic uncinate process ➡.

AMPULLA OF VATER CARCINOMA

Stage IIB (T3 N1 M0)

Stage IIB (T3 N1 M0)

(Left) Axial CECT in an 86-year-old man who presented with painless jaundice shows dilatation of the common bile duct ➡ and the pancreatic duct ➡ with mild intrahepatic biliary dilatation ➡. *(Right)* Axial CECT in the same patient shows the dilated common bile duct ➡ with a slightly heterogeneous mass ➡ invading the pancreatic head.

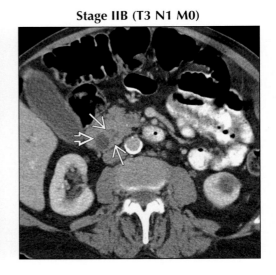

Stage IIB (T3 N1 M0)

Stage IIB (T3 N1 M0)

(Left) Axial CECT in the same patient shows the main bulk of the ampullary mass ➡ invading into the duodenal lumen ➡. *(Right)* Coronal CECT in the same patient shows dilatation of the common bile duct ➡ with a large obstructing ampullary mass ➡ invading into the duodenum ➡.

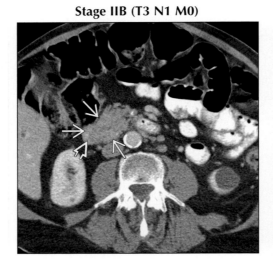

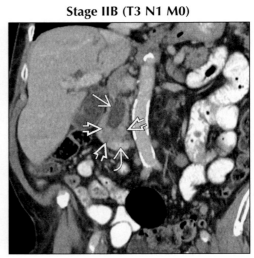

Stage IIB (T3 N1 M0)

Stage IIB (T3 N1 M0)

(Left) Coronal CECT in the same patient shows common bile duct ➡ and intrahepatic biliary ➡ dilatation. Multiple enlarged periaortic lymph nodes ➡ are present. *(Right)* Axial CECT in the same patient obtained 2 months after the initial examination and after placement of a biliary stent ➡ shows the ampullary tumor ➡ invading into the pancreatic head.

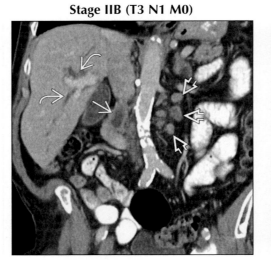

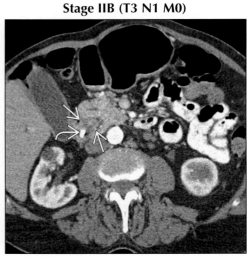

AMPULLA OF VATER CARCINOMA

Stage III (T4 N1 M0)

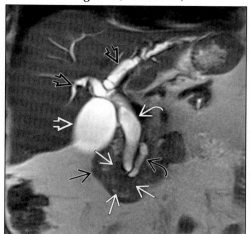

Stage III (T4 N1 M0)

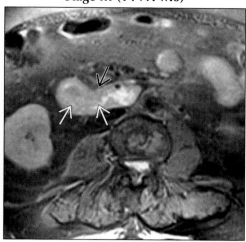

(Left) Coronal MRCP shows dilatation of the hepatic ducts ⮂, common bile duct ⮕, and pancreatic duct ⮕ with distention of the gallbladder ⮂. There is a low signal intensity mass ➡ at the region of the ampulla and protruding into the duodenum ⮕. *(Right)* Axial T2WI FS MR in the same patient shows the mass ➡ invading the wall of the duodenum ⮕.

Stage III (T4 N1 M0)

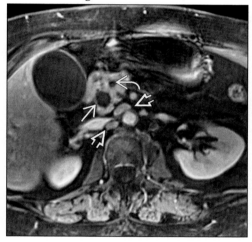

Stage III (T4 N1 M0)

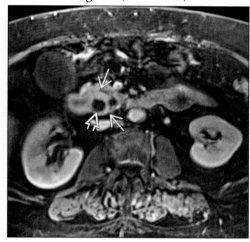

(Left) Axial T1WI C+ FS MR in the same patient shows dilatation of the common bile duct ➡ and pancreatic duct ⮕ within the head of the pancreas. Multiple enlarged periaortic lymph nodes ⮂ are also seen on this image. *(Right)* Axial T1WI C+ FS MR in the same patient shows, in addition to ductal dilatation, an enhancing tumor ➡ within the pancreatic head surrounding the distal common bile duct ⮂.

Stage III (T4 N1 M0)

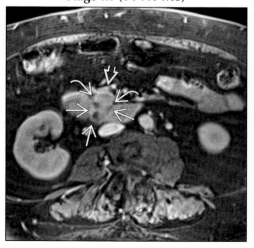

Stage III (T4 N1 M0)

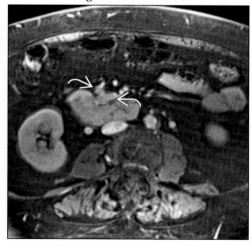

(Left) Axial T1WI C+ FS MR in the same patient shows the enhancing ampullary mass ➡ invading the wall of the duodenum ⮕ and extending beyond the duodenum and pancreatic head into the peripancreatic fat ⮂. *(Right)* Axial T1WI C+ FS MR in the same patient shows the lower end of the tumor ➡ infiltrating the peripancreatic fat. Tumors invading the peripancreatic soft tissue or other adjacent organs are classified T4.

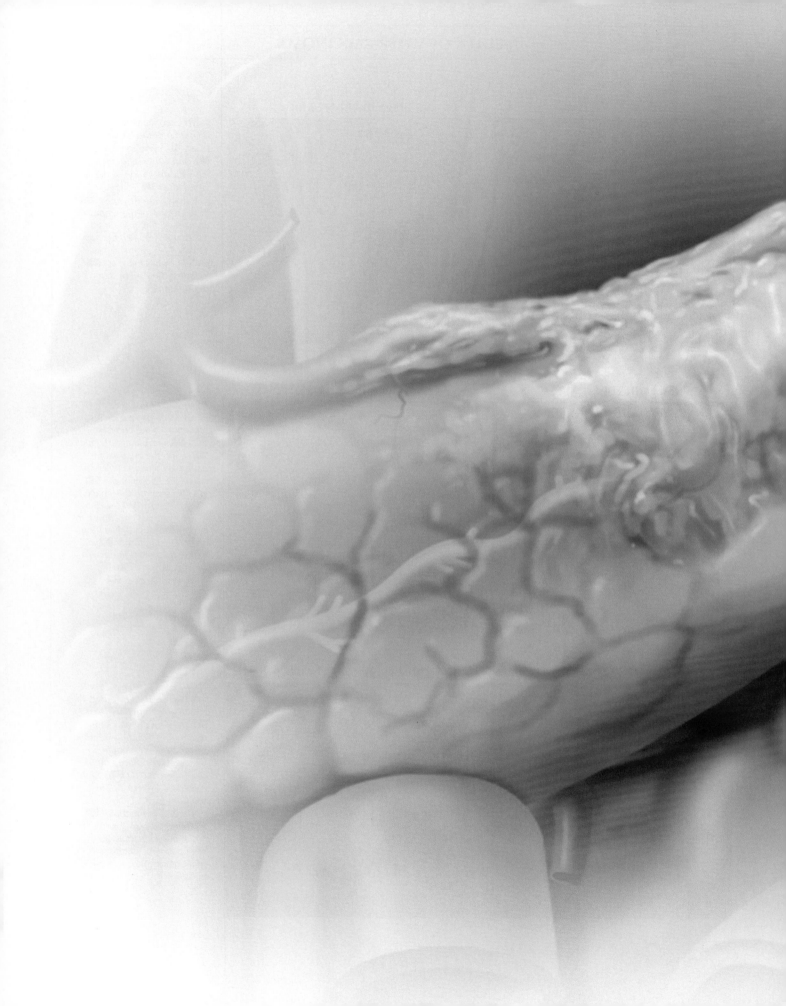

Endocrine Pancreatic Carcinoma

ENDOCRINE PANCREATIC CARCINOMA

(T) Primary Tumor

Adapted from 7th edition AJCC Staging Forms.

TNM	Definitions
TX	Primary tumor cannot be assessed
T0	No evidence of primary tumor
Tis	Carcinoma in situ*
T1	Tumor limited to the pancreas, ≤ 2 cm in greatest dimension
T2	Tumor limited to the pancreas, > 2 cm in greatest dimension
T3	Tumor extends beyond the pancreas but without involvement of the celiac axis or the superior mesenteric artery
T4	Tumor involves the celiac axis or the superior mesenteric artery (unresectable primary tumor)

(N) Regional Lymph Nodes

NX	Regional lymph nodes cannot be assessed
N0	No regional lymph node metastasis
N1	Regional lymph node metastasis

(M) Distant Metastasis

M0	No distant metastasis
M1	Distant metastasis

This also includes the "PanInIII" classification.

AJCC Stages/Prognostic Groups

Adapted from 7th edition AJCC Staging Forms.

Stage	T	N	M
0	Tis	N0	M0
IA	T1	N0	M0
IB	T2	N0	M0
IIA	T3	N0	M0
IIB	T1	N1	M0
	T2	N1	M0
	T3	N1	M0
III	T4	Any N	M0
IV	Any T	Any N	M1

ENDOCRINE PANCREATIC CARCINOMA

T1

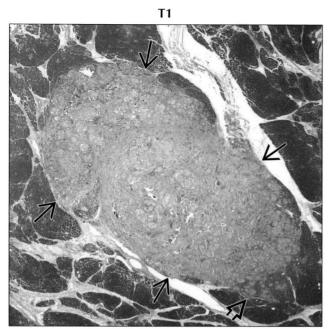

H&E stained section of a pancreatic resection specimen shows a 1.1 cm pancreatic neuroendocrine tumor ⇥ that invades the relatively well-demarcated surrounding pancreatic lobules ⇥. (Original magnification 20x.)

T1

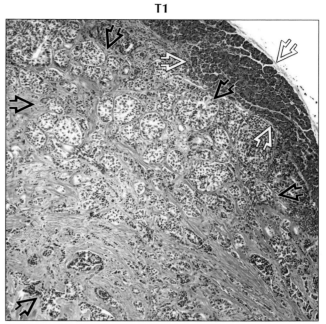

Higher magnification of the previous image shows ribbons and irregular islands of neoplastic cells ⇥ with a large amount of dense eosinophilic stroma. Note the normal pancreatic exocrine cells in the right upper corner of the slide ⇥. (Original magnification 100x.)

T3

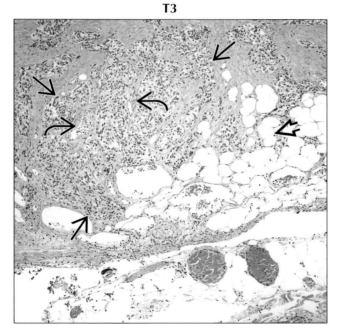

H&E stained section shows tumor extending beyond the pancreas. The nests and sheets of neoplastic cells ⇥ sit in a prominent fibrous stroma with numerous small blood vessels ⇥ and infiltrate into the peripancreatic fatty tissue ⇥. (Original magnification 40x.)

T3

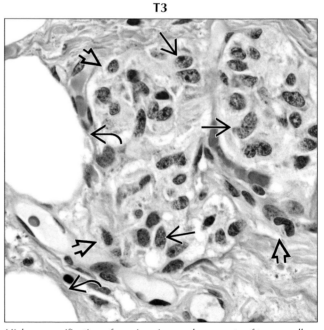

Higher magnification of previous image shows nests of tumor cells ⇥ in close proximity to fat cells ⇥. The neoplastic cells have somewhat elongated nuclei with "salt and pepper" chromatin and numerous forms showing prominent nucleoli ⇥. (Original magnification 500x.)

ENDOCRINE PANCREATIC CARCINOMA

T1

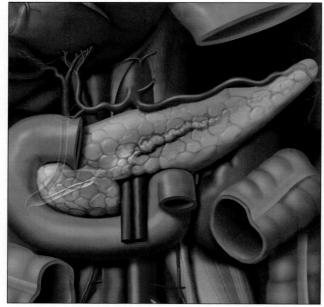

Graphic illustrates T1 disease, with tumor confined to the pancreas and is ≤ 2 cm in greatest dimension.

T2

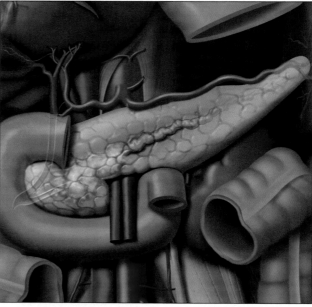

Graphic illustrates T2 disease. Tumor is confined to the pancreas and is > 2 cm in greatest dimension.

T3

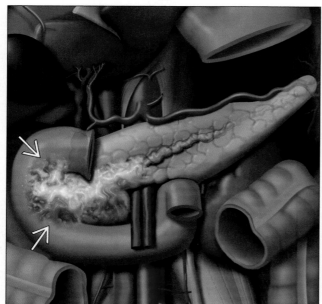

Graphic illustrates tumor involving the duodenum ➡, consistent with T3 disease. T3 tumors extend beyond the pancreas but without involvement of the celiac axis or superior mesenteric artery.

T3

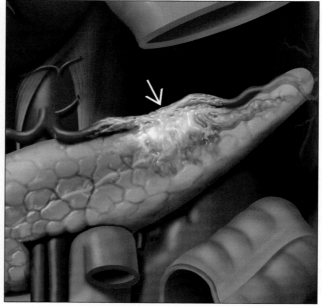

Graphic illustrates tumor invading the splenic artery ➡, which is also consistent with T3 disease. Tumor extends beyond the pancreas but without involvement of the celiac axis or superior mesenteric artery.

T4

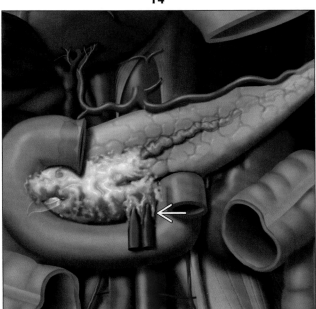

Graphic illustrates tumor involving the superior mesenteric artery ➡️*, consistent with T4 disease. Any tumor that involves the celiac axis or superior mesenteric artery is considered T4.*

Peripancreatic Lymph Node Groups

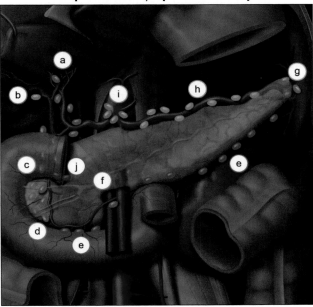

Graphic depicts peripancreatic lymph node groups: a) hepatic, b) cystic duct, c) posterior pancreaticoduodenal, d) anterior pancreaticoduodenal, e) inferior, f) superior mesenteric, g) splenic hilar, h) superior, i) celiac, and j) pyloric.

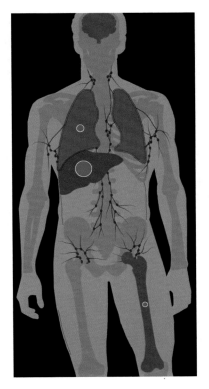

METASTASES, ORGAN FREQUENCY

Liver	60%*
Lung	17%
Bone	7-15%

*Percentage of patients with malignant pancreatic neuroendocrine tumors (PNET) who present with liver metastases. Since histological examination is not reliable in differentiating benign from malignant tumors, it is the presence of metastases, whether nodal or hepatic, that classifies a PNET as malignant. Other reported sites of metastases include the mediastinum, skin, and heart.

ENDOCRINE PANCREATIC CARCINOMA

OVERVIEW

General Comments

- Single pancreatic staging system is now used for both pancreatic adenocarcinoma and pancreatic neuroendocrine tumors (PNET)
- PNETs are presented separately because their imaging features are distinct from those of pancreatic adenocarcinoma
- PNETs are also called islet cell tumors
  - Endocrine pancreatic tumors originate from islet cells of Langerhans that make up endocrine pancreas
    - Less than 5% of total pancreatic mass consists of endocrine cells

Classification

- All endocrine tumors are hormonally active to variable degree
- Typically divided depending on clinical and biochemical manifestations into
  - Syndromic (hyperfunctioning, 65-70%)
    - Insulinoma
    - Gastrinoma
    - Glucagonoma
    - VIPoma
    - Somatostatinoma
    - Others
  - Nonsyndromic (nonhyperfunctioning, 30-35%)
- Classification of PNET as benign or malignant is not consistent
  - All PNET irrespective of benign or malignant classification should be staged using this system
- Carcinoid tumors of pancreas are also included in this staging schema
  - Carcinoid tumor
  - Atypical carcinoid
  - Composite carcinoid (combined with adenocarcinoma)
  - Adenocarcinoid

PATHOLOGY

Routes of Spread

- Local spread
  - Very unusual in syndromic tumors due to early detection
  - More likely in nonsyndromic tumors
  - Local spread to peripancreatic structures including
    - Retroperitoneum, duodenum, adrenal gland, kidney, and spleen
    - Vascular involvement of superior mesenteric vessels, celiac artery and its branches, portal and splenic veins
- Nodal metastases
  - Unusual in syndromic PNET and when tumor is small
  - Regional lymph nodes include
    - Head and neck of pancreas
      - Nodes along common bile duct
      - Nodes along common hepatic artery
      - Nodes along portal vein
      - Nodes along posterior and anterior pancreaticoduodenal arcade
      - Nodes along superior mesenteric vein
      - Nodes along right side of superior mesenteric artery
    - Body and tail of pancreas
      - Nodes along common hepatic artery
      - Nodes along celiac axis
      - Nodes along splenic artery
      - Nodes within splenic hilum
- Distant metastases
  - Liver is most common site for metastatic PNET
  - Other sites include lung, bone, mediastinum, skin, and heart

General Features

- Comments
  - High rate of malignancy (60-92%)
    - Malignant potential of insulinoma is low (6-10%)
    - Other syndromic tumors are more frequently malignant
  - Insulinoma
    - Arises from islet β cells
    - Most common functioning PNET
    - Usually solitary
    - Equal distribution in head, body, and tail
    - 10% are associated with multiple endocrine neoplasia type 1 (MEN1)
    - 6-10% are malignant
    - 10% of patients with clinical syndrome will have "islet cell hyperplasia" rather than discrete insulinoma
  - Gastrinoma
    - Located in gastrinoma triangle
      - Formed by cystic duct confluence, junction of pancreatic neck and body, and junction of 2nd and 3rd parts of duodenum
    - 2nd most common syndromic PNET
    - Most common PNET in patients with MEN1
    - Many patients will have Zollinger-Ellison syndrome
      - Excess production of gastrin
    - Usually multiple
    - Frequently malignant
      - 60-90% are malignant
      - Approximately 30% of patients presenting with liver metastases
  - Glucagonoma
    - Uncommon PNET
    - Typically manifests in middle-aged patients and affects men and women equally
    - 60% are malignant
  - VIPoma
    - Can be extrapancreatic in 10–20% of cases
    - 80% are malignant
      - Usually accompanied by liver metastases at time of diagnosis
    - Secrete variety of hormones, including vasoactive intestinal peptide (VIP)
  - Somatostatinoma
    - Duodenal in 50% of cases
- Genetics
  - Usually occur sporadically
  - May be associated with genetic syndromes, such as
    - MEN1

ENDOCRINE PANCREATIC CARCINOMA

- Inherited condition characterized by synchronous or metachronous tumors of parathyroid glands, anterior pituitary, pancreas, and gastrointestinal tract
- 75% gastrinomas, 25% insulinomas
- 40-70% of MEN patients develop PNET
- Germline mutation in 1 copy of gene located on centromeric portion of long arm of chromosome 11 (11q13), known as *mu* gene
  - von Hippel–Lindau (VHL) disease
    - PNETs develop in 10-17% of patients with VHL
    - Almost invariably nonsyndromic PNETs
  - Neurofibromatosis type 1
  - Tuberous sclerosis
- Epidemiology & cancer incidence
  - Rare tumors
    - 1–2% of all primary pancreatic malignancies
    - Crude annual incidence of 0.22 per 100,000 in USA
    - PNETs can be found in 0.8–10% of autopsies
      - Discrepancy between incidence in population and incidence at autopsy suggests that people frequently harbor asymptomatic PNETs
    - Slightly higher incidence among males
    - Incidence increases with age and peaks in 6th and 7th decade
      - Early age of onset in patients with genetic syndromes

Gross Pathology & Surgical Features

- Tumor size is variable
  - 90% of insulinomas are smaller than 2 cm in diameter
    - Most patients with insulinoma have early and obvious clinical symptoms and present with relatively small tumors
  - Glucagonoma usually is large (mean diameter is 6.5 cm)
- Small tumors are homogeneous, and larger tumors are cystic, necrotic, or hemorrhagic
- Round or ovoid
- Well demarcated
- Expansile growth pattern
- Calcifications may be found in larger tumors
- Smaller tumors are unencapsulated and larger tumors have fibrous pseudocapsule
  - Pseudocapsule is often incomplete and should not be mistaken for invasive behavior
- Soft to firm or rubbery in consistency, depending on relative content of fibrous stroma

Microscopic Pathology

- Both benign and malignant PNETs have similar appearance
  - Determination of benign vs. malignant is primarily by finding additional metastatic sites in liver and lymph nodes
- Majority show histologic patterns that reflect relatively high level of cellular differentiation
  - Cells are composed of sheets or nests of monomorphic medium-sized cells
  - May be arranged in 3 different patterns
    - Trabecular ± gyriform arrangement
    - Acinar or glandular pattern, often surrounding lumen

- Medullary or solid pattern
  - Nuclei are relatively uniform in size and shape, with dispersed chromatin, inconspicuous nucleoli
    - Mitoses are unusual, even in tumors that behave aggressively
- Rare type of PNET appears as poorly differentiated neoplasms that are virtually identical to small cell carcinomas of lung
  - More likely to exhibit infiltrative growth pattern similar to pancreatic adenocarcinoma

IMAGING FINDINGS

Detection

- Diagnosis depends on laboratory tests, which are beyond scope of this text
- Radiological localization of PNET
  - Most pancreatic VIPomas, glucagonomas, and somatostatinomas are large and therefore detectable with conventional studies
  - Many gastrinomas and insulinomas are frequently < 1 cm and may be difficult to detect
- Ultrasound
  - Transabdominal ultrasound
    - Sensitivity in detecting PNET ranges from 9-64%
    - Sonographic appearance
      - Small lesions are usually homogeneous and hypoechoic
      - Larger lesions are more heterogeneous reflecting presence of hemorrhage, necrosis, and calcifications
  - Endoscopic ultrasound (EUS)/FNA
    - EUS is able to identify PNETs in approximately 90% of cases
    - FNA is useful for pathologic confirmation
- CT
  - Overview
    - Dual phase MDCT shows sensitivity > 80%
    - Necessity of obtaining images during more than 1 phase of enhancement
      - Most tumors show increased enhancement in at least 1 phase
  - Imaging features
    - Syndromic PNETs
      - Tumor detection is difficult because of their small size
      - Typically intense and prolonged enhancement
      - Some are hypoattenuating relative to enhancing pancreas, best seen during portal venous or pancreatic phase
      - Can be homogeneous, heterogeneous, or cystic in appearance
      - Cystic degeneration, calcification, and necrosis are more common in larger syndromic PNETs
    - Nonsyndromic PNETs
      - Tend to be large at initial presentation (average tumor size is 5.2 cm)
      - May show calcifications, cysts, necrosis
      - Hypervascular, enhancing during both arterial and venous phases
    - Cystic neuroendocrine tumors
      - Uncommon appearance of PNET
      - May be syndromic or nonsyndromic

ENDOCRINE PANCREATIC CARCINOMA

- Typically solid and well vascularized with central cystic component
- Cystic components were found in 17% of PNETs
- More likely to occur in patients with MEN1 syndrome
- Believed to be secondary to tumor degeneration
- Predominantly well circumscribed
- MR
  - Sensitivity of MR has been reported to be 74-100%
  - T1WI
    - Low signal intensity compared to bright pancreas
    - May be best sequence to detect subtle tumors
  - T2WI
    - Usually bright
    - Lesions with intermediate or low T2W signal intensity may be seen
      - Due to abundant fibrous tissue may show low signal intensity on T2WI
  - Gadolinium-enhanced T1WI
    - Typical hyperenhancing during arterial phase
    - Degree, uniformity, and timing of enhancement can be highly variable
      - Tumors may be discernible on only 1 contrast-enhanced phase
      - May be seen best on venous phase images
      - May even be seen only on unenhanced images
    - Larger, more malignant lesions usually show more heterogeneous enhancement
  - Diffusion-weighted imaging (DWI)
    - Can be added to MR imaging protocol to detect lesions in patients with clinical suspicion for PNET with negative or suspicious imaging findings
    - Restricted water diffusion → ↓ signal on ADC maps and ↑ signal intensity on diffusion-weighted images
- Octreotide scintigraphy
  - Somatostatin receptor scintigraphy is useful for localization of PNET
  - Not all neuroendocrine tumors express enough somatostatin receptors to be detected
    - Negative scan cannot exclude gastrinoma or insulinoma
  - Diagnostic sensitivity of In-111 DTPA-octreotide scans is 80-90% and varies among different types of PNETs
    - Glucagonomas (100%)
    - VIPomas (88%)
    - Carcinoids (87%)
    - Gastrinomas (73%)
    - Insulinomas (< 25%)
  - Single photon emission tomography (SPECT imaging) is essential to achieve high sensitivity
    - To isolate possible lesions from renal background
  - Octreotide scan has been used for prediction of octreotide therapeutic response
    - Positive result suggests likely therapeutic benefit
- Percutaneous transhepatic portal venous sampling (PTPVS)
  - Performed by transhepatic catheterization of portal vein
    - Invasive procedure with significant complication rate and mortality
  - Samples for hormonal analysis are obtained from splenic vein, superior and inferior mesenteric veins, and portal and pancreatic veins
  - Exact location of tumor cannot be pinpointed in same way as in imaging study
    - PTPVS only localizes tumors to region of pancreas
    - Problems of localization may arise
      - When there are multiple tumors
      - If hormone gradient is low
- Arterial stimulation with venous sampling (ASVS)
  - Invasive technique for detection of insulinomas and gastrinomas
    - Should only be used if noninvasive techniques fail to reveal tumor
  - Rationale
    - Tumor cells differ from normal β cells in their insulin response to intraarterial calcium injection
    - Intraarterial calcium is potent stimulator of insulin production from islet β cells
  - Catheter placed selectively in splenic, superior mesenteric, and gastroduodenal arteries with infusion of calcium gluconate followed by venous sampling from hepatic vein
  - Localize discrete insulin-secreting PNETs to regions of pancreas
  - ≥ 2x step-up in right hepatic vein insulin concentration from baseline at 20, 40, &/or 60 sec after arterial calcium injection constitutes positive response
    - Positive response when gastroduodenal artery or superior mesenteric artery is injected → head/neck lesion
    - Positive response after proximal or midsplenic artery injection → body and tail lesion
    - Positive response after proper hepatic artery injection → liver metastases
  - Sensitivity > 90% for detection and localization of insulinoma

Staging
- Local staging
  - CT and MR have comparable accuracy in evaluation of local disease
  - Radiological staging
    - T1: Tumor confined to pancreas ≤ 2 cm in size
    - T2: Tumor confined to pancreas > 2 cm in size
    - T3: Tumor extends beyond pancreas with involvement of surrounding structures (potentially resectable)
      - May involve superior mesenteric, splenic, or portal vein
      - May involve duodenum, stomach, or spleen
      - May extend to retroperitoneum and involve adrenal and kidney
    - T4: Tumor involving celiac axis or superior mesenteric artery (unresectable)
      - Tumor encasing or invading into celiac or superior mesenteric artery
- Nodal staging
  - Regional nodes are involved based on primary tumor location as described above
- Liver metastases
  - Most common site for metastatic disease

- Multiphase contrast-enhanced CT and MR are useful for detection of liver metastases
  - Sensitivity of up to 94%
- CT appearance
  - Hypoattenuating to liver on NECT
    - May shows areas of increased attenuation due to hemorrhage
  - Typically hypervascular and often best seen on early arterial phase images
- MR appearance
  - T1WI: Hypointense or isointense compared with normal liver
  - T2WI: Hyperintense compared with normal liver
  - Variable enhancement patterns of liver metastases parallel variability of primary tumor
    - Typically early, transient, and without peripheral nodularity
    - Typically hypervascular and often are seen on early arterial phase images
    - Sometimes are best appreciated on portal venous phase images because of rapid washout
- Bone metastases are usually sclerotic or mixed osteolytic and sclerotic pattern on standard radiography
  - 10% are purely osteolytic
- Octreotide scintigraphy
  - Octreoscan is highly sensitive in detection of metastases from PNET
    - Sensitivity varies depending on presence and density of somatostatin receptors in tumor as well as tumor size
      - Sensitivity of 90% for detection of gastrinoma metastases
  - Increased uptake indicates presence of high-affinity somatostatin receptors, located on most tumoral endocrine cells
  - Helpful in predicting benefit of somatostatin analogue therapy

Restaging

- CT or MR can be used for follow-up of patients following tumor resection
  - Detection of local recurrence
  - Detection of hepatic metastases
  - Detection of new tumors in patients with MEN1
- Variable enhancement pattern of liver metastases can make it difficult to assess treatment response
  - Unenhanced images on CT and MR can be useful for measuring lesions
    - Independent of variability between studies in timing of contrast enhancement

CLINICAL ISSUES

Presentation

- Insulinoma
  - Classic clinical triad (Whipple triad) includes
    - Fasting serum glucose levels < 50 mg/dL
    - Symptoms of hypoglycemia
    - Relief of symptoms after glucose administration
  - Symptoms related to catecholamine release
    - Palpitations, sweating, and headache
- Gastrinoma
  - Most patients present with epigastric pain

    - Due to recurrent or intractable peptic ulcer disease
    - Ulcers in unusual locations (e.g., postbulbar)
  - Patients may also have diarrhea due to excessive delivery of acid to small bowel
  - ↑ serum gastrin levels
- Glucagonoma
  - Characteristic migratory rash called necrolytic migratory erythema
    - Usually affects genitals
  - Stomatitis, diarrhea, anemia, weight loss, depression, and deep vein thrombosis
    - 4D syndrome: **D**ermatosis, **d**iarrhea, **d**epression, and **d**eep vein thrombosis
  - ↑ glucagon level
  - Levels of associated hormones, such as insulin, serotonin, or gastrin may also be elevated
- VIPoma
  - WDHA syndrome: **W**atery **d**iarrhea, **h**ypokalemia, and **a**chlorhydria

Cancer Natural History & Prognosis

- Better survival compared to pancreatic adenocarcinoma
  - Overall 5-year survival rate is 29.2% for all patients
    - 55.4% for patients with resected tumor
    - Only 15.6% for patients with unresected tumor
  - 5-year survival for PNET according to stage
    - Stage I (61%)
    - Stage II (52%)
    - Stage III (41%)
    - Stage IV (16%)

Treatment Options

- Major treatment alternatives
  - Surgical treatment
    - Patients with localized, regional, and metastatic PNETs who are reasonable operative candidates should be considered for resection of their primary tumors
      - Survival benefit was demonstrated even for patients with metastatic disease
    - Choice of procedure depends on
      - Tumor location
      - Number of tumors
      - Risk of malignancy based on parameters such as type, size, and tumor features
    - Enucleation
      - Preserves pancreatic parenchyma, reducing risk of pancreatic insufficiency
      - Lymphadenectomy is not usually performed
      - Particularly for insulinomas since majority are benign and for small nonfunctioning tumors
      - Feasible when tumor is single, < 4 cm, and separated from pancreatic duct by 2-3 mm
    - Distal pancreatectomy
    - Pancreaticoduodenectomy
    - Resection of hepatic metastases whenever possible
    - Debulking in advanced local tumors
      - Possibility of treating residual tumor with locoregional therapies
      - Better control of symptoms due to hypersecretion
      - Improved survival
  - Interventional procedures

- Mainly directed at treatment of hepatic or extrahepatic metastases
- Possible interventions include
  - Transcatheter arterial embolization (TAE)
  - Transcatheter arterial chemoembolization (TACE)
  - Radiofrequency ablation (RFA)
- Medical treatment
  - Gastrinoma
    - Symptoms of acid hypersecretion can be controlled by proton pump inhibitors in virtually all patients with Zollinger–Ellison syndrome
    - Histamine H2 receptor antagonists or somatostatin analogues are also effective
  - Insulinoma
    - Prior to surgery and for rare patients with malignant disease
    - Treatment for hypoglycemia
    - Frequent small feedings
    - Diazoxide, a benzothiadiazide, which directly inhibits insulin release and causes adrenergic stimulation promoting glycogenolysis
  - Glucagonoma
    - Combination chemotherapy for unresectable tumor
    - Somatostatin analogue therapy
    - Necrotizing erythema of glucagonoma: Somatostatin analogue, with nearly complete disappearance within 1 week

REPORTING CHECKLIST

T Staging

- Tumor localization
  - Best seen during arterial phase of contrast enhancement
    - Some are best seen during portal venous phase
  - If tumor is not seen on cross-sectional imaging
    - Consider octreotide scintigraphy, percutaneous transhepatic portal venous sampling, or arterial stimulation with venous sampling
- Tumor size determines T designation of tumor confined to pancreas
  - Tumor ≤ 2 cm: T1
  - Tumor > 2 cm: T2
- Involvement of celiac or superior mesenteric arteries determines T designation of tumor extending outside pancreas
  - No involvement of celiac or superior mesenteric arteries: T3
  - Involvement of celiac or superior mesenteric arteries: T4

N Staging

- Nodal location depends on site of primary tumor

M Staging

- Commonly to liver, lungs, and bones
- Liver metastases are usually hypervascular
- Bone metastases are usually sclerotic

SELECTED REFERENCES

1. American Joint Committee on Cancer: AJCC Cancer Staging Manual. 7th ed. New York: Springer. 241-9, 2010
2. Bakir B et al: Diffusion weighted MR imaging of pancreatic islet cell tumors. Eur J Radiol. 74(1):214-20, 2010
3. Anaye A et al: Successful preoperative localization of a small pancreatic insulinoma by diffusion-weighted MRI. JOP. 10(5):528-31, 2009
4. Guettier JM et al: Localization of insulinomas to regions of the pancreas by intraarterial calcium stimulation: the NIH experience. J Clin Endocrinol Metab. 94(4):1074-80, 2009
5. Hill JS et al: Pancreatic neuroendocrine tumors: the impact of surgical resection on survival. Cancer. 115(4):741-51, 2009
6. Kalb B et al: MR imaging of cystic lesions of the pancreas. Radiographics. 29(6):1749-65, 2009
7. Halfdanarson TR et al: Pancreatic neuroendocrine tumors (PNETs): incidence, prognosis and recent trend toward improved survival. Ann Oncol. 19(10):1727-33, 2008
8. Metz DC et al: Gastrointestinal neuroendocrine tumors: pancreatic endocrine tumors. Gastroenterology. 135(5):1469-92, 2008
9. Bilimoria KY et al: Application of the pancreatic adenocarcinoma staging system to pancreatic neuroendocrine tumors. J Am Coll Surg. 205(4):558-63, 2007
10. Tamm EP et al: Imaging of neuroendocrine tumors. Hematol Oncol Clin North Am. 21(3):409-32; vii, 2007
11. Chung EM et al: Pancreatic tumors in children: radiologic-pathologic correlation. Radiographics. 26(4):1211-38, 2006
12. Falconi M et al: Surgical strategy in the treatment of pancreatic neuroendocrine tumors. JOP. 7(1):150-6, 2006
13. Debray MP et al: Imaging appearances of metastases from neuroendocrine tumours of the pancreas. Br J Radiol. 74(887):1065-70, 2001
14. Wick MR et al: Pancreatic neuroendocrine neoplasms: a current summary of diagnostic, prognostic, and differential diagnostic information. Am J Clin Pathol. 115 Suppl:S28-45, 2001

ENDOCRINE PANCREATIC CARCINOMA

Stage IA (T1 N0 M0)

Stage IA (T1 N0 M0)

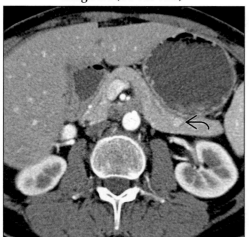

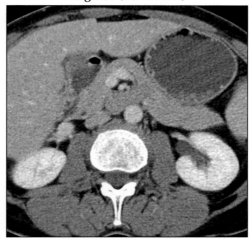

(Left) Axial CECT obtained during the arterial phase in a 52-year-old woman with history of hypoglycemia shows a 1 cm enhancing pancreatic tail mass ➶. (Right) Axial CECT obtained during a more delayed phase of contrast enhancement does not show any evidence of the small insulinoma. This case emphasizes the importance of obtaining arterial phase images when examining the pancreas for PNETs, since these tumors are often subtle and only seen during the arterial phase.

Stage IA (T1 N0 M0)

Stage IA (T1 N0 M0)

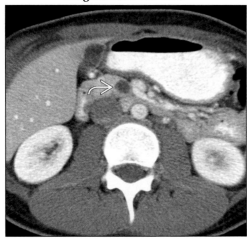

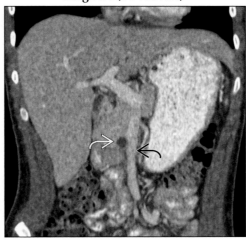

(Left) Axial CECT in a 25-year-old woman with history of MEN1 and symptoms of hypoglycemia shows a well-defined hypoattenuating 1.2 cm lesion ➶ within the pancreatic head. No enhancement is seen, and the lesion was thought to represent pancreatic cyst or pseudocyst. (Right) Coronal CECT in the same patient shows a well-defined hypoattenuating lesion ➶ adjacent to the superior mesenteric vein ➶.

Stage IA (T1 N0 M0)

Stage IA (T1 N0 M0)

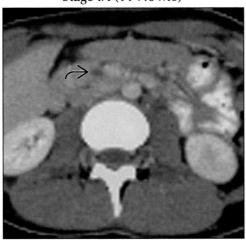

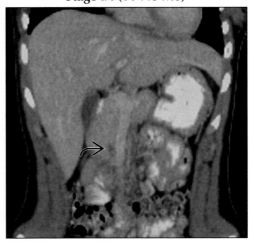

(Left) Axial PET/CT in the same patient shows the pancreatic head lesion ➶ without increase in metabolic activity. (Right) Coronal PET/CT in the same patient shows pancreatic head lesion ➶ without increase in metabolic activity. Because of the high clinical concern, endoscopic ultrasound and FNA were performed and revealed PNET. Cystic PNET is more common in patients with MEN, but there is usually a rim of enhancement around the tumor.

ENDOCRINE PANCREATIC CARCINOMA

Stage IB (T2 N0 M0)

Stage IB (T2 N0 M0)

(Left) Axial CECT in a 34-year-old man with abdominal pain shows a 2.5 cm peripherally enhancing exophytic pancreatic neck mass ⮞ with central necrosis. The mass does not invade the portal vein confluence ⮕. *(Right)* Coronal CECT in the same patient shows the enhancing pancreatic neck mass ⮞ without invasion of the surrounding structures.

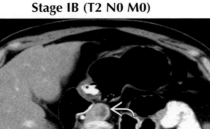

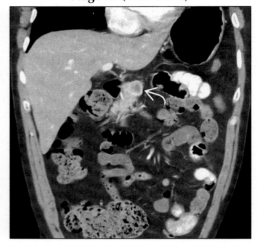

Stage IB (T2 N0 M0)

Stage IB (T2 N0 M0)

(Left) Axial CECT in a 22-year-old woman with MEN1 who presented with severe watery diarrhea shows a 3 cm enhancing mass ⮕ confined to the pancreas. *(Right)* Axial CECT in the same patient shows another 2 cm enhancing mass ⮞ in the tail of the pancreas without evidence of extension beyond the pancreas.

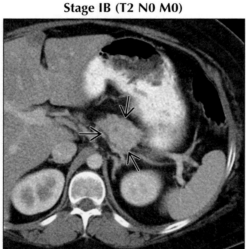

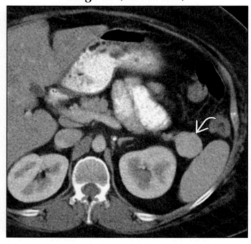

Stage IB (T2 N0 M0)

Stage IB (T2 N0 M0)

(Left) Axial CECT in the same patient shows the pancreatic tail mass ⮞ and a 3rd mass ⮞ at the junction of the body and tail. *(Right)* Frontal indium-111 pentetreotide scan in the same patient shows tracer accumulation in all 3 lesions ⮞ seen on the abdominal CT.

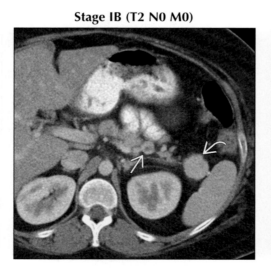

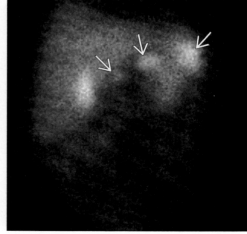

ENDOCRINE PANCREATIC CARCINOMA

Stage IB (T2 N0 M0)

Stage IB (T2 N0 M0)

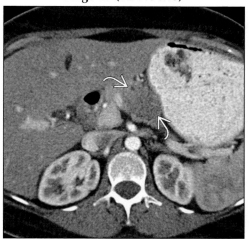
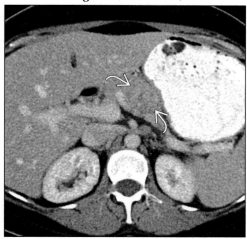

(Left) Axial CECT during the arterial phase in a 38-year-old woman shows a poorly enhancing 3 cm pancreatic body mass ➡. (Right) Axial CECT in the same patient during the portal venous phase shows increased enhancement of the pancreatic mass ➡ compared to the arterial phase. This illustrates the importance of obtaining images during both the arterial and venous phases of contrast enhancement since some tumors may not be seen on both phases.

Stage IB (T2 N0 M0)

Stage IB (T2 N0 M0)

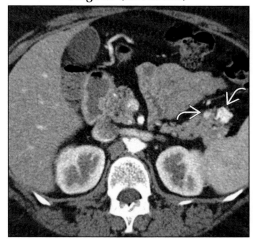
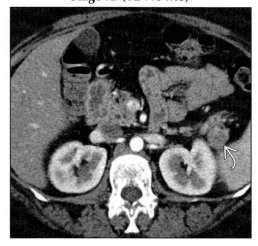

(Left) Axial CECT in a 30-year-old woman with MEN1 syndrome shows 2 enhancing pancreatic tail masses ➡. (Right) Axial CECT in the same patient during the arterial phase of contrast enhancement shows a 3rd pancreatic tail mass ➡ that enhances less than the 2 lesions seen previously. PNETs in patients with MEN1 can show variable enhancement patterns even in the same patient.

Stage IB (T2 N0 M0)

Stage IB (T2 N0 M0)

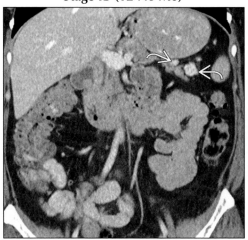
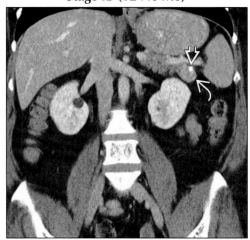

(Left) Coronal CECT in the same patient shows 2 pancreatic tail enhancing lesions ➡. (Right) Coronal CECT in the same patient during the portal venous phase shows increased enhancement of the 3rd lesion ➡ compared to the arterial phase. Focal area of calcification ➡ is seen in this lesion. Calcifications can occur in PNET and are more common in larger lesions.

ENDOCRINE PANCREATIC CARCINOMA

Stage IB (T2 N0 M0)

Stage IB (T2 N0 M0)

(Left) Axial CECT arterial phase in a 45-year-old woman with history of MEN1 and recurrent peptic ulcer disease shows a single 2.5 cm heterogeneously and intensely enhancing mass ➡ in the pancreatic tail representing a gastrinoma. *(Right)* Axial CECT portal venous phase in the same patient shows contrast retention within the pancreatic tail mass ➡.

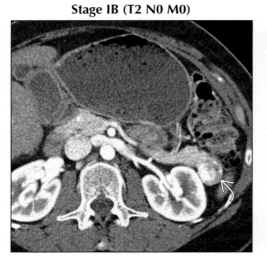

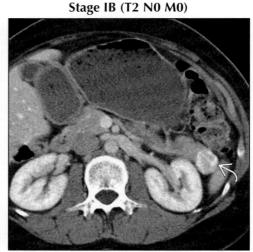

Stage IIA (T3 N0 M0)

Stage IIA (T3 N0 M0)

(Left) Axial CECT in a 62-year-old man shows a heterogeneous mass ➡ with cystic areas ➡ that is contiguous with the head of pancreas ➡ and anterior to the duodenum ➡. *(Right)* Axial CECT in the same patient shows the mixed solid/cystic mass ➡ with extension into the duodenum ➡. Tumors extending beyond the pancreas without involvement of the celiac or superior mesenteric arteries are considered T3 disease.

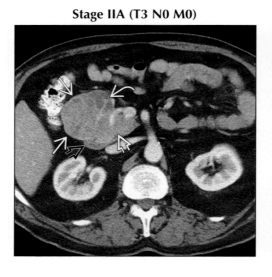

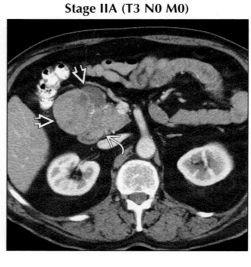

Stage IIA (T3 N0 M0)

Stage IIA (T3 N0 M0)

(Left) Coronal CECT in the same patient shows exophytic tumor ➡ arising from the head of pancreas ➡. *(Right)* Coronal CECT in the same patient shows small nodular extension into the wall of the duodenum ➡. Duodenal invasion was confirmed during surgery. On imaging, it may be difficult to differentiate tumors arising in this location from duodenal or ampullary carcinoids.

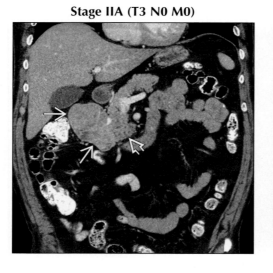

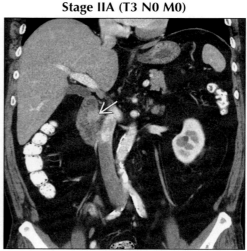

ENDOCRINE PANCREATIC CARCINOMA

Stage IIB (T2 N1 M0)

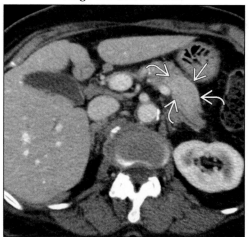

Stage IIB (T2 N1 M0)

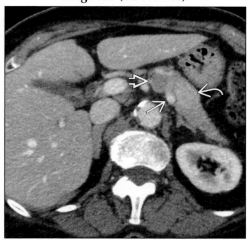

(Left) Axial CECT in a 77-year-old woman who underwent a CT for lower abdominal pain shows an incidental enhancing pancreatic tail mass ➡ that measured 3 cm. The pancreatic contour ➡ is smooth with no evidence of extension beyond the pancreas. (Right) Axial CECT in the same patient shows the upper end of the pancreatic mass ➡ as well as a poorly enhancing peripancreatic lymph node ➡. The pancreatic mass is clear of the splenic artery ➡.

Stage IIB (T2 N1 M0)

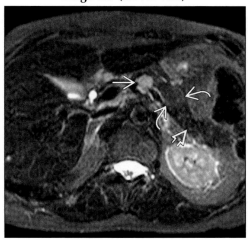

Stage IIB (T2 N1 M0)

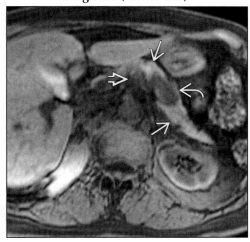

(Left) Axial T2WI FS MR in the same patient shows the pancreatic tail mass ➡ that is slightly hyperintense relative to the normal pancreas ➡. Note the high signal intensity peripancreatic node ➡. (Right) Axial pre-contrast VIBE in the same patient shows that the pancreatic tail mass ➡ is hypointense relative to the high signal intensity of the normal pancreas ➡. The peripancreatic node ➡ is also hypointense relative to the pancreas.

Stage IIB (T2 N1 M0)

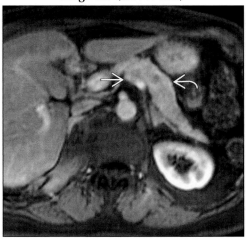

Stage IIB (T2 N1 M0)

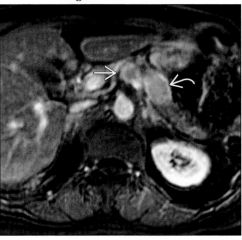

(Left) Axial T1WI C+ FS MR in the same patient during an early phase of contrast enhancement shows early enhancement of the pancreatic tail mass ➡, which is difficult to distinguish from the normal pancreas on this image. The peripancreatic node ➡ is also enhancing. (Right) Axial T2WI FS MR during a more delayed phase of contrast enhancement shows persistent enhancement of the pancreatic mass ➡ and peripheral enhancement of the peripancreatic node ➡.

ENDOCRINE PANCREATIC CARCINOMA

Stage III (T4 N1 M0)

Stage III (T4 N1 M0)

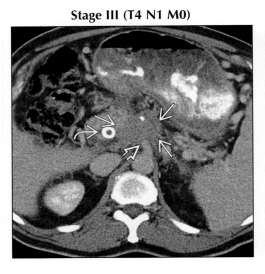 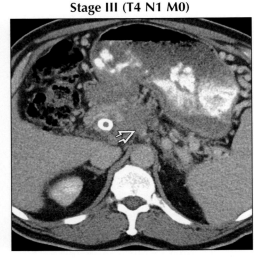

(Left) Axial CECT shows a poorly enhancing tumor ➡ that involves the celiac axis ➡ in a 59-year-old man who was found to have jaundice following cholecystectomy. ERCP and EUS were performed and revealed a tumor obstructing the common bile duct, and a biliary stent ➡ was placed. Biopsy showed a poorly differentiated PNET. *(Right)* Axial CECT in the same patient shows tumor involving the celiac axis ➡.

Stage III (T4 N1 M0)

Stage III (T4 N1 M0)

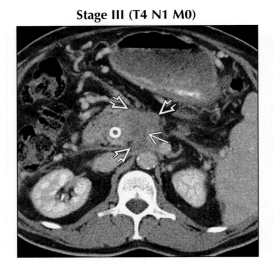 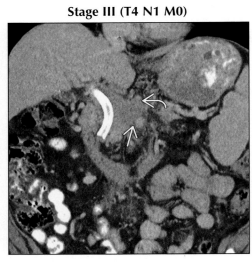

(Left) Axial CECT in the same patient shows tumor ➡ involving the superior mesenteric artery ➡. *(Right)* Coronal CECT in the same patient shows tumor invading the celiac artery ➡ and abutting the superior mesenteric artery ➡. The infiltrative pattern of this tumor is unusual for PNETs, which are usually well defined, and is likely due to the undifferentiated histological appearance.

Stage IV (T3 N0 M1)

Stage IV (T3 N0 M1)

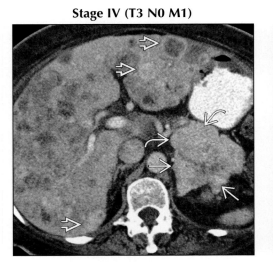 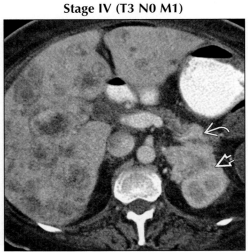

(Left) Axial CECT in a 50-year-old man who presented with abdominal pain shows a large, enhancing pancreatic tail mass ➡ that invades the retroperitoneum and the left adrenal gland ➡. Multiple liver metastatic lesions are present ➡, which show the characteristic peripheral pattern of enhancement. *(Right)* Axial CECT in the same patient shows the pancreatic tail mass ➡ invading the upper pole of the left kidney ➡.

ENDOCRINE PANCREATIC CARCINOMA

Stage IV (T2 N0 M1)

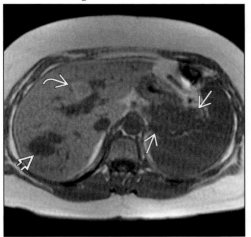

Stage IV (T2 N0 M1)

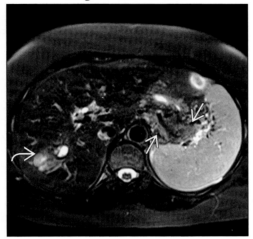

(Left) Axial T1WI MR in a 64-year-old woman who presented with right upper quadrant abdominal pain shows an intermediate signal intensity (relative to skeletal muscles), 5 cm, pancreatic body and tail mass ➡. Low signal intensity ➡ and slightly high signal intensity ➡ hepatic lesions are also seen. *(Right)* Axial T2WI FS MR in the same patient shows the pancreatic mass ➡ exhibiting low signal intensity. A heterogeneous liver lesion ➡ is present.

Stage IV (T2 N0 M1)

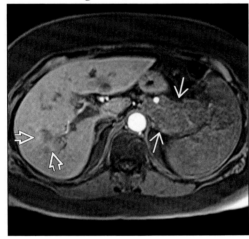

Stage IV (T2 N0 M1)

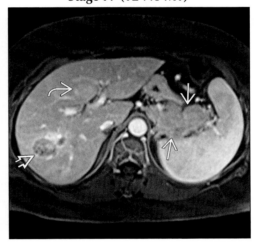

(Left) Axial T1WI C+ FS MR in the same patient shows the pancreatic mass ➡ with poor arterial enhancement. The liver lesion ➡ is starting to show enhancement during the arterial phase. *(Right)* Axial T1WI C+ FS MR in the same patient shows modest enhancement of the pancreatic mass ➡ and heterogeneous, mainly peripheral enhancement of 1 hepatic lesion ➡ and more diffuse enhancement of the other lesion ➡.

Stage IV (T2 N0 M1)

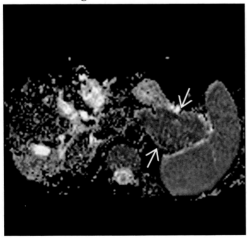

Stage IV (T2 N0 M1)

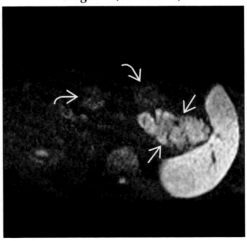

(Left) Axial DWI MR shows the pancreatic mass ➡ to be dark on the ADC map. *(Right)* Axial DWI MR using a b value of 800 shows the pancreatic mass ➡ as well as multiple hepatic lesions ➡ to be bright. This can be useful in detection of small lesions and may be helpful in staging by detection of metastatic liver lesions or lymph nodes.

ENDOCRINE PANCREATIC CARCINOMA

Stage IV (T3 N0 M1)

Stage IV (T3 N0 M1)

(Left) Coronal CECT in a different patient shows tumor invading the left adrenal gland ⇗ and multiple liver metastases ⇲. *(Right)* Coronal CECT in the same patient shows tumor invading the upper pole of the left kidney ⇗. Tumors extending beyond the pancreas without involvement of the celiac axis or the superior mesenteric artery are designated as T3.

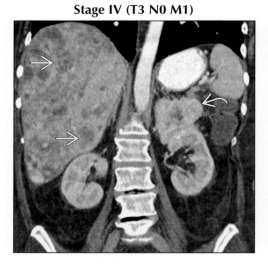
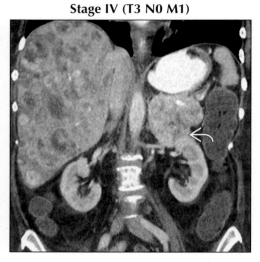

Stage IV (T3 N1 M1)

Stage IV (T3 N1 M1)

(Left) Axial CECT in a 25-year-old woman who presented with abdominal pain shows a heterogeneous pancreatic body and tail mass ⇗ with tumor filling the splenic vein ⇗ and extending into the portal vein at the confluence ⇲. *(Right)* Axial CECT in the same patient shows multiple liver metastases ⇲ and multiple enlarged celiac lymph nodes ⇗.

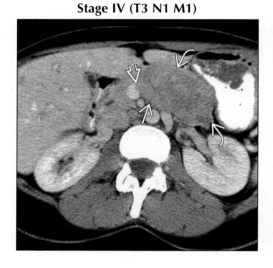
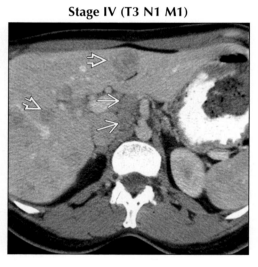

Stage IV (T3 N1 M1)

Stage IV (T3 N1 M1)

(Left) Axial PET/CT in the same patient shows increased metabolic activity in the pancreatic mass ⇗ and aortocaval lymph node ⇲. *(Right)* Axial PET/CT in the same patient shows increased metabolic activity in liver metastatic lesions ⇗ and gastrohepatic lymph node ⇗.

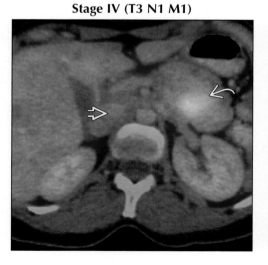
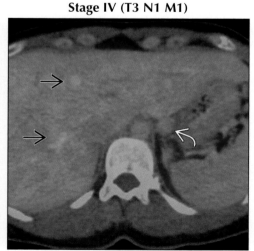

ENDOCRINE PANCREATIC CARCINOMA

Stage IV (T3 N1 M1)

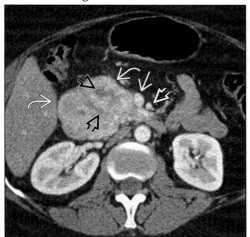

Stage IV (T3 N1 M1)

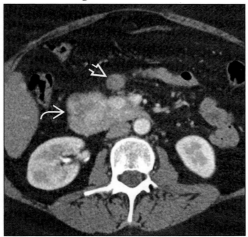

(Left) Axial CECT in a 48-year-old woman who presented with abdominal pain shows a large, intensely enhancing pancreatic head mass ➡. Areas of necrosis ⮂ are seen scattered within the mass. The mass does not involve the superior mesenteric vein ➡ or the superior mesenteric artery ⮂. (Right) Axial CECT in the same patient shows the pancreatic head mass ➡ and an enlarged peripancreatic lymph node ⮂.

Stage IV (T3 N1 M1)

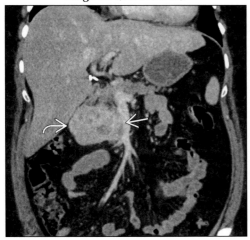

Stage IV (T3 N1 M1)

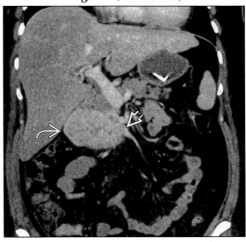

(Left) Coronal CECT in the same patient shows the pancreatic head enhancing mass ➡ abutting the superior mesenteric vein ➡ without actual invasion. (Right) Coronal CECT in the same patient shows the pancreatic head mass ➡ invading 1 of the tributaries of the superior mesenteric vein ⮂. Tumors extending beyond the pancreas without involvement of the celiac axis or the superior mesenteric artery are considered T3.

Stage IV (T3 N1 M1)

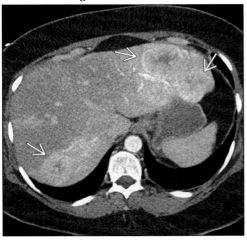

Stage IV (T3 N1 M1)

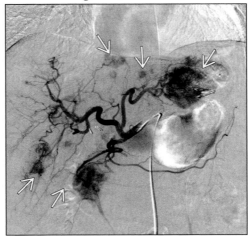

(Left) Axial CECT in the same patient shows multiple enhancing hepatic metastases ➡. The metastatic lesions morphologically resemble the primary tumor. (Right) Hepatic arteriogram obtained during chemoembolization of the hepatic lesions shows multiple highly vascular masses ➡ involving both lobes of the liver.

Stage IV (T3 N1 M1)

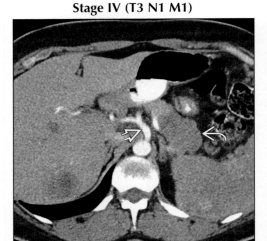

Stage IV (T3 N1 M1)

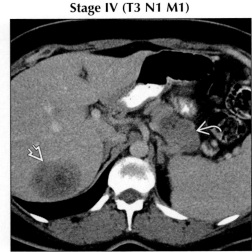

(Left) Axial CECT during the arterial phase in a 41-year-old woman shows a hypovascular mass ➡ in the tail of pancreas. The mass does not involve the celiac artery ➡. A subtle lesion is present in segment 7 of the right lobe of the liver. *(Right)* Axial CECT during the portal venous phase in the same patient again shows the pancreatic tail mass ➡. The hepatic metastatic lesion ➡ is better seen during the portal venous phase.

Stage IV (T3 N1 M1)

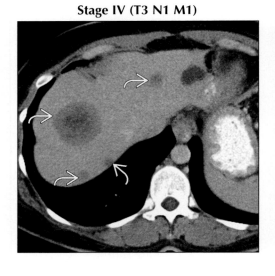

Stage IV (T3 N1 M1)

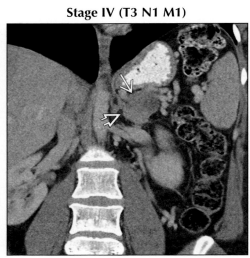

(Left) Axial CECT during the portal venous phase in the same patient shows multiple hepatic lesions ➡. The lesions are hypoattenuating relative to the liver during the portal venous phase. *(Right)* Coronal CECT in the same patient shows pancreatic tail mass ➡ invading the splenic vein ➡.

Stage IV (T3 N1 M1)

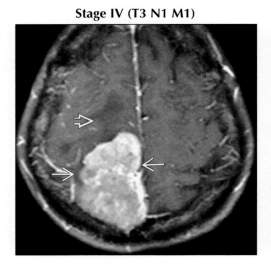

Stage IV (T3 N1 M1)

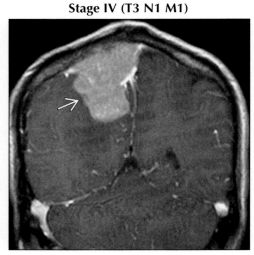

(Left) Axial T1WI C+ FS MR in the same patient, presenting with headache 2 years after the initial presentation, shows a dural-based extraaxial intensely enhancing right parietal mass ➡ surrounded by vasogenic edema ➡. *(Right)* Coronal T1WI C+ FS MR in the same patient shows the dural-based extraaxial mass ➡. The lesion was found to represent metastatic neuroendocrine tumor during surgery.

ENDOCRINE PANCREATIC CARCINOMA

Late Metastases from PNET

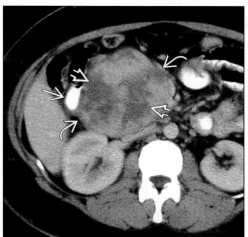

Late Metastases from PNET

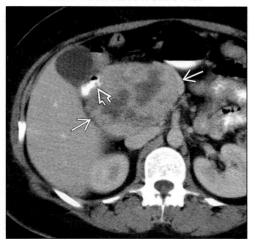

(Left) Axial CECT in a 22-year-old woman who presented with abdominal pain shows a large enhancing pancreatic head mass ➡ with areas of necrosis ➡. The mass is inseparable from the duodenum ➡. *(Right)* Axial CECT in the same patient shows the pancreatic head mass ➡ involving the duodenum ➡. No liver metastases were present at the initial presentation. Initial staging was stage IIB (T3 N0 M0).

Late Metastases from PNET

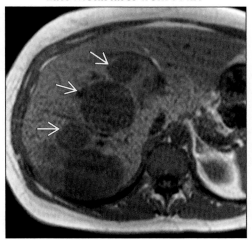

Late Metastases from PNET

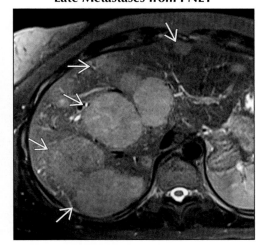

(Left) Axial T1WI MR in the same patient 2 years later during a routine follow-up shows multiple low signal intensity liver lesions ➡. *(Right)* Axial T2WI FS MR in the same patient shows multiple hepatic lesions ➡ with increased signal intensity relative to the liver.

Late Metastases from PNET

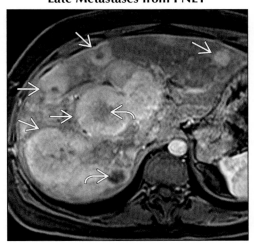

Late Metastases from PNET

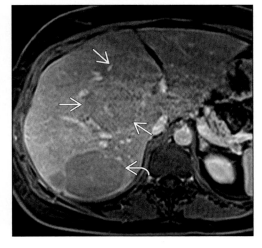

(Left) Axial T1WI C+ FS MR during the arterial phase in the same patient shows arterially enhancing hepatic lesions ➡ with central low signal intensity ➡. *(Right)* Axial T1WI C+ FS MR during the portal venous phase in the same patient shows that most of the lesions ➡ are isointense relative to the liver, and the larger lesion ➡ in segment 7 is hypointense relative to the liver. Biopsy showed metastatic neuroendocrine tumor.

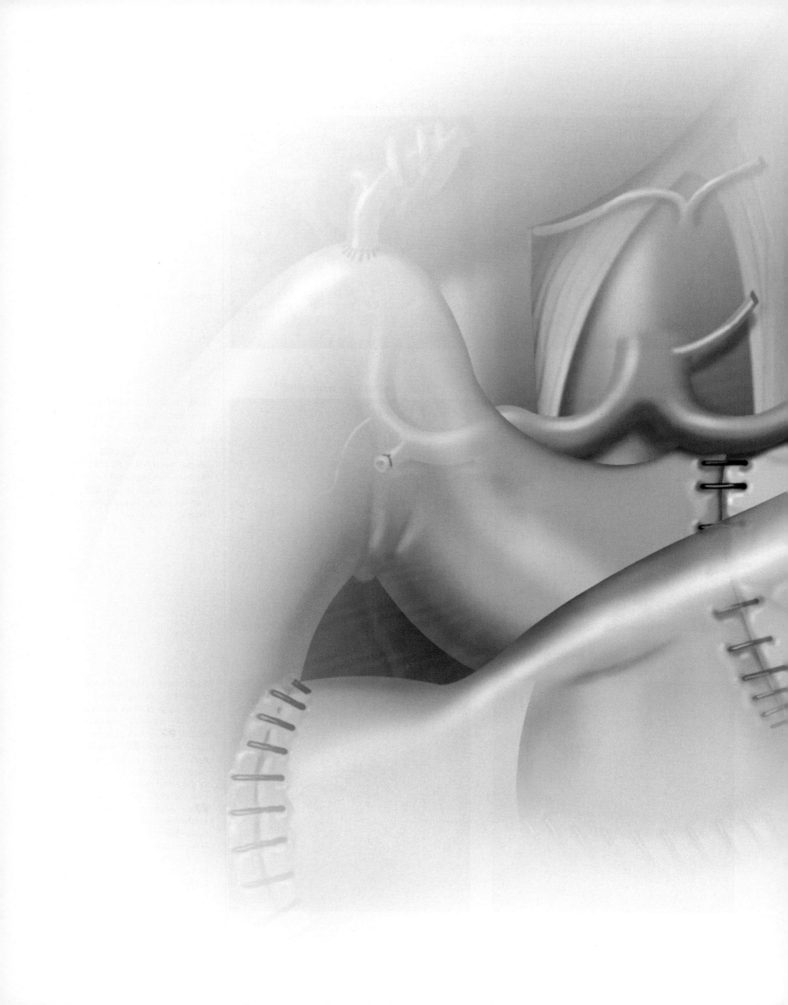

Exocrine Pancreatic Carcinoma

EXOCRINE PANCREATIC CARCINOMA

(T) Primary Tumor

Adapted from 7th edition AJCC Staging Forms.

TNM	Definitions
TX	Primary tumor cannot be assessed
T0	No evidence of primary tumor
Tis	Carcinoma in situ*
T1	Tumor limited to the pancreas, ≤ 2 cm in greatest dimension
T2	Tumor limited to the pancreas, > 2 cm in greatest dimension
T3	Tumor extends beyond the pancreas but without involvement of the celiac axis or the superior mesenteric artery
T4	Tumor involves the celiac axis or the superior mesenteric artery (unresectable primary tumor)

(N) Regional Lymph Nodes

NX	Regional lymph nodes cannot be assessed
N0	No regional lymph node metastasis
N1	Regional lymph node metastasis

(M) Distant Metastasis

M0	No distant metastasis
M1	Distant metastasis

This also includes the "PanInIII" classification.

AJCC Stages/Prognostic Groups

Adapted from 7th edition AJCC Staging Forms.

Stage	T	N	M
0	Tis	N0	M0
IA	T1	N0	M0
IB	T2	N0	M0
IIA	T3	N0	M0
IIB	T1	N1	M0
	T2	N1	M0
	T3	N1	M0
III	T4	Any N	M0
IV	Any T	Any N	M1

Tis

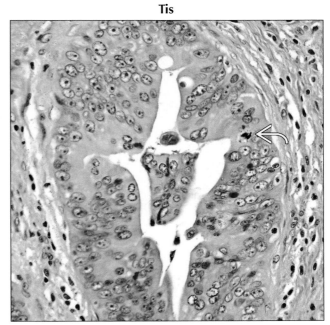

H&E stained section shows carcinoma in situ (Tis) involving an interlobular duct ➡ with surrounding fibrosis. The portion of the duct in the upper right portion of the image ⏩ demonstrates high-grade dysplasia without invasion of the basement membrane. (Original magnification 100x.)

Tis

High-power view (400x) of the right upper portion of the previous image shows neoplastic epithelial cells, which are characterized by increased nuclear to cytoplasmic ratio and haphazard arrangement of atypical nuclei. Additionally, the atypical nuclei are conspicuous, vesicular, and chromatic. Mitotic figures ➡ are easily found.

T1

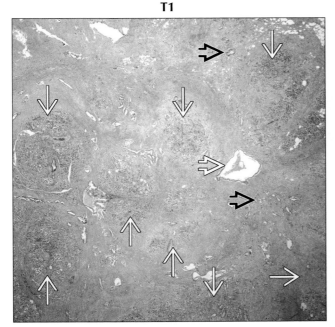

H&E stained section shows chronic pancreatitis with considerable loss of unevenly distributed acinar tissue ➡ with intervening fibrosis and a few dilated ducts with inspissated secretions ⏩. Scattered foci of well-differentiated ductal adenocarcinoma ⏩ are present. (Original magnification 20x.)

T1

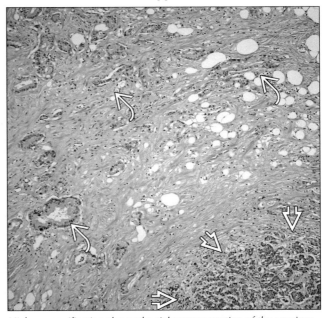

Higher magnification shows the right upper portion of the previous image. The left upper portion of this image demonstrates invasive well-differentiated ductal adenocarcinoma ➡. Pancreatic islet cells ⏩ are seen in the lower right portion of this image. (Original magnification 100x.)

EXOCRINE PANCREATIC CARCINOMA

T1

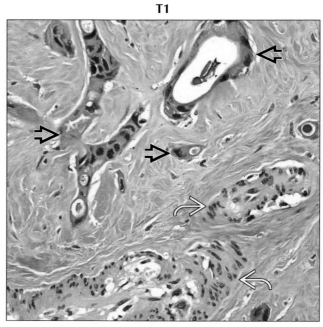

H&E stained section shows a ≤ 2 cm pancreatic adenocarcinoma in the left upper portion of the image that is confined to the pancreas, consistent with T1 disease. Note the interface between the pancreas and the peripancreatic fat ▣. (Original magnification 40x.)

T1

Higher power view of the previous image shows neoplastic cells arranged in irregular glands ▣ invading into a densely fibrotic stroma (wavy pink areas). Several nerves are seen in the lower portion of the image ▣. (Original magnification 400x.)

T3

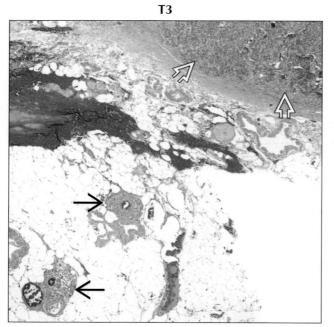

Low-power H&E stained section shows pancreatic tissue ▣ in the right upper portion of the image. Two small foci of pancreatic adenocarcinoma ▣ are present in the peripancreatic fat. (Original magnification 20x.)

TX

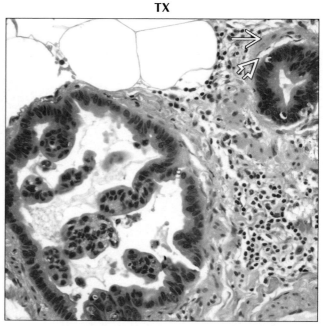

High-power view (400x) of pancreatic adenocarcinoma shows neoplastic glands expanding the lumina of 2 vessels. A slit-like space ▣ represents a portion of the lumen lined by endothelial cells ▣. Lymphatic and venous invasion have been combined into lymphovascular invasion for collection by cancer registrars.

EXOCRINE PANCREATIC CARCINOMA

T1

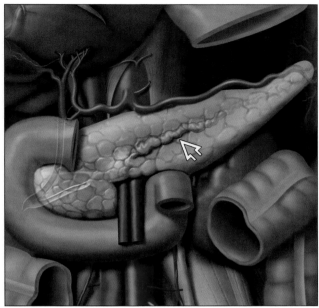

Graphic depicts a tumor ≤ 2 cm without extension beyond the pancreas, consistent with T1 disease. In this case, there is upstream pancreatic dilation ⮞. This is a resectable tumor.

T2

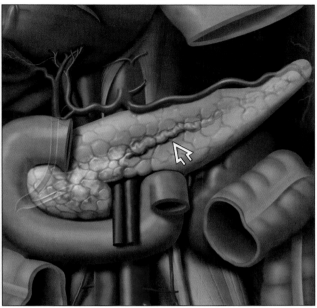

Graphic depict a tumor measuring > 2 cm confined to the pancreas, consistent with T2 disease. Note upstream pancreatic ductal dilation ⮞. This is a resectable tumor.

T3

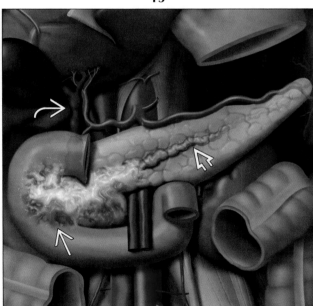

Graphic depicts a resectable tumor that invades into the duodenum ➡ and produces a "double duct" sign by obstructing and distending the pancreatic ⮞ and common bile ducts ➡. Tumors that extend beyond the pancreas but do not involve the superior mesenteric or celiac arteries are designated T3.

T3

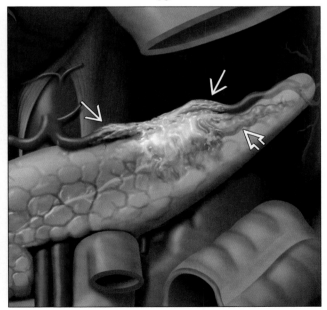

This pancreatic tail tumor extends beyond the pancreas and invades the splenic artery. Tumor tracks along the perivascular, perineural, &/or perilymphatic tissues toward the splenic hilum and celiac axis ⮞. There is upstream pancreatic ductal dilation ⮞. This is a borderline resectable tumor.

EXOCRINE PANCREATIC CARCINOMA

T3

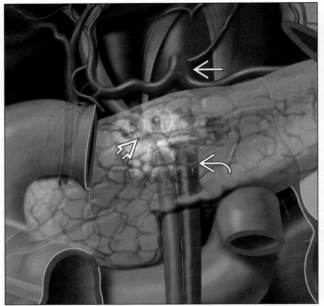

Graphic depicts tumor that extends beyond the pancreas posteriorly and invades the confluence of the superior mesenteric, splenic, and main portal veins ➡. Tumors that extend beyond the pancreas but do not involve the superior mesenteric ➡ or celiac ➡ arteries, such as this borderline resectable tumor, are designated T3.

T3

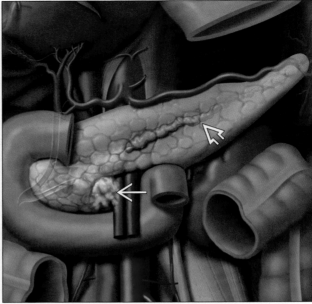

This pancreatic head tumor extends beyond the pancreas and invades the upper superior mesenteric vein ➡. However, because the superior mesenteric and celiac arteries are spared, this borderline resectable tumor is classified as T3. Upstream pancreatic ductal dilation is present ➡.

T4

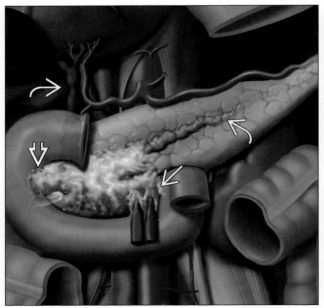

Graphic depicts tumor invading the superior mesenteric artery and vein ➡. Additionally, there is invasion of the duodenum ➡ and a "double duct" sign ➡. This unresectable tumor is classified as T4, as any tumors that invade the superior mesenteric or celiac arteries are designated T4.

T4

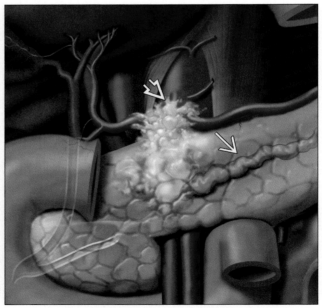

Graphic depicts tumor that extends beyond the pancreas and invades the celiac axis ➡, as well as the proximal common hepatic and splenic arteries. Upstream pancreatic ductal dilation is present ➡. Involvement of the celiac axis results in a T4 classification. This is an unresectable tumor.

EXOCRINE PANCREATIC CARCINOMA

Peripancreatic Lymph Node Groups

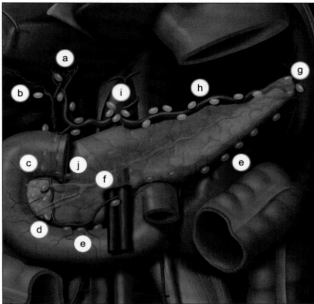

Graphic depicts peripancreatic lymph node groups: a) hepatic, b) cystic duct, c) posterior pancreaticoduodenal, d) anterior pancreaticoduodenal, e) inferior, f) superior mesenteric, g) splenic hilar, h) superior, i) celiac, and j) pyloric.

Whipple Anatomy

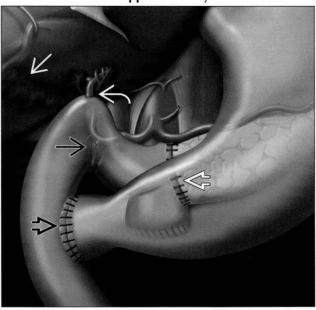

Graphic depicts Whipple anatomy: Pancreaticojejunostomy ▣, choledochojejunostomy ▣, gastrojejunostomy or duodenojejunostomy ▣, and cholecystectomy ▣. The pylorus may be removed or preserved, depending on extent of disease and surgeon preference. Note the ligated gastroduodenal artery ▣.

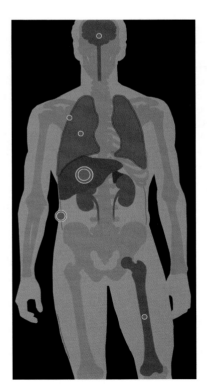

METASTASES, ORGAN FREQUENCY

Liver	43-62%
Peritoneum	27-43%
Other (bone, brain, pleura, lung, etc.)	27%

EXOCRINE PANCREATIC CARCINOMA

OVERVIEW

General Comments
- Exocrine pancreatic cancer: Histopathologically heterogeneous group of carcinomas

Classification
- Ductal origin (> 95%)
  - Ductal adenocarcinoma (> 85%)
  - Cystic mucinous carcinoma
  - Noncystic mucinous carcinoma (colloid carcinoma)
    - Associated with more protracted course
  - Undifferentiated carcinoma
    - Sarcomatoid (spindle cell)
    - Anaplastic giant cell
    - Carcinosarcoma
    - Undifferentiated carcinoma with osteoclast-like giant cells
  - Adenosquamous carcinoma
  - Intraductal papillary mucinous carcinoma
  - Signet ring cell carcinoma
  - Serous cystadenocarcinoma (very rare)
  - Medullary carcinoma (very rare)
- Acinar origin (1-2%)
  - Acinar cell carcinoma
- Mixed origin
  - Mixed ductal-endocrine carcinoma (rare)
    - Behaves similar to ductal carcinoma
  - Mixed ductal-acinar carcinoma (rare)
    - Behaves similar to ductal carcinoma
  - Mixed acinar-endocrine carcinoma
    - Behaves similar to acinar carcinoma
  - Pancreatoblastoma
    - Typically includes all 3 cell types (endocrine, ductal, acinar) but composed of cells of acinar origin
    - Typically in children (peak age: 4 years) with small 2nd peak in 4th decade of life
- Supportive element origin
  - Squamous cell carcinoma (very rare)
- Unknown origin
  - Solid pseudopapillary carcinoma
- Borderline, indolent, or premalignant neoplasms (up to 2% of exocrine pancreatic cancers arise from these)
  - Intraductal papillary mucinous neoplasm (IPMN)
  - Pancreatic intraepithelial neoplasia III (PanInIII)
  - Mucinous cystadenoma
  - Intraductal oncocytic papillary neoplasm (very rare)
  - Solid pseudopapillary tumor
- According to 2010 AJCC staging guidelines, pancreatic exocrine and endocrine tumors now utilize same staging system, which was previously reserved for exocrine pancreatic carcinoma

PATHOLOGY

Routes of Spread
- **Local invasion**
  - Vascular invasion
    - Celiac trunk
    - Superior mesenteric artery (SMA)
    - Common and proper hepatic artery
    - Gastroduodenal artery (GDA)
    - Splenic artery
    - Portal vein
    - Superior mesenteric vein (SMV)
    - Splenic vein
  - Primary tumor in pancreatic head &/or uncinate
    - Duodenum
    - Stomach
    - Inferior vena cava
    - Aorta
    - Right renal artery
  - Primary tumor in pancreatic body &/or tail
    - Transverse colon and mesocolon
    - Stomach
    - Left renal vein
    - Left adrenal gland
    - Superior pole of left kidney
    - Spleen
    - Splenic flexure of colon
    - Inferior vena cava
    - Aorta
- **Lymphatic spread**
  - Pancreatic head and uncinate tumors
    - Anterior and superior pancreatic head
      - Drain along anterior superior pancreaticoduodenal vessels to pyloric and celiac axis nodes
    - Posterior and superior pancreatic head
      - Drain along posterior superior pancreaticoduodenal vessels to pyloric and celiac axis nodes or along common bile duct to portal vein and to hepatic hilar nodes
    - Inferior pancreatic head and uncinate
      - Drain along inferior pancreaticoduodenal vessels to superior mesenteric and paraaortic nodes
  - Pancreatic body and tail tumors
    - Drain either along splenic artery to celiac axis nodes or splenic hilar nodes
- **Perineural/perivascular spread**
  - Pathways similar to lymphatic spread of tumor
  - 80% of pancreatic carcinomas demonstrate perineural invasion on pathology
- **Hematogenous spread**
  - Occurs late in disease, but common for patients to have hematogenous metastases at time of presentation
  - Hepatic metastases are common
    - Pancreas drained by portal venous structures
    - Hepatic sinusoids lack basement membrane and are relatively porous, which is thought to allow metastases to permeate into space of Disse
  - Distant hematogenous metastases are less common and generally only seen in advanced disease (lung, pleura, adrenal glands, brain, bone, other)
- **Peritoneal spread**
  - Common location of metastatic disease

General Features
- Comments
  - Majority of pancreatic carcinomas arise from ductal structures
    - Ductal tissue represents 15% of volume of pancreas, remaining 85% is acinar tissue
    - Ductal tissue is only pancreatic tissue exposed to external carcinogens

EXOCRINE PANCREATIC CARCINOMA

- ○ Primary tumor location
  - Head (60%)
  - Body (20%)
  - Tail (5%)
  - Diffuse (15%)
- Etiology
  - ○ Risk factors
    - Tobacco
      - 2-3x increased risk
      - Smoking responsible for 20-35% of pancreatic carcinomas
    - Increased BMI
    - Occupational exposure
      - β-naphthylamine, benzidine (used in dye production)
      - Metal-refining chemicals
    - Family history
    - Hereditary syndromes
      - BRCA2, Peutz-Jeghers (STK1 gene), atypical multiple mole-melanoma syndrome (p16 gene), hereditary nonpolyposis colorectal cancer (MLH1 and MSH2 genes), familial pancreatic cancer (PALLD gene)
      - 40-75% lifetime risk for pancreatic carcinoma in patients with familial chronic pancreatitis
    - Chronic pancreatitis
    - Diabetes mellitus (type 2)
    - Beckwith-Wiedemann or familial polyposis coli syndromes (pancreatoblastoma)
- Epidemiology & cancer incidence
  - ○ 4th leading cause of cancer death in USA
  - ○ Estimated 37,680 new cases in 2008; estimated 34,290 deaths in 2008
  - ○ Age-adjusted incidence
    - 11.3/100,000 (2000-2003)
    - Lifetime risk of 1.3%
  - ○ Racial incidence
    - African-American 14.9/100,000
    - Caucasian-American 11.2/100,000
    - Native-American 10.8/100,000
    - Hispanic-American 10.3/100,000
    - Asian-American 9.0/100,000
  - ○ M = F
  - ○ Median age at diagnosis: 72 years

Gross Pathology & Surgical Features

- Scirrhous mass with ill-defined borders
- Difficult to differentiate macroscopically from benign scar tissue within pancreas (i.e., chronic pancreatitis)

Microscopic Pathology

- H&E
  - ○ Ductal adenocarcinoma
    - Often well differentiated with recognizable ductal structures that are occasionally difficult to distinguish from benign ductal epithelium
      - May be poorly differentiated with no recognizable ductal structures
    - Ductal adenocarcinoma cells are usually cuboidal with nuclear atypia and form duct-like structures
    - Highly infiltrative
      - Desmoplastic stroma with abundant fibrosis and inflammation is characteristic
      - Tumors often have more stromal than ductal tissue

- Up to 80% of tumors have microscopic perineural invasion
- Vascular invasion is common
  - May manifest as well-formed ductal elements within vascular spaces, which is rare with other tumors
- Squamous differentiation may rarely occur in ductal adenocarcinoma
  - Pure squamous cell carcinoma without ductal elements is very rare
- Undifferentiated carcinomas may be composed of epithelioid &/or spindle cells
  - May rarely include bone or cartilage components
  - May include nonneoplastic osteoclast-like giant cells
  - ○ Acinar cell carcinoma
    - Monotonous and highly cellular tumor arranged in solid sheets and nests with foci of acinar or glandular cells
    - Lacks desmoplastic stroma seen in ductal adenocarcinoma
    - Cells classically demonstrate apical eosinophilic granularity secondary to zymogen granules (trypsin, lipase, and chymotrypsin)
  - ○ Polyphenotypic carcinoma
    - Mixed acinar-endocrine, mixed ductal-acinar, mixed ductal-endocrine, and pancreatoblastoma are rare tumors
    - Pancreatoblastoma is predominantly composed of cells of acinar lineage
      - "Squamoid nest" is a characteristic finding
- Special stains
  - ○ Immunohistochemical stains for trypsin, lipase, and chymotrypsin are useful for diagnosing acinar cell carcinoma

IMAGING FINDINGS

Detection

- **Abdominal ultrasound**
  - ○ Primary tumor
    - Generally ill defined and hypoechoic but can be heterogeneous or echogenic
    - May have increased color Doppler signal
    - May efface or obliterate normal planes between pancreas and vessels in setting of vascular invasion
    - Enlarged lymph nodes may be present
  - ○ May present as pancreatic &/or biliary ductal dilation without mass
- **NECT**
  - ○ Generally isodense to normal pancreatic parenchyma unless extensive necrosis or cystic changes are present
    - Cystic changes are uncommon
    - Occasionally pseudocysts may be present
  - ○ Calcifications are rare
- **Pancreatic protocol CECT**
  - ○ Primary tumor
    - Typically ill-defined margins and delayed enhancement

- Isoenhancing or avid early arterial enhancing lesions are less common
  - Detection rate for tumors ≤ 2 cm (71%), > 2 cm (89%)
  - Invasion of extrapancreatic structures
  - "Double duct" sign
    - Nonspecific for pancreatic mass
    - Suggestive of pancreatic head or ampullary mass
    - Pancreatic ductal dilation may be absent in setting of pancreas divisum
  - Distended pancreatic duct distal to tumor
    - Tumor itself may be difficult to appreciate if isoattenuating &/or small
    - Often seen in conjunction with pancreatic atrophy distal to tumor
  - Massively distended gallbladder
    - Courvoisier sign
  - Disruption of normal pancreatic architecture or contour abnormalities
    - Abnormal focal increased tissue density in patients with fatty atrophy of pancreas
  - Diffuse pancreatic carcinoma can mimic acute pancreatitis
  - Acinar cell carcinoma imaging characteristics
    - Well marginated (90%)
    - Partially or completely exophytic (80%)
    - Typically homogeneously hypoenhancing to pancreas on venous phase imaging; reports of early arterial enhancement
    - Oval or round
    - Solid when small, can have large areas of cystic necrosis if tumor is large
    - May have calcifications
    - Often larger than ductal adenocarcinoma at time of diagnosis
  - Vascular involvement
    - Distended mesenteric venous collaterals in setting of superior mesenteric, portal, or splenic venous obstruction or occlusion
    - Perivascular soft tissue cuffs indicating perineural, perivascular, or lymphatic disease
    - Irregular narrowing of normal contours of arteries or veins (SMA, celiac, portal vein, SMV, gastroduodenal artery [GDA], hepatic arteries)
      - Teardrop morphology of SMV implies venous involvement
  - Local nodal involvement
    - Should be identified, but CT is poor at prognosticating presence of metastatic disease
    - Hepatic artery lymph node (at origin of gastroduodenal artery) is important to identify if present, regardless of size
      - If diseased at pathology, associated survival rate is similar to patients with liver or peritoneal metastases
  - Metastatic disease
    - Regional lymphadenopathy
      - Lymphadenopathy beyond surgical bed is considered metastatic disease
    - Hepatic metastases
    - Peritoneal metastases
    - Other distant metastases are uncommon (lung, brain, pleura, adrenal gland, bone)

- **MR**
  - T1WI: Hypointense relative to bright pancreas
  - T2WI: Variable signal relative to pancreas but often hypointense and difficult to visualize unless there is substantial necrosis
  - "Duct penetrating" sign to distinguish inflammatory mass from pancreatic cancer
    - Seen more often in pancreatitis (85%) than pancreatic cancer (4%)
    - Defined as either normal or stenotic main pancreatic duct without ductal wall irregularity penetrating pancreatic mass
    - Pancreatic cancer tends to obstruct duct or demonstrate ductal irregularity of intratumoral main pancreatic duct
  - Post-contrast images: Similar enhancement characteristics to CT
    - Tumor margins are generally ill defined and infiltrative
    - Typically tumors demonstrate delayed enhancement compared to pancreatic parenchyma secondary to extensive desmoplastic reaction
- **Endoscopic ultrasound (EUS)**
  - Useful in cases where pancreatic or biliary ductal dilation is present but no mass is identified on CT or MR
  - More sensitive than CT for small masses
    - EUS reported to have nearly 100% detection of tumors < 1.6 cm, whereas CT may miss up to 33%
- **PET/CT**
  - Generally demonstrates increased FDG uptake, although highly mucinous tumors may have areas without significant uptake
  - False-negatives with lesions < 8 mm
  - Blood glucose > 150 mg/dL may result in false-negatives
- **ERCP**
  - Irregular, nodular, rat-tailed eccentric obstruction
  - "Double duct" sign
  - Generally used for stenting and biliary decompression
  - Intraductal brushings can provide tissue diagnosis, but yield is significantly lower than EUS

Staging
- General principles
  - Staging is based on size of primary tumor, extrapancreatic invasion, local nodal involvement, vascular invasion, and distant metastatic disease
  - Staging is designated by modality (CT, EUS, MR, surgical) to convey inherent advantages and limitations of each method
  - Biopsy proof of malignancy is not necessary prior to surgical resection if there is high index of suspicion and should not delay definitive therapy
  - Biopsy of metastatic lesion is preferred over sampling of primary tumor, if possible
  - Endoscopic ultrasound-guided FNA tissue sampling is preferred to percutaneous biopsy to decrease risk of peritoneal seeding
- **Pancreatic protocol CT**

EXOCRINE PANCREATIC CARCINOMA

○ Primary method of staging due to wide availability and ability to assess local tumor invasion, presence of lymph nodes, vascular involvement, and distal metastases

○ Excellent at determining unresectability of tumors (89-100%) but less accurate for predicting tumor resectability (45-79%)

○ Good for identifying regional lymph nodes, but poor at prognosticating whether they are malignant

○ Allows for concurrent evaluation of metastatic disease
  ■ However, CT is unable to resolve low volume peritoneal or hepatic metastatic disease
    – Found intraoperatively in up to 20% of cases deemed resectable by CT

○ CT angiography can by used for presurgical planning and to identify variant vascular anatomy

○ If distant metastases are present, there is no need for diagnostic endoscopic ultrasound

○ Pancreatic protocol CECT for staging should ideally be performed prior to biliary decompression
  ■ Eliminate confounding post-procedure inflammatory findings that can mimic local invasion or lymphatic/perineural spread of tumor

• **Endoscopic ultrasound**
  ○ Complementary with CT for diagnosis and staging
  ○ Good for evaluation of venous involvement
    ■ 80% sensitive and 85% specific for involvement of portal and superior mesenteric veins
  ○ Better at prognosticating malignancy in regional lymph nodes than CT
    ■ Findings of malignancy
      – Size (> 1 cm)
      – Distinct margins
      – Hypoechogenicity
      – Round shape
    ■ If all 4 findings are present in same lymph node, there is 80% likelihood of malignant involvement
  ○ Allows for fine needle aspiration to establish tissue diagnosis
  ○ Limited availability and operator dependent
  ○ Limited evaluation of superior mesenteric artery and uncinate process of pancreas in some patients
  ○ Celiac plexus neurolysis can be performed

• **MR**
  ○ Rarely used as primary modality for staging unless patient has renal disease or contrast allergy
  ○ Occasionally used for staging if MRCP desired
  ○ Used as problem-solving tool
    ■ Improved tissue contrast may identify primary tumor in cases where it is isoattenuating to pancreas on CT
    ■ MR is slightly more accurate (94%) than CT (87%) in identifying hepatic metastases
  ○ Poor at evaluating peritoneal metastases

• **PET/CT**
  ○ Rarely used as primary staging tool but may be used for evaluating for recurrence
  ○ Generally used as problem-solving tool
  ○ Good for evaluating regional lymphadenopathy and findings suspicious for distant metastasis

• **Staging laparoscopy ± ultrasound**

○ Occasionally performed to rule out subradiologic metastatic disease in patients at a high risk of disseminated disease, as indicated by
  ■ Borderline resectable disease
  ■ Markedly elevated CA-19.9 (> 150)
  ■ Body or tail tumors
  ■ Large primary tumor

○ Can be used to further evaluate questionable hepatic or peritoneal lesions on cross-sectional imaging or in setting of low volume ascites

○ Malignant cytology from peritoneal washings is considered M1 disease

○ Detects occult metastases not seen on staging CT in 24-31%
  ■ 7% had positive cytology from intraoperative peritoneal washings as only evidence of occult metastatic disease

• **Exploratory laparotomy**
  ○ Performed if tumor deemed resectable or following neoadjuvant therapy for borderline resectable tumors
  ○ Allows for palliative procedures in tumors deemed unresectable at time of laparotomy

Restaging

• Following resection and adjuvant therapy, surveillance recommended every 3-6 months for 2 years and yearly thereafter
  ○ Surveillance includes
    ■ CECT
    ■ CA-19.9 levels
    ■ History and physical exam
    ■ PET/CT or MR may be used for problem solving in certain cases

• Findings of recurrence
  ○ Local tumor recurrence in surgical bed
  ○ Metastatic disease (regional lymphadenopathy, liver, and peritoneum are most common)
  ○ Increasing periarterial soft tissue
    ■ Must distinguish from post-treatment scarring
    ■ May represent recurrent local tumor or perineural/lymphatic disease progression

Criteria for Resectability

• **Resectable**
  ○ Clean fat plane surrounding superior mesenteric and celiac arteries and patent superior mesenteric and portal veins
  ○ No distant metastatic disease

• **Borderline resectable**
  ○ If high likelihood of tumor resection resulting in R1 (microscopic disease at surgical margins) or R2 (gross disease at margins), neoadjuvant chemoradiation is recommended prior to attempted resection
  ○ Head or body tumors
    ■ Severe unilateral (< 180°) SMV &/or PV abutment
    ■ Tumor abuts (< 180°) SMA
      – More likely to be resectable if this abutment manifests as soft tissue stranding or has convex margin with SMA
    ■ GDA encased up to origin from common hepatic artery
    ■ Short segment involvement of hepatic artery without celiac involvement

- – Criterion is only used at some very select high volume centers
  - ▪ Limited tumor involvement of inferior vena cava
  - ▪ Short segment SMV occlusion if SMV is patent both proximally and distally
  - ▪ Short segment occlusion of SMV, portal vein (PV), or SMV-PV confluence if involvement is amenable to vascular reconstruction
    - – Criterion is used at some high volume centers
    - – Venous structures proximal and distal to occlusion must be patent and amenable to reconstruction
    - – If splenic vein is preserved and < 2 cm of vein is resected, anastomosis can usually be performed without interposition graft
    - – If splenic vein is ligated and < 2-3 cm of vein is resected, anastomosis can usually be performed without interposition graft
    - – If primary anastomosis cannot be performed, interposition graft (internal jugular vein) may be placed
  - ▪ Colon or mesocolon invasion
  - ○ Tail tumors
    - ▪ Adrenal, colon, mesocolon, or renal invasion
- **Unresectable**
  - ○ Pancreatic head tumors
    - ▪ Distant metastases
    - ▪ SMA or celiac encasement
    - ▪ SMV &/or PV occlusion
    - ▪ Aortic or IVC invasion
    - ▪ SMV invasion below transverse mesocolon
  - ○ Pancreatic body tumors
    - ▪ Distant metastases
    - ▪ SMA or celiac encasement
    - ▪ SMV &/or PV occlusion
    - ▪ Aortic invasion
  - ○ Pancreatic tail tumors
    - ▪ Distant metastases
    - ▪ SMA or celiac encasement
    - ▪ Rib or vertebral body invasion
  - ○ Nodal status
    - ▪ Metastatic disease to lymph nodes beyond field of resection

CLINICAL ISSUES

Presentation
- Jaundice
  - ○ Courvoisier's law: Jaundice and palpable gallbladder
- Back pain
- Weight loss
- Dark urine
- Abdominal pain
- Light or floating stools
- Nausea
- Venous thromboembolic disease
- Lipase hypersecretion syndrome
  - ○ May be seen in acinar cell carcinoma secondary to lipase secretion
  - ○ Subcutaneous fat necrosis, polyarthralgia, and eosinophilia

Cancer Natural History & Prognosis
- Pancreatic adenocarcinoma

- ○ Overall median survival is 3-6 months with 5-year survival rate of 3-6%
- ○ Median survival in resected patients is 15-19 months with 5-year survival rate of 10-25%
  - ▪ Only 10-15% of patients have resectable tumors
- Acinar cell carcinoma
  - ○ More indolent course than ductal carcinomas
  - ○ Tend to present at younger age (56 vs. 70)
  - ○ Overall 5-year survival rate (43%)
  - ○ Resected 5-year survival rate (72%)
  - ○ Unresectable disease 5-year survival rate (22%)

Treatment Options
- Major treatment alternatives
  - ○ Surgical resection
  - ○ Chemoradiation
  - ○ Systemic chemotherapy
- Treatment options by stage
  - ○ Stage I or II: Resectable or borderline resectable
    - ▪ Treatment is guided by resectability
      - – Resectable: Surgical resection followed by adjuvant therapy
      - – Borderline resectable: Neoadjuvant chemoradiation followed by laparotomy with intent to resect
    - ▪ Surgical resection
      - – Whipple (pancreaticoduodenectomy) for pancreatic head and uncinate tumors
      - – Distal pancreatectomy ± splenectomy for pancreatic body and tail tumors
      - – Total pancreatectomy is rarely necessary to achieve negative margins
    - ▪ Adjuvant therapy following resection
      - – Chemoradiation (5-FU based) and systemic chemotherapy (gemcitabine)
      - – Clinical trial
      - – Chemotherapy alone (gemcitabine)
    - ▪ Neoadjuvant chemoradiation (5-FU based) prior to attempted resection for borderline resectable tumors
  - ○ Stage III: Locally unresectable disease
    - ▪ Clinical trial **or** chemoradiation with chemotherapy (gemcitabine) **or** chemotherapy alone (gemcitabine or combination)
    - ▪ Endoscopic biliary stenting, surgical bypass, &/or celiac neurolysis as needed
  - ○ Stage IV: Metastatic disease
    - ▪ Clinical trial **or** chemotherapy (gemcitabine or combination)
    - ▪ Endoscopic biliary stenting, surgical bypass, &/or celiac neurolysis as needed
  - ○ Recurrent disease
    - ▪ Treatment is guided by tumor resectability status (resectable, borderline, or unresectable)
- Surgical considerations
  - ○ Pancreaticoduodenectomy (Whipple)
    - ▪ Pylorus sparing vs. traditional
    - ▪ Retroperitoneal margin
      - – Most important surgical margin adjacent to proximal 3-4 cm of SMA
    - ▪ Variant vascular anatomy
      - – Replaced or accessory right hepatic arteries arising from SMA course through retroperitoneal surgical margin

- Replaced common hepatic artery arising from SMA is rare but important, as ligation may lead to fatal hepatic necrosis
  - Celiac axis stenosis
    - May result in liver predominantly being supplied by collaterals from SMA
    - Concurrent presence of replaced right hepatic artery from SMA may result in impaired arterial flow to proximal bile ducts (generally supplied by right hepatic artery)
  - Venous reconstruction
    - Requires patency of distal and proximal PV, SMV, or PV-SMV confluence for reconstruction
    - Primary venous anastomosis may be performed if splenic vein is preserved and < 2 cm is resected **or** if splenic vein is ligated/cut and 2-3 cm is resected
    - Interposition graft is needed (usually internal jugular vein) for larger resections
- Complications
  - Disease related
    - Hemorrhage
    - Bowel or stomach obstruction
    - Fistula formation
    - Pseudoaneurysm
    - Venous invasion or thrombosis
  - Surgery related
    - Infection
      - Abscess
    - Hemorrhage
      - Ruptured pseudoaneurysm
      - Vascular stump leak (i.e., GDA)
    - Anastomotic leak or fistula
      - Pancreatic (3-30%) or biliary
  - Other
    - Radiation ulcers
    - Delayed gastric emptying
    - Biliary stent obstruction

REPORTING CHECKLIST

T Staging
- Size
- Location
- Extrapancreatic extension
- Invasion of adjacent organs

N Staging
- Location (with regard to potential resection margins)
- Size

M Staging
- Liver
- Peritoneal
- Other (lung, bone, brain, pleura, lymph nodes beyond surgical field, etc.)

Vascular Involvement
- SMA and celiac axis involvement
- SMV, PV, splenic vein involvement including occlusion or presence of thrombus
- Length of venous involvement and distal venous patency
- Hepatic artery and gastroduodenal artery involvement

Anomalous Anatomy
- Replaced or accessory hepatic arteries
- Celiac or SMA stenosis

Complications
- Biliary dilation
- Pseudoaneurysms
- Gastric or duodenal obstruction
- Fistulas or leaks

SELECTED REFERENCES

1. American Joint Committee on Cancer: AJCC Cancer Staging Manual. 7th ed. New York: Springer. 241-9, 2010
2. Lowy AM et al: Pancreatic Cancer. M.D. Anderson Solid Tumor Oncology Series. New York: Springer, 2008
3. NCCN Clinical Practice Guidelines in Oncology: Pancreatic Adenocarcinoma. V.I.2008
4. Wisnoski NC et al: 672 patients with acinar cell carcinoma of the pancreas: a population-based comparison to pancreatic adenocarcinoma. Surgery. 144(2):141-8, 2008
5. Brennan DD et al: Comprehensive preoperative assessment of pancreatic adenocarcinoma with 64-section volumetric CT. Radiographics. 27(6):1653-66, 2007
6. Varadhachary GR et al: Borderline resectable pancreatic cancer: definitions, management, and role of preoperative therapy. Ann Surg Oncol. 13(8):1035-46, 2006
7. Tatli S et al: CT and MRI features of pure acinar cell carcinoma of the pancreas in adults. AJR Am J Roentgenol. 184(2):511-9, 2005
8. Soriano A et al: Preoperative staging and tumor resectability assessment of pancreatic cancer: prospective study comparing endoscopic ultrasonography, helical computed tomography, magnetic resonance imaging, and angiography. Am J Gastroenterol. 99(3):492-501, 2004
9. Roche CJ et al: CT and pathologic assessment of prospective nodal staging in patients with ductal adenocarcinoma of the head of the pancreas. AJR Am J Roentgenol. 180(2):475-80, 2003
10. Tamm EP et al: Diagnosis, staging, and surveillance of pancreatic cancer. AJR Am J Roentgenol. 180(5):1311-23, 2003
11. Ichikawa T et al: Duct-penetrating sign at MRCP: usefulness for differentiating inflammatory pancreatic mass from pancreatic carcinomas. Radiology. 221(1):107-16, 2001
12. Diederichs CG et al: Values and limitations of 18F-fluorodeoxyglucose-positron-emission tomography with preoperative evaluation of patients with pancreatic masses. Pancreas. 20(2):109-16, 2000
13. Tabuchi T et al: Tumor staging of pancreatic adenocarcinoma using early- and late-phase helical CT. AJR Am J Roentgenol. 173(2):375-80, 1999
14. Legmann P et al: Pancreatic tumors: comparison of dual-phase helical CT and endoscopic sonography. AJR Am J Roentgenol. 170(5):1315-22, 1998
15. Lu DS et al: Local staging of pancreatic cancer: criteria for unresectability of major vessels as revealed by pancreatic-phase, thin-section helical CT. AJR Am J Roentgenol. 168(6):1439-43, 1997
16. Griffin JF et al: Patterns of failure after curative resection of pancreatic carcinoma. Cancer. 66(1):56-61, 1990

EXOCRINE PANCREATIC CARCINOMA

Stage IA (T1 N0 M0)

Stage IA (T1 N0 M0)

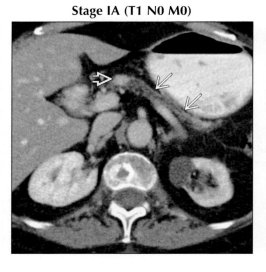

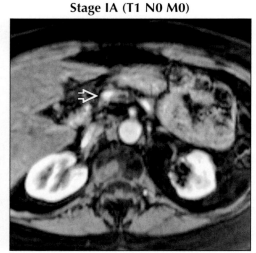

(Left) Axial CECT demonstrates a ≤ 2 cm early arterial enhancing mass ⮞ and distal pancreatic atrophy ➔. There is no extrapancreatic extension, local lymph nodes, metastatic disease, or vascular involvement. *(Right)* Axial T1WI C+ FS MR in the same patient and plane shows similar findings ⮞. Distinct margins and early arterial enhancement are atypical for ductal adenocarcinoma. Surgical pathology was acinar cell carcinoma.

Stage IA (T1 N0 M0)

Stage IA (T1 N0 M0)

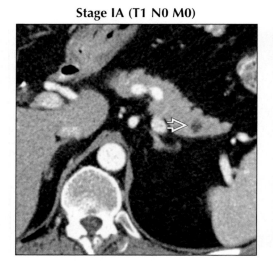

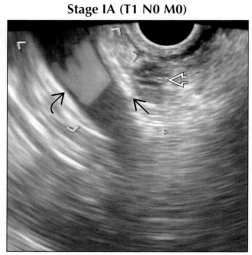

(Left) Axial CECT shows a ≤ 2 cm hypoenhancing mass confined to the pancreatic body with mildly indistinct margins ⮞. This is a classic appearance for ductal adenocarcinoma, which was the pathological diagnosis. *(Right)* Endoscopic ultrasound (EUS) shows a hypoechoic 0.7 cm pancreatic head mass ⮞. Note the distinct echogenic plane ➔ between the mass and the portal vein ➔. EUS is more sensitive than CT for detection of pancreatic masses < 1.6 cm.

Stage IB (T2 N0 M0)

Stage IB (T2 N0 M0)

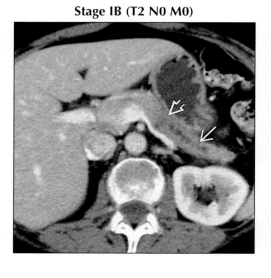

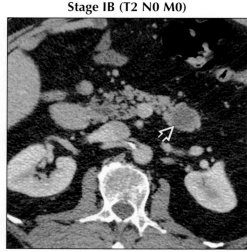

(Left) Axial CECT shows a > 2 cm, poorly marginated, mildly hypoenhancing pancreatic body mass ⮞ with distal ductal dilation ➔. Abrupt distal pancreatic ductal dilation, even in the absence of a definite lesion, is highly suspicious for a pancreatic mass. Pathology was ductal adenocarcinoma. *(Right)* Axial CECT shows a well-marginated, hypoenhancing acinar cell carcinoma ⮞ in the pancreatic tail. These are characteristic features for this pathology.

EXOCRINE PANCREATIC CARCINOMA

Stage IB (T2 N0 M0)

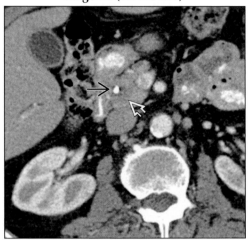

Stage IB (T2 N0 M0)

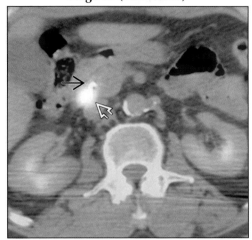

(Left) Axial CECT shows a subtle, nearly isoenhancing > 2 cm ductal adenocarcinoma ➡ in the pancreatic head. Note the temporary biliary stent ➡ within the common bile duct. (Right) Axial PET/ CT at the same level shows prominent FDG uptake in the pancreatic head ➡. PET can be used to identify subtle tumors, metabolic nodes, or metastatic lesions. Biliary stents ➡ produce local inflammatory changes and confound interpretation of PET and CT findings.

Stage IIA (T3 N0 M0)

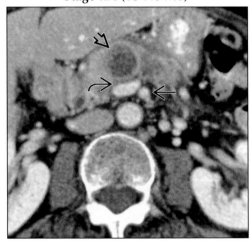

Stage IIA (T3 N0 M0)

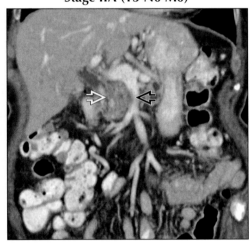

(Left) Axial CECT shows a > 2 cm ductal adenocarcinoma ➡ abutting (< 180°) the SMV ➡. The SMA ➡ is not involved, evidenced by presence of a circumferentially intact fat plane. This is a borderline resectable lesion. (Right) Coronal CECT from the same study shows the tumor ➡ abutting the SMV ➡ with short segment narrowing. Patency of the SMV proximal and distal to the abutment is important in resections requiring venous reconstruction.

Stage IIA (T3 N0 M0)

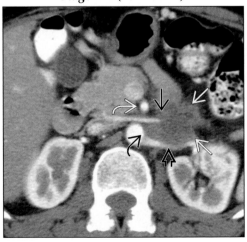

Stage IIA (T3 N0 M0)

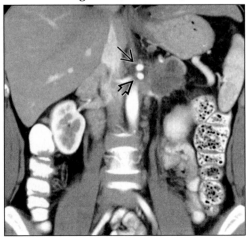

(Left) Axial CECT shows an infiltrative ductal adenocarcinoma ➡ in the pancreatic tail invading the left renal vein ➡, aorta ➡, and left renal artery ➡. The superior mesenteric artery (SMA) ➡ and celiac axis were not involved. Presence of aortic involvement makes this locally unresectable. (Right) Coronal CECT in the same patient shows the SMA ➡ and celiac axis ➡ with some surrounding fat stranding but no clear encasement or abutment.

EXOCRINE PANCREATIC CARCINOMA

Stage IIB (T2 N1 M0)

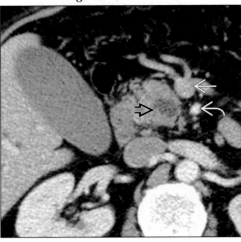

Stage IIB (T2 N1 M0)

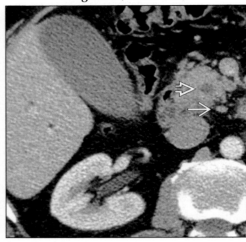

(Left) Axial CECT shows a > 2 cm hypoenhancing mixed ductal-endocrine carcinoma in the uncinate process ⇨ without evidence of extrapancreatic extension. The SMV ➡ and SMA ➡ have clean surrounding fat planes. *(Right)* Axial CECT inferior to the previous image shows the primary tumor ⇨ and a small lymph node ➡. CT is poor at prognosticating the presence of tumor within a node and all nodes should be mentioned. Surgical pathology showed nodal disease.

Stage IIB (T3 N1 M0)

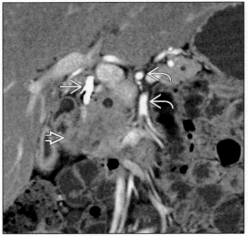

Stage IIB (T3 N1 M0)

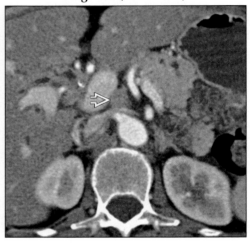

(Left) Coronal CECT shows a hypoenhancing pancreatic head adenocarcinoma that invades the duodenum ⇨. The SMA and celiac axis ➡ are not involved. A temporary biliary stent is present ➡. Staging CT should be performed prior to stenting to minimize confusion between inflammatory changes related to stenting and local tumor extent. *(Right)* Axial CECT shows an enlarged celiac lymph node ⇨. Pathology confirmed N1 disease. This is a resectable tumor.

Stage IIB (T3 N1 M0)

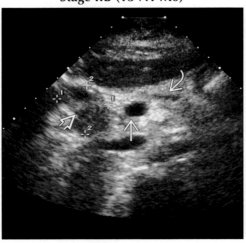

Stage IIB (T3 N1 M0)

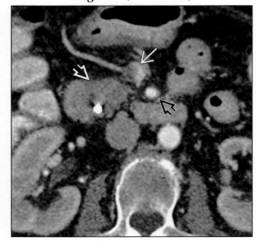

(Left) Transverse transabdominal ultrasound shows a hypoechoic pancreatic head ductal adenocarcinoma ⇨ without sonographic evidence of SMV abutment ➡. Note the mild distal pancreatic ductal dilation ➡. *(Right)* Axial CECT through the pancreatic head shows an isoenhancing mass ⇨ with SMV involvement ➡, evidenced by a teardrop configuration of the vein. The SMA ⇨ is uninvolved. EUS-guided lymph node FNA was positive for cancer.

EXOCRINE PANCREATIC CARCINOMA

Stage IIB (T3 N1 M0)

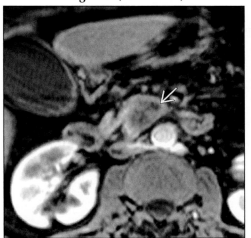

Stage IIB (T3 N1 M0)

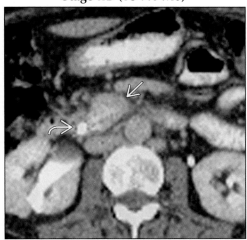

(Left) Axial T1WI C+ FS MR shows a heterogeneously hypoenhancing ductal adenocarcinoma in the pancreatic head ➡. Although there is no imaging evidence of extrapancreatic spread, surgical pathology staged this as a T3 N1 tumor. *(Right)* Axial PET/CT at the same level demonstrates marked FDG avidity within the pancreatic head mass ➡. A temporary biliary stent is noted in the common bile duct ➡. This is a resectable cancer.

Stage IIB (T3 N1 M0)

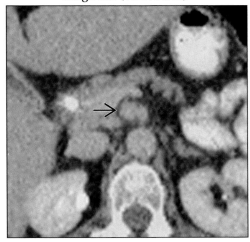

Stage IIB (T3 N1 M0)

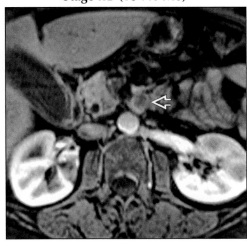

(Left) Axial PET/CT shows a small lymph node adjacent to the celiac axis with increased FDG uptake ➡. This is a good example that lymph node size and morphology on CT are poor predictors of the presence of disease within a node. PET/CT can be applied to further evaluate for nodal or metastatic disease. However, false-negatives can occur with lesions < 8 mm in size. *(Right)* Axial T1WI C+ MR shows a centrally hypoenhancing lymph node ➡. Surgical staging was T3 N1.

Stage IIB (T3 N1 M0)

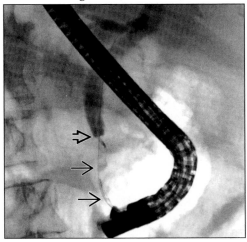

Stage IIB (T3 N1 M0)

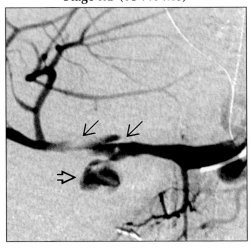

(Left) ERCP shows irregularity of the distal common bile duct ➡ with associated shouldering ➡. This is concerning for malignancy. ERCP is generally performed for biliary decompression, but brushings can provide a diagnosis. *(Right)* Coronal digital subtraction angiography (DSA) after Whipple shows extravasation from the gastroduodenal artery stump ➡. Dissection of the hepatic artery is noted ➡. The stump was coiled and the artery stented.

EXOCRINE PANCREATIC CARCINOMA

Stage III (T4 NX M0)

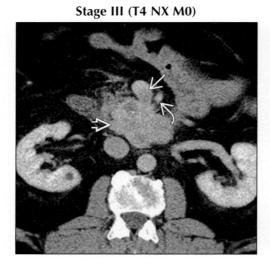

(Left) Axial CECT shows an acinar cell carcinoma ➡ arising from the uncinate process and invading the posterior wall of the SMV ➡. The SMA is not involved on this image ➡. *(Right)* Axial PET/CT at the same level shows FDG-avid tumor invading the SMV ➡. Acinar cell carcinoma is often larger than ductal adenocarcinoma at the time of diagnosis, but it carries a better prognosis when compared by stage.

Stage III (T4 NX M0)

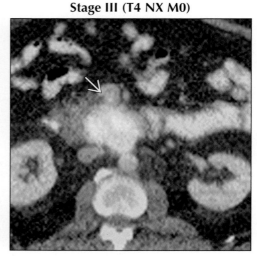

Stage III (T4 NX M0)

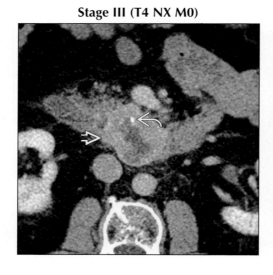

(Left) Axial CECT in the same patient shows a well-marginated, partially exophytic tumor in the uncinate process ➡. A dystrophic calcification ➡ is present. This is not uncommon in acinar cell carcinoma but is rare in ductal adenocarcinoma. *(Right)* Coronal CECT in the same patient shows the large uncinate process mass ➡ abutting (< 180°) the SMA ➡. This is borderline resectable or unresectable, depending on the institution.

Stage III (T4 NX M0)

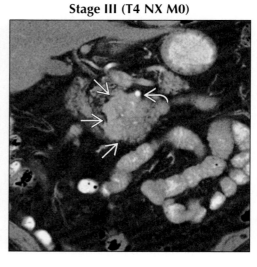

Stage III (T4 N0 M0)

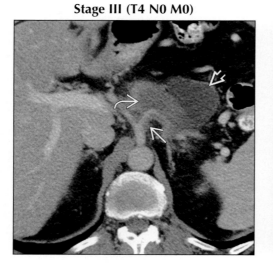

(Left) Axial CECT shows a hypoenhancing ductal adenocarcinoma ➡ invading the splenic, hepatic, and celiac arteries ➡. A large cystic component is seen anterior to the body ➡. Both inflammatory cysts and cystic tumor components can be present in pancreatic cancer. *(Right)* Coronal T2WI MR shows tumor abutting (< 180°) the celiac axis ➡ and SMA ➡ and encasing the splenic artery ➡. The cystic component seen on the previous image is T2 bright ➡.

Stage III (T4 N0 M0)

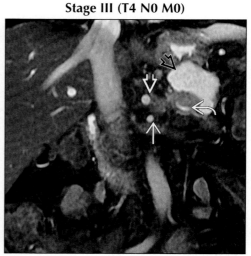

EXOCRINE PANCREATIC CARCINOMA

Stage IV (T4 N1 M1)

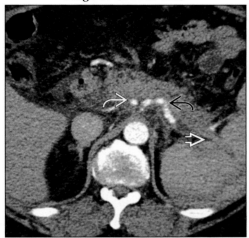

Stage IV (T4 N1 M1)

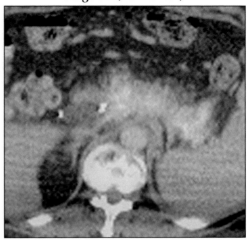

(Left) Axial CECT demonstrates a diffusely infiltrative pancreatic adenocarcinoma encasing the splenic ⇗, common hepatic ⇘, and celiac arteries. Diffusely infiltrative pancreatic adenocarcinoma can mimic acute pancreatitis, but this patient had normal serum enzymes. Invasion of the splenic hilum is present ⇒. This is an unresectable tumor. *(Right)* Axial PET/CT shows diffuse FDG uptake. This finding can be seen with pancreatitis or cancer.

Stage IV (T4 N1 M1)

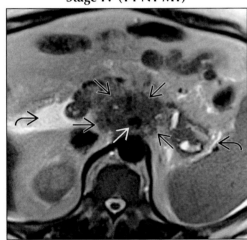

Stage IV (T4 N1 M1)

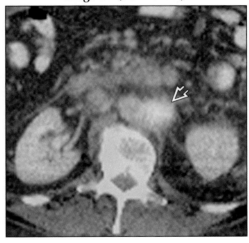

(Left) Axial T2WI MR in the same patient shows a diffusely infiltrative T2 hypointense mass ⇒ encasing (> 180°) the celiac axis ⇒. Areas of peripancreatic inflammation and edema are present ⇗. *(Right)* Axial PET/CT shows an FDG-avid paraaortic lymph node ⇒. Percutaneous biopsy showed adenocarcinoma. Diseased lymph nodes beyond the surgical field are considered metastatic (M1). Biopsy of a metastatic lesion is preferred to biopsy of the primary tumor.

Stage IV (T4 N1 M1)

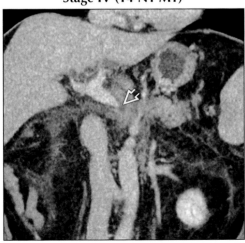

Stage IV (T4 N1 M1)

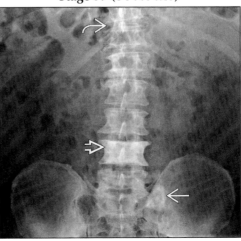

(Left) Coronal CECT in the same patient shows encasement of the portal vein ⇒. The confluence of superior mesenteric vein and portal vein is nearly occluded by tumor invasion. *(Right)* Coronal abdominal radiograph shows blastic osseous metastases including an ivory L4 vertebral body ⇒ and a left sacral lesion ⇒. Distant hematogenous metastases usually occur after hepatic or peritoneal metastases, late in the disease process. A permanent common bile duct stent is also seen ⇗.

EXOCRINE PANCREATIC CARCINOMA

Stage IV (T4 N1 M1)

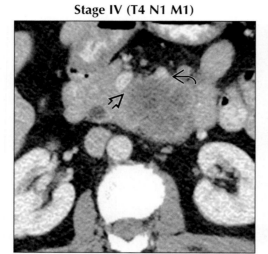

Stage IV (T4 N1 M1)

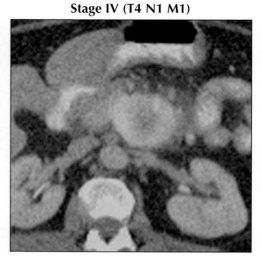

(Left) Axial CECT shows a well-marginated, centrally hypoenhancing ductal adenocarcinoma in the uncinate process abutting (< 180°) the superior mesenteric artery ⇗ and superior mesenteric vein ⇙. *(Right)* Axial PET/CT of the same mass shows peripheral FDG avidity with a central area of decreased uptake, consistent with necrosis. This mass is unresectable.

Stage IV (T4 N1 M1)

Stage IV (T4 N1 M1)

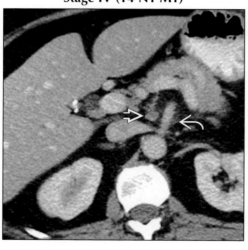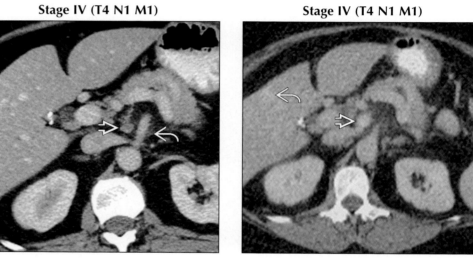

(Left) Axial CECT in the same patient shows fat stranding around the SMA ⇗. Perineural, perivascular, or perilymphatic spread of tumor can have this appearance, which is nonspecific. A lymph node is present ⇙. *(Right)* Axial PET/CT at the same level shows increased FDG uptake in the small lymph node ⇙ at the SMA origin. A focus of FDG avidity ⇗, not evident on CT, is seen in the liver. PET is useful for evaluation of local nodal or metastatic disease.

Stage IV (T4 NX M1)

Stage IV (T4 NX M1)

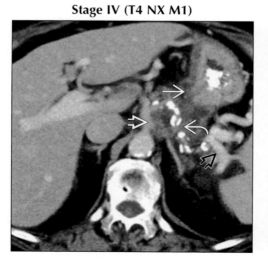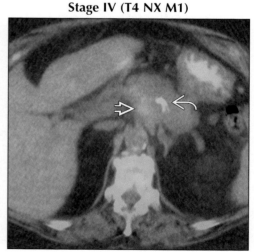

(Left) Axial CECT shows an infiltrative mucinous cystadenocarcinoma in the pancreatic body encasing the splenic artery ⇗ and celiac axis ⇙. The mass invades the posterior wall of the gastric body ⇘. Distention of the mesenteric veins are secondary to splenic vein occlusion ⇙. *(Right)* Axial PET/CT shows areas of increased ⇙ and decreased ⇗ FDG uptake. Mucinous adenocarcinoma can have little or no FDG uptake, resulting in false-negatives on PET.

EXOCRINE PANCREATIC CARCINOMA

Stage IV (T4 NX M1)

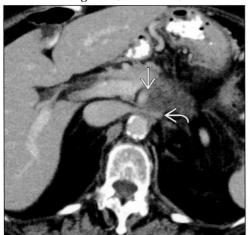

Stage IV (T4 NX M1)

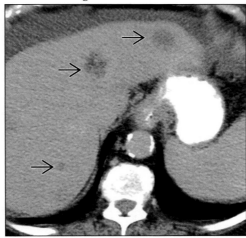

(Left) Axial CECT of the same mass shows an infiltrative mucinous cystadenocarcinoma encasing the SMA ➡ and left renal vein ➡. *(Right)* Axial CECT shows multiple hypoattenuating, ill-defined hepatic metastatic lesions ➡. Liver and peritoneum are the most common sites of metastatic pancreatic cancer. Note the presence of perihepatic ascites, which is suspicious for subradiological peritoneal metastases.

Stage IV (T2 N1 M1)

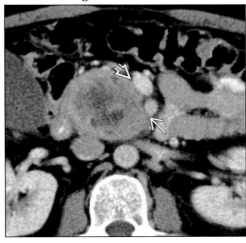

Stage IV (T2 N1 M1)

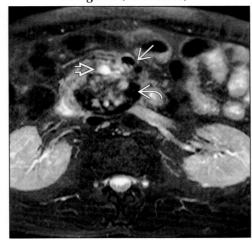

(Left) Axial CECT demonstrates an undifferentiated carcinoma with osteoclast-like giant cells in the pancreatic head. A thin fat plane separates the SMV ➡ and SMA ➡ from the mass. Surgical pathology showed T2 N1 M1 disease. *(Right)* Axial T2WI MR through the same mass shows areas of T2 hyper- ➡ and hypointensity ➡. These likely represent necrosis or cysts and microscopic dystrophic calcifications, respectively. Note displacement of SMA and SMV ➡.

Stage IV (T2 N1 M1)

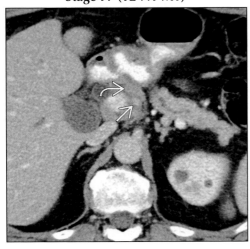

Stage IV (T2 N1 M1)

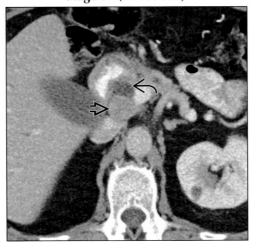

(Left) Axial CECT of the same patient shows an enlarged hepatic artery lymph node ➡. This node is located adjacent to the hepatic artery ➡ at the origin of the gastroduodenal artery. Reports in the literature state that presence of disease in the hepatic artery node carries the same prognosis as metastatic disease to the liver. *(Right)* Axial CECT shows an enlarged lymph node ➡ posterior to a dilated common bile duct ➡.

EXOCRINE PANCREATIC CARCINOMA

Stage IV (T4 NX M1)

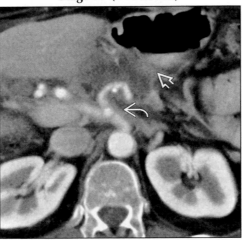

Stage IV (T4 NX M1)

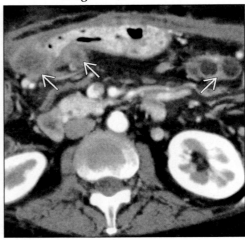

(Left) Axial CECT shows an infiltrative ductal adenocarcinoma encasing (> 180°) the splenic, common hepatic, and celiac arteries ➡️. Additionally, there is invasion of the posterior wall of the gastric body ➡️. This is an unresectable primary tumor. *(Right)* Axial CECT in the same patient shows multiple peripherally enhancing peritoneal metastases ➡️. Along with the liver, the peritoneum is the most common site of metastatic disease in pancreatic cancer.

Stage IV (T3 N1 M1)

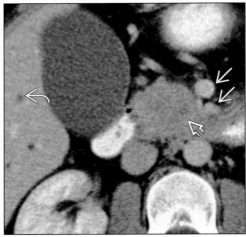

Stage IV (T3 N1 M1)

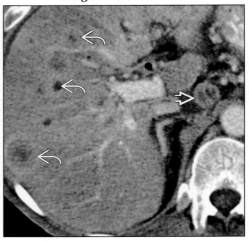

(Left) Axial CECT shows an ill-defined, slightly hypoenhancing mixed ductal-acinar cell carcinoma ➡️ without involvement of the SMV or SMA ➡️. Note the mildly distended intrahepatic bile ducts ➡️. *(Right)* Axial CECT in the same patient shows multiple hypoattenuating liver metastases ➡️. An enlarged lymph node ➡️ with central hypoattenuation is consistent with N1 disease.

Stage IV (T3 N1 M1)

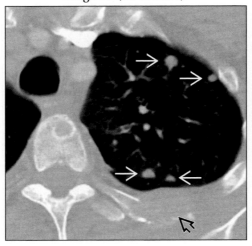

Stage IV (T3 N1 M1)

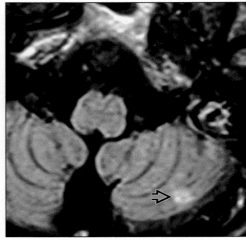

(Left) Axial NECT in the same patient shows multiple pulmonary metastases ➡️ and a large destructive osseous lesion in a posterior left-sided rib ➡️. Distant hematogenous metastases are rarely seen in the absence of either hepatic or peritoneal metastases and occur late in the disease process. *(Right)* Axial T1WI C+ MR in the same patient shows an enhancing metastasis to the left cerebellum ➡️. Brain metastases are rare.

EXOCRINE PANCREATIC CARCINOMA

Stage IV (T4 NX M1)

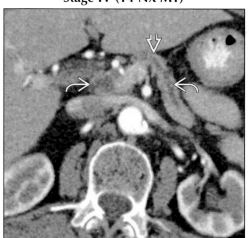

Stage IV (T4 NX M1)

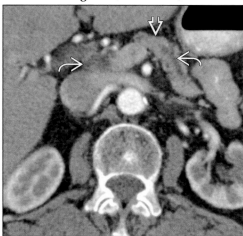

(Left) Axial CECT shows a hypoattenuating lesion in the pancreatic head and associated ductal dilation ➡, consistent with a mixed type intraductal papillary mucinous neoplasm (IPMN). Note the unremarkable appearance of the pancreatic body at this time ➡. *(Right)* Axial CECT for surveillance of the IPMN ➡ in the same patient 6 months later shows a new filling defect in the dilated main pancreatic duct ➡.

Stage IV (T4 NX M1)

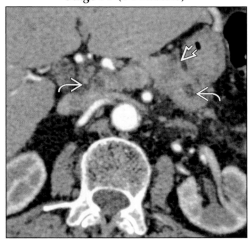

Stage IV (T4 NX M1)

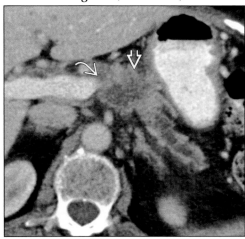

(Left) Axial CECT in the same patient 12 months after the initial CT shows an infiltrative hypoenhancing mass in the pancreatic body ➡, consistent with ductal adenocarcinoma. The IPMN is again seen ➡. *(Right)* Axial CECT in the same patient 15 months after the initial CT shows continued progression of the ductal adenocarcinoma ➡. This is an example of malignant transformation of a mixed-type IPMN into adenocarcinoma. The portal vein is encased ➡.

Stage IV (T4 NX M1)

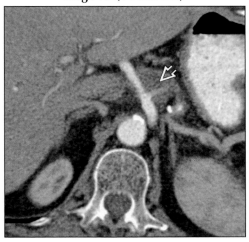

Stage IV (T4 NX M1)

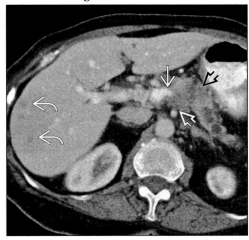

(Left) Axial CECT in the same patient shows encasement ➡ of the celiac axis and proximal splenic and common hepatic arteries, consistent with T4 disease. This is unresectable. *(Right)* Axial CECT from the same study shows the invasive ductal adenocarcinoma ➡ invading the portal vein ➡ and abutting the SMA ➡. Small, ill-defined, hypoattenuating metastatic lesions are seen in the periphery of the liver ➡.

EXOCRINE PANCREATIC CARCINOMA

Stage IV (T3 NX M1)

Stage IV (T3 NX M1)

(Left) Axial CECT shows a hypoenhancing ductal adenocarcinoma centered in the uncinate process and infiltrating beyond the pancreatic parenchyma ⮞. Note the intact fat plane between the mass and the SMA ⮞, making this a T3 lesion. *(Right)* Axial CECT from the same study shows a "double duct" sign with distention of the common bile duct ⮞ and pancreatic duct ⮞. The presence of a subcentimeter celiac lymph node is important to note ⮞.

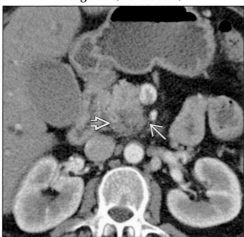
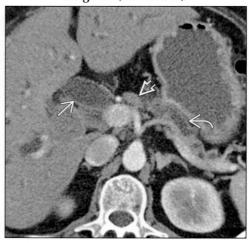

Stage IV (T3 NX M1)

Stage IV (T3 NX M1)

(Left) Frontal chest x-ray from the same patient shows a large cavitary mass in the left lung ⮞. A 2nd solid mass is seen in the right infrahilar lung ⮞. *(Right)* Axial NECT from the same patient confirms the presence of multiple cavitary pulmonary masses ⮞. Numerous smaller pulmonary nodules are seen throughout the lungs. These were biopsy-proven metastases. Pancreatic cancer metastases to the lungs are very rarely cavitary.

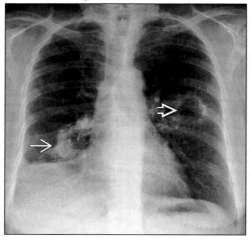
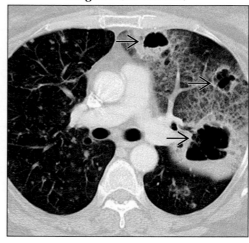

Stage IV (T3 N0 M1)

Stage IV (T3 N0 M1)

(Left) Axial CECT following neoadjuvant chemotherapy for a T3 cancer shows progression of disease. At the time of diagnosis, the mass encased the left renal artery and abutted the aorta. Now the mass has invaded the left renal artery ⮞, resulting in infarction of the left kidney ⮞. A small focus of gas ⮞ within the mass was secondary to fistulization with the duodenum. *(Right)* Axial CECT shows a peritoneal metastasis ⮞ in the same patient.

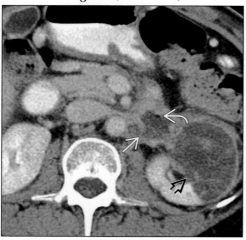
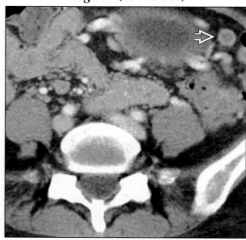

EXOCRINE PANCREATIC CARCINOMA

Stage IV (T3 NX M1)

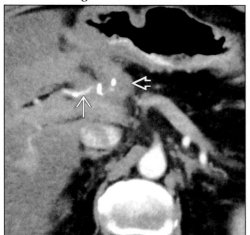

Stage IV (T3 NX M1)

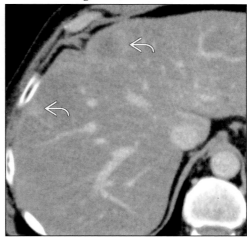

(Left) Axial CECT following a Whipple procedure shows local recurrence around the surgical clips ⮞ with encasement of the proper hepatic artery ➡. The demonstrated soft tissue mass had progressed from prior studies. Post-treatment scarring can have a similar appearance but should not progress. *(Right)* Axial CECT in the same patient shows development of peripherally enhancing liver metastases ⮫ following surgical resection.

Stage IV (T4 NX M1)

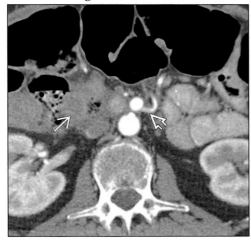

Stage IV (T4 NX M1)

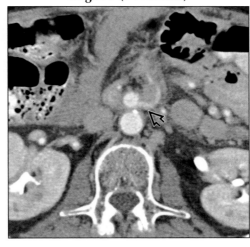

(Left) Axial CECT in a different patient shows a study performed soon after surgical resection (Whipple). Note the postoperative changes ➡ and clean fat planes around the SMA and proximal jejunal branch ⮞. *(Right)* Axial CECT in the same patient at follow-up shows development of encasement of the proximal jejunal branch to the level of the SMA ⮞. This is consistent with local perineural, perivascular, or lymphatic disease recurrence.

Stage IV (T4 NX M1)

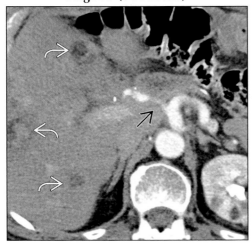

Stage IV (T4 NX M1)

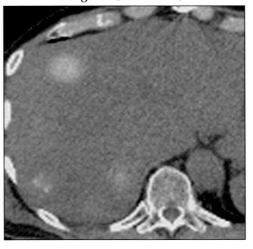

(Left) Axial CECT in the same patient demonstrates development of multiple hypoattenuating liver metastases ⮫ and encasement and narrowing of the proximal common hepatic artery ➡ following Whipple resection of the primary tumor. *(Right)* Axial PET/CT in the same patient shows multiple FDG-avid liver metastases. The most common patterns of failure in pancreatic cancer are local recurrence or development of peritoneal or hepatic metastatic disease.

INDEX

A

Acinar cell carcinoma, pancreatic, 315
Adenocarcinoma
    esophageal. *See* Esophageal carcinoma.
    gastric. *See* Stomach carcinoma.
Adenomatous polyposis, familial (FAP), 103
Adenomatous polyps, colorectal carcinoma
    related to, 102
Ampulla of vater carcinoma, 270–287
    classification, 276
    clinical issues, 277–278
    images, 279–287
        Stage IA (T1 N0 M0), 279–281
        Stage IB (T2 N0 M0), 282–285
        Stage IIA (T3 N0 M0), 285
        Stage IIB (T3 N1 M0), 286
        Stage III (T4 N1 M0), 287
    imaging findings, 277
    metastases, organ frequency, 275
    overview, 276
    pathology, 276–277
    reporting checklist, 278
    routes of spread, 276
    staging examples, 271–275
        N1, 275
        N1 and M1, 275
        T1, 271, 273
        T2, 272, 273
        T3, 272, 274
        T4, 272, 274
        Tis, 271
    staging systems
        AJCC stages/prognostic grouping, 270
        (M) distant metastasis, 270
        (T) primary tumor, 270
        (N) regional lymph nodes, 270
    treatment options, 278
Anal canal carcinoma, 118–133
    classification, 124
    clinical issues, 125–126
    images, 127–133
        recurrent anal carcinoma, 133
        Stage II (T2 N0 M0), 127–128
        Stage IIIA (T4 N0 M0), 128–130
        Stage IIIB (T1 N2 M0), 131
        Stage IIIB (T4 N3 M0), 131–132
        Stage IV (T2 N0 M1), 132–133
    imaging findings, 124–125
        detection, 124–125
    staging and restaging, 125
    metastases, organ frequency, 123
    overview, 124
    pathology, 124
    reporting checklist, 126
    routes of spread, 124
    staging examples, 119–123
        N1, 122
        N2, 122
        N3, 122–123
        T1, 119–120, 121
        T2, 120, 121
        T3, 121
        T4, 121
        Tis, 119
    staging systems
        AJCC stages/prognostic groups, 118
        (M) distant metastasis, 118
        (T) primary tumor, 118
        (N) regional lymph nodes, 118
    treatment options, 125–126
Appendiceal carcinoid, 86–93
    classification, 90
    clinical issues, 91
    images, 92–93
        Stage I (T1a N0 M0), 92
        Stage II (T2 N0 M0), 92–93
        Stage III (T1a N1 M0), 93
    imaging findings, 90
    metastases, organ frequency, 89
    overview, 90
    pathology, 90
    reporting checklist, 91
    routes of spread, 90
    staging examples, 87–89
        nodal drainage, 89
        T1a, 87, 88
        T1b, 88
        T2, 87, 88
        T3, 88
        T4, 89
    staging systems
        AJCC stages/prognostic groups, 86
        (M) distant metastasis, 86
        (T) primary tumor, 86
        (N) regional lymph nodes, 86
        (R) residual tumor, 86
    treatment options, 91

Appendiceal carcinoma, 66–85
  classification, 72
  clinical issues, 74–75
  images, 76–85
    Stage I (T2 N0 M0), 76
    Stage IIA (T3 N0 M0), 76
    Stage IIC (T4b N0 M0), 77
    Stage IIIA (T2 N1 M0), 78
    Stage IIIB (T3 N1 M0), 78–79
    Stage IIIB (T4a N1 M0), 79–80
    Stage IVA (T4a N0 M1a G1), 80–81
    Stage IVC (T3 N0 M1b), 81
    Stage IVC (T4a N0 M1b), 82–84
    Stage IVC (T4b N0 M1b), 85
  imaging findings, 73–74
    detection, 73
    restaging, 74
    staging, 73–74
  metastases, organ frequency, 71
  overview, 72
  pathology, 72–73
  reporting checklist, 75
  routes of spread, 72
  staging examples, 68–71
    nodal drainage, 71
    T1, 68, 70
    T2, 68, 70
    T3, 69, 70
    T4a, 69, 70
    T4b, 71
  staging systems, 66–67
    AJCC stages/prognostic groups, 67
    (M) distant metastasis, 66
    (G) histologic grade, 66
    (T) primary tumor, 66
    (N) regional lymph nodes, 66
    (R) residual tumor, 67
  treatment options, 74–75

B

Bile duct carcinoma, distal, 258–269
  classification, 262
  clinical issues, 264–265
  images, 266–269
    Stage IA (T1 N0 M0), 266–267
    Stage IB (T2 N0 M0), 268
    Stage IIB (T3 N1 M0), 269
  imaging findings, 263–264
    detection, 263
    staging, 263–264
  metastases, organ frequency, 261
  overview, 262
  pathology, 262–263
  reporting checklist, 265
  routes of spread, 262
  staging examples, 259–261
    M1, 261

    N1, 261
    T1, 259, 260
    T2, 260
    T3, 259, 260
    T4, 260
    Tis, 259
  staging systems
    AJCC stages/prognostic grouping, 258
    (M) distant metastasis, 258
    (T) primary tumor, 258
    (N) regional lymph nodes, 258
  treatment options, 265
Bile duct carcinoma, intrahepatic, 224–237
  classification, 230
  clinical issues, 232–233
  images, 234–237
    Stage I (T1 N0 M0), 234
    Stage II (T2a N0 M0), 234
    Stage II (T2b N0 M0), 235
    Stage III (T3 N0 M0), 235–236
    Stage IVA (T2a N1 M0), 237
    Stage IVA (T4 N0 M0), 236
  imaging findings, 231–232
  metastases, organ frequency, 229
  overview, 230
  pathology, 230–231
  reporting checklist, 233
  routes of spread, 230
  staging examples, 225–229
    N1, 229
    T1, 225, 227
    T2a, 226, 227
    T2b, 227–228
    T3, 226, 228
    T4, 228
  staging systems
    AJCC stages/prognostic grouping, 224
    (M) distant metastasis, 224
    (T) primary tumor, 224
    (N) regional lymph nodes, 224
  treatment options, 233
Bile duct carcinoma, perihilar, 238–257
  classification, 244
  clinical issues, 247–248
  images, 249–257
    Bismuth-Corlette type I, 256
    Bismuth-Corlette type II, 256
    Bismuth-Corlette type IIIa, 257
    Bismuth-Corlette type IIIb, 257
    Bismuth-Corlette type IV, 257
    recurrence, 255–256
    Stage II (T2a N0 M0), 249–250
    Stage II (T2b N0 M0), 250
    Stage IIIA (T3 N0 M0), 251
    Stage IIIB (T2b N1 M0), 251
    Stage IVA (T4 N0 M0), 251–254
    Stage IVB (T3 N2 M0), 254

Stage IVB (T4 N0 M1), 254–255
Stage IVB (T4 N2 M0), 254
imaging findings, 245–247
detection, 245–246
staging, 246–247
metastases, organ frequency, 243
overview, 244
pathology, 244–245
reporting checklist, 248
routes of spread, 244
staging examples, 239–243
N1, 243
N2, 243
T1, 239, 240
T2a, 239, 240
T2b, 239, 241
T3, 241
T4, 242
staging systems
AJCC stages/prognostic grouping, 238
(M) distant metastasis, 238
(T) primary tumor, 238
(N) regional lymph nodes, 238
treatment options, 247–248

C

Carney triad, gastrointestinal stromal tumor
associated with, 140
Cholangitis, primary sclerosing
distal bile duct carcinoma associated with, 262
intrahepatic bile duct carcinoma associated
with, 230
perihilar bile duct carcinoma associated with,
244
Choledochal cysts
distal bile duct carcinoma associated with, 262
intrahepatic bile duct carcinoma associated
with, 230
perihilar bile duct carcinoma associated with,
244
Colonic-type (nonmucinous) adenocarcinoma,
appendiceal, 72, 73
Colorectal carcinoma
classification, 102
clinical issues, 106–107
images, 108–117
recurrent metastatic disease, 117
Stage 0 (Tis N0 M0), 108
Stage I (T2 N0 M0), 108–109
Stage IIB (T4a N0 M0), 109–110
Stage IIC (T4b N0 M0), 110
Stage IIIA (T2 N1b M0), 111
Stage IIIB (T3 N1b M0), 111
Stage IIIB (T4a N1b M0), 111
Stage IIIC (T3 N2b M0), 113–114
Stage IIIC (T4a N2a M0), 112

Stage IIIC (T4a N2b M0), 114
Stage IIIC (T4b N2a M0), 113
Stage IVA (T4b N2b M1a), 115
Stage IVB (T3 N0 M1b), 115–117
Stage IVB (T3 N2b M1b), 117
imaging findings, 103–106
detection, 103–104
restaging, 106
staging, 104–105
metastases, organ frequency, 101
overview, 102
pathology, 102–103
reporting checklist, 107
routes of spread, 102
staging examples, 96–101
adenoma-carcinoma sequence, 99
N1a and N1b, 101
N2, 101
nodal drainage
cecum, ascending and transverse colon,
100
descending and sigmoid colon, 100
T1, 96, 99
T2, 96–97, 99
T3, 99
T4a, 97, 100
T4b, 100
Tis, 96
staging systems
AJCC stages/prognostic groups, 95
(M) distant metastasis, 94
(G) histologic grade, 95
(T) primary tumor, 94
(N) regional lymph nodes, 94
surgical treatment, 98
treatment options, 106–107
Colorectal gastrointestinal stromal tumor. See
Gastrointestinal stromal tumor (GIST).
Colorectal neuroendocrine tumors
classification, 162
clinical issues, 165–166
images
colonic carcinoid
Stage IIIA (T4 N0 M0), 169
Stage IV (T4 N1 M1), 177
rectal carcinoid
Stage IIIB (T2 N1 M0), 170
Stage IV (T4 N1 M1), 179
imaging findings, 164–165
overview, 162
pathology, 163
reporting checklist, 167
routes of spread, 162
staging examples
colorectal NET
nodal drainage, 161
T1a and T1b, 160
T2, 160

T3, 160
T4, 160
lymphatic drainage of rectum, 161
rectal NET: T1a, 157
staging systems, 154–155
treatment options, 166–167
Crohn disease, associated with small intestine
carcinoma, 58

D

Distal bile duct carcinoma. *See* Bile duct carcinoma,
distal.
Ductal adenocarcinoma, pancreatic, 315
Duodenal gastrointestinal stromal tumor. *See*
Gastrointestinal stromal tumor (GIST).
Duodenal neuroendocrine tumors
classification, 162
clinical issues, 165–166
images
duodenal carcinoid
Stage I (T1 N0 M0), 168
Stage IIA (T2 N0 M0), 169
malignant carcinoid in duodenal duplication
cyst, Stage IV (T3 N0 M1), 176
imaging findings, 164–165
overview, 162
pathology, 162, 163
reporting checklist, 167
routes of spread, 162
staging examples, duodenal NET: T1, 156
staging systems, 154–155
treatment options, 166–167

E

Endocrine pancreatic carcinoma. *See* Pancreatic
carcinoma, endocrine.
Esophageal carcinoma, 2–27
anatomical divisions of esophagus, 11
classification, 10
clinical issues, 14–15
images, 16–27
adenocarcinoma
Stage IA (T1 N0 M0 G2), 16
Stage IB (T2 N0 M0 G2), 16
Stage IIB (T2 N1 M0), 19
Stage IIB (T3 N0 M0), 17–18
Stage IIIB (T3 N2 M0), 20
Stage IIIC (T3 N3 M0), 22
Stage IIIC (T4b N0 M0), 21
metastatic disease following esophagectomy,
26
recurrent esophageal carcinoma, 25
recurrent local and metastatic disease
following esophagectomy, 27
squamous cell carcinoma

Stage IIA (T3 N0 M0 G2), 17
Stage IIB (T2 N1 M0), 20
Stage IIIC (T4b N1 M0), 21
Stage IV (T2 N1 M1), 23
Stage IV (T3 N2 M1), 24
Stage IV (T4b N0 M1), 24
imaging findings, 12–14
detection, 12
restaging, 14
staging, 12–14
metastases, organ frequency, 9
overview, 10
pathology, 10–12
reporting checklist, 15
routes of spread, 10
staging examples, 4–9
regional nodal drainage, 8–9
T1a, 4, 6
T1b, 6
T2, 5, 6
T3, 5, 6–7
T4a, 7
T4b, 5, 8
Tis, 4
staging systems
AJCC stages/prognostic groups
adenocarcinoma, 3
squamous cell carcinoma, 3
(M) distant metastasis, 2
(G) histologic grade, 2
(T) primary tumor, 2
(N) regional lymph nodes, 2
treatment options, 14–15
Esophageal gastrointestinal stromal tumor. *See*
Gastrointestinal stromal tumor (GIST).
Exocrine pancreatic carcinoma. *See* Pancreatic
carcinoma, exocrine.

F

Familial adenomatous polyposis (FAP), 103
Fibrolamellar carcinoma, hepatocellular carcinoma
associated with, 186

G

Gallbladder carcinoma, 202–223
classification, 208
clinical issues, 210–211
images, 213–223
Stage I (T1 N0 M0), 213
Stage II (T2 N0 M0), 213
Stage IIIA (T3 N0 M0), 214
Stage IIIB (T3 N1 M0), 215–217
Stage IVA (T4 N0 M0), 218
Stage IVB (T3 N1 M1), 220
Stage IVB (T3 N2 M0), 219

INDEX

Stage IVB (T3 N2 M1), 221–223
Stage IVB (T4 N2 M0), 219–220
imaging findings, 209–210
detection, 209–210
staging and restaging, 210
metastases, organ frequency, 207
overview, 208
pathology, 208–209
reporting checklist, 211–212
routes of spread, 208
staging examples, 203–207
N1, 207
N2, 207
T1a, 203, 205
T1b, 204, 205
T2, 204, 205
T3, 204, 206
T4, 206
Tis, 203
staging systems
AJCC stages/prognostic grouping, 202
(M) distant metastasis, 202
(T) primary tumor, 202
(N) regional lymph nodes, 202
treatment options, 211
Gastric carcinoma. *See* Stomach carcinoma.
Gastric gastrointestinal stromal tumor. *See*
Gastrointestinal stromal tumor (GIST).
Gastric neuroendocrine tumors
classification, 162
clinical issues, 165–166
images, gastric carcinoid
Stage IIA (T2 N0 M0), 168
Stage IV (T3 N1 M1), 177
type III, Stage IIIA (T4 N0 M0), 170
imaging findings, 164–165
overview, 162
pathology, 162–164
types I-IV gastric carcinoids, 163
reporting checklist, 167
routes of spread, 162
staging examples, stomach NET
nodal drainage, 158
T1, 156, 158
T2 and T3, 158
T4, 158
Tis, 158
staging systems, 154–155
treatment options, 166–167
Gastrinoma, 292
Gastrointestinal stromal tumor (GIST), 134–153
classification, 140
clinical issues, 143
images, 145–153
duodenal GIST, Stage I (T2 N0 M0 G1), 145
esophageal GIST
Stage IIIB (T3 N0 M0 G2), 148

Stage IV (T2 N0 M1 G2), 153
gastric GIST
recurrent, Stage IIIB (T4 N0 M0 G2), 150
Stage IA (T2 N0 M0 G1), 145
Stage IB (T3 N0 M0 G1), 146
Stage II (T4 N0 M0 G1), 146
Stage IIIA (T3 N0 M0 G2), 147
Stage IIIB (T4 N0 M0 G2), 148–149
Stage IV (T2 N0 M1 G2), 152, 153
after therapy, 153
recurrence after therapy, 153
Stage IV (T3 N0 M1 G2), 151
after therapy, 151
liver metastases, Stage IV, 152
after therapy, 152
rectal GIST, Stage IIIB (T4 N0 M0 G2), 149
after therapy, 149
sigmoid colon GIST, Stage IIIA (T4 N0 M0
G1), 147
small bowel GIST
Stage II (T3 N0 M0 G1), 146–147
Stage IV, 152
Stage IV (T3 N0 M1 G2), 150
after therapy, 150
imaging findings, 141–142
detection, 141
restaging, 142
staging, 141–142
metastases, organ frequency, 139
overview, 140
pathology, 140–141
reporting checklist, 143–144
routes of spread, 140
staging examples, 136–139
esophageal GIST, Stage I-III, 138
extragastrointestinal GIST, Stage I-III, 138
gastric GIST
metastatic, Stage IV, 137
Stage I-III, 137
metastatic small bowel GIST
Stage IV, 137–138
treated, 138
rectal GIST
Stage I-III, 139
treated, 139
T2, 136
staging systems, 134–135
AJCC stages/prognostic groups
gastric GIST, 134
small intestinal GIST, 135
(M) distant metastasis, 134
gastrointestinal stromal tumor prognostic
grouping, 135
(G) histologic grade, 134
(T) primary tumor, 134
(N) regional lymph nodes, 134
treatment options, 143
Glucagonoma, 292

INDEX

Goblet cell carcinoids, appendiceal, 73

H

Hepatobiliary flukes
    distal bile duct carcinoma associated with, 262
    intrahepatic bile duct carcinoma associated
        with, 230
    perihilar bile duct carcinoma associated with,
        244
Hepatocellular carcinoma, 180–201
    classification, 186
    clinical issues, 189–191
    Edmondson grading system, 187
    images, 192–201
        fibrolamellar HCC, Stage IIIA (T3a N0 M0),
          198
        Stage I (T1 N0 M0), 192–194
        Stage II (T2 N0 M0), 195–197
        Stage IIIA (T3a N0 M0), 198–199
        Stage IIIB (T3b N0 M0), 199–200
        Stage IIIC (T4 N0 M0), 200
        Stage IVA (T1 N1 M0), 201
        Stage IVB (T2 N1 M1), 201
        Stage IVB (T3a N1 M1), 201
    imaging findings, 187–189
        detection, 187–188
        staging, 188–189
    metastases, organ frequency, 185
    overview, 186
    pathology, 186–187
    reporting checklist, 191
    routes of spread, 186
    staging examples, 181–185
        regional lymphadenopathy, 185
        T1, 181, 183
        T2, 181–182, 183
        T3a, 182, 183
        T3b, 182, 184
        T4, 184
        thoracic lymphadenopathy, 185
    staging systems
        AJCC stages/prognostic grouping, 180
        (M) distant metastasis, 180
        (G) histologic grade, 180
        (T) primary tumor, 180
        (N) regional lymph nodes, 180
    treatment options, 190–191
Hepatolithiasis
    distal bile duct carcinoma associated with, 262
    intrahepatic bile duct carcinoma associated
        with, 230
    perihilar bile duct carcinoma associated with,
        244–245
Hereditary nonpolyposis colorectal cancer (Lynch
    syndrome), 103
Hyperplastic polyposis syndrome (HPS), 103

I

Ileal neuroendocrine tumors. *See* Jejunoileal
    neuroendocrine tumors.
Insulinoma, 292
Intrahepatic bile duct carcinoma. *See* Bile duct
    carcinoma, intrahepatic.

J

Jejunoileal neuroendocrine tumors
    classification, 162
    clinical issues, 165–166
    images, ileal carcinoid
        Stage IIIB (T3 N1 M0), 171
        Stage IIIB (T4 N1 M0), 172–173
        Stage IIIB (TX N1 M0), 173
        Stage IV (T4 N1 M1), 178
        Stage IV (TX N1 M1), 174–175
    imaging findings, 164–165
    overview, 162
    pathology, 162, 163
    reporting checklist, 167
    routes of spread, 162
    staging examples, ileal NET: T2, 157
    staging systems, 154–155
    treatment options, 166–167

L

Lynch syndrome (hereditary nonpolyposis
    colorectal cancer), 103

M

Metastases, organ frequency
    ampulla of vater carcinoma, 275
    anal canal carcinoma, 123
    appendiceal carcinoid, 89
    appendiceal carcinoma, 71
    bile duct carcinoma
        distal, 261
        intrahepatic, 229
        perihilar, 243
    colorectal carcinoma, 101
    esophageal carcinoma, 9
    gallbladder carcinoma, 207
    gastrointestinal stromal tumor (GIST), 139
    hepatocellular carcinoma, 185
    neuroendocrine tumors, 161
    pancreatic carcinoma
        endocrine, 291
        exocrine, 313
    small intestine carcinoma, 57
    stomach carcinoma, 35
Mucinous carcinoma. *See* Stomach carcinoma.
Mucocele, appendiceal, 72–73

Index

INDEX

N

NET. *See* Neuroendocrine tumors.
Neuroendocrine tumors, 154–179
  classification, 162
  clinical issues, 165–167
  images, 168–179
    colonic carcinoid
      Stage IIIA (T4 N0 M0), 169
      Stage IV (T4 N1 M1), 177
    duodenal carcinoid
      Stage I (T1 N0 M0), 168
      Stage IIA (T2 N0 M0), 169
    gastric carcinoid
      Stage IIA (T2 N0 M0), 168
      Stage IV (T3 N1 M1), 177
      type III, Stage IIIA (T4 N0 M0), 170
    ileal carcinoid
      Stage IIIB (T3 N1 M0), 171
      Stage IIIB (T4 N1 M0), 172–173
      Stage IIIB (TX N1 M0), 173
      Stage IV (T4 N1 M1), 178
      Stage IV (TX N1 M1), 174–175
    malignant carcinoid in duodenal duplication
      cyst, Stage IV (T3 N0 M1), 176
    rectal carcinoid
      Stage IIIB (T2 N1 M0), 170
      Stage IV (T4 N1 M1), 179
  imaging findings, 164–165
    detection, 164
    staging and restaging, 165
  metastases, organ frequency, 161
  natural history & prognosis, 166
  overview, 162
  pathology, 162–164
  reporting checklist, 167
  routes of spread, 162
  staging examples, 156–161
    colorectal NET
      nodal drainage, 161
      T1a and T1b, 160
      T2, 160
      T3, 160
      T4, 160
    duodenal NET: T1, 156
    ileal NET: T2, 157
    lymphatic drainage of rectum, 161
    rectal NET: T1a, 157
    small intestinal NET
      mesenteric metastasis, 159
      T1 and T2, 159
      T3, 159
      T4, 159
    stomach NET
      nodal drainage, 158
      T1, 156, 158
      T2 and T3, 158
      T4, 158
      Tis, 158
  staging systems, 154–155
    AJCC stages/prognostic grouping, 155
    (M) distant metastasis, 155
    (T) primary tumor
      colon or rectum, 154
      duodenum/ampulla/jejunum/ileum, 154
      stomach, 154
    (N) regional lymph nodes, 155
  treatment options, 166–167
Neurofibromatosis type 1, gastrointestinal stromal
  tumor associated with, 140

P

Pancreatic carcinoma, endocrine, 288–307
  classification, 292
  clinical issues, 295–296
  images, 297–307
    late metastases from PNET, 307
    Stage IA (T1 N0 M0), 297
    Stage IB (T2 N0 M0), 298–300
    Stage IIA (T3 N0 M0), 300
    Stage IIB (T2 N1 M0), 301
    Stage III (T4 N1 M0), 302
    Stage IV (T2 N0 M1), 303
    Stage IV (T3 N0 M1), 302, 304
    Stage IV (T3 N1 M1), 304–306
  imaging findings, 293–295
    detection, 293–294
    restaging, 295
    staging, 294–295
  metastases, organ frequency, 291
  overview, 292
  pathology, 292–293
  reporting checklist, 296
  routes of spread, 292
  staging examples, 289–291
    peripancreatic lymph node groups, 291
    T1, 289, 290
    T2, 290
    T3, 289, 290
    T4, 291
  staging systems
    AJCC stages/prognostic grouping, 288
    (M) distant metastasis, 288
    (T) primary tumor, 288
    (N) regional lymph nodes, 288
  treatment options, 295–296
Pancreatic carcinoma, exocrine, 308–331
  classification, 314
  clinical issues, 318–319
  images, 320–331
    Stage IA (T1 N0 M0), 320
    Stage IB (T2 N0 M0), 320–321
    Stage IIA (T3 N0 M0), 321
    Stage IIB (T2 N1 M0), 322
    Stage IIB (T3 N1 M0), 322–323

Stage III (T4 N0 M0), 324
Stage III (T4 NX M0), 324
Stage IV (T2 N1 M1), 327
Stage IV (T3 N0 M1), 330
Stage IV (T3 N1 M1), 328
Stage IV (T3 NX M1), 330, 331
Stage IV (T4 N1 M1), 325–326
Stage IV (T4 NX M1), 326–327, 328, 329, 331
imaging findings, 315–318
criteria for resectability, 317–318
detection, 315–316
restaging, 317
staging, 316–317
metastases, organ frequency, 313
overview, 314
pathology, 314–315
reporting checklist, 319
routes of spread, 314
staging examples, 309–313
peripancreatic lymph node groups, 313
T1, 309–310, 311
T2, 311
T3, 310, 311–312
T4, 312
Tis, 309
TX, 310
Whipple anatomy, 313
staging systems
AJCC stages/prognostic grouping, 308
(M) distant metastasis, 308
(T) primary tumor, 308
(N) regional lymph nodes, 308
treatment options, 318–319
Papillary adenocarcinoma. *See* Stomach carcinoma.
Perihilar bile duct carcinoma. *See* Bile duct
carcinoma, perihilar.
PNETs. *See* Pancreatic carcinoma, endocrine.
Polyphenotypic carcinoma, pancreatic, 315
Pseudomyxoma peritonei (jelly belly), appendiceal,
72, 73–74

R

Rectal carcinoma. *See* Colorectal carcinoma.
Rectal gastrointestinal stromal tumor. *See*
Gastrointestinal stromal tumor (GIST).
Rectal neuroendocrine tumors. *See* Colorectal
neuroendocrine tumors.

S

Sigmoid colon gastrointestinal stromal tumor. *See*
Gastrointestinal stromal tumor (GIST).
Signet ring cell carcinoma. *See* Stomach carcinoma.
Small intestine carcinoma, 52–65. *See also* Small
intestine neuroendocrine tumors.

classification, 58
clinical issues, 60–61
images, 62–65
Stage I (T2 N0 M0), 62
Stage IIA (T3 N0 M0), 62–63
Stage IIB (T4 N0 M0), 63
Stage IIIA (T3 N1 M0), 64–65
Stage IIIA (T4 N1 M0), 63
Stage IV (T4 N2 M1), 65
imaging findings, 59–60
detection, 59–60
restaging, 60
staging, 60
metastases, organ frequency, 57
overview, 58
pathology, 58–59
reporting checklist, 61
routes of spread, 58
staging examples, 53–57
N1, 57
N2, 57
regional lymph nodes
duodenum, 56
jejunum, ileum, and terminal ileum, 56
T1a, 53, 54
T1b, 54
T2, 54
T3, 53, 54–55
T4, 55–56
Tis, 53
staging systems
AJCC stages/prognostic groups, 52
(M) distant metastasis, 52
(T) primary tumor, 52
(N) regional lymph nodes, 52
treatment options, 61
Small intestine gastrointestinal stromal tumor. *See*
Gastrointestinal stromal tumor (GIST).
Small intestine neuroendocrine tumors
classification, 162
clinical issues, 165–166
imaging findings, 164–165
overview, 162
pathology, 162–164
reporting checklist, 167
routes of spread, 162
staging examples, small intestinal NET
mesenteric metastasis, 159
T1 and T2, 159
T3, 159
T4, 159
staging systems, 154–155
Somatostatinoma, 292
Squamous cell carcinoma, esophageal. *See*
Esophageal carcinoma.
Stomach carcinoma, 28–51
Bormannthis morphological classification, 37

INDEX

classification, 36
clinical issues, 39
images, 41–51
    Stage IA (T1a N0 M0), 41
    Stage IIA (T2 N1 M0), 41
    Stage IIA (T3 N0 M0), 41
    Stage IIB (T2 N2 M0), 42
    Stage IIB (T4a N0 M0), 42
    Stage IIIA (T4a N1 M0), 43–44
    Stage IIIB (T4b N1 M0), 44
    Stage IIIC (T4b N2 M0), 45–46
    Stage IV (T3 N0 M1), 47
    Stage IV (T3 N2 M1), 48
    Stage IV (T3 N3a M1), 48
    Stage IV (T4a N1 M1), 48–49
    Stage IV (T4a N2 M1), 49–51
imaging findings, 37–39
    detection, 37
    restaging, 39
    staging, 37–39
metastases, organ frequency, 35
overview, 36
pathology, 36–37
reporting checklist, 40
routes of spread, 36
staging examples, 30–35
    M1, 35
    N1, 34
    N2, 34
    N3a, 34
    N3b, 35
    nodal stations of stomach, 34
    T1, 30–31
    T1a, 32
    T1b, 32
    T2, 31, 32
    T3, 32–33
    T4, 31
    T4a, 33
    T4b, 33
    Tis, 30
staging systems
    AJCC stages/prognostic groups, 29
    (M) distant metastasis, 28
    (T) primary tumor, 28
    (N) regional lymph nodes, 28
treatment options, 39
Stomach neuroendocrine tumors. *See* Gastric
    neuroendocrine tumors.

T

Tubular carcinoma. *See* Stomach carcinoma.

V

VIPoma, 292